D1521044

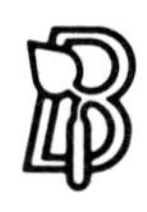

AIDS Epidemiology
Methodological Issues

Nicholas P. Jewell
Klaus Dietz
Vernon T. Farewell
Editors

Birkhäuser
Boston · Basel · Berlin

Nicholas P. Jewell
Dept. of Statistics
University of California
Berkeley, CA 94720

Vernon T. Farewell
Dept. of Statistics
University of Waterloo
Waterloo, Ontario N2L 3G1,
Canada

Klaus Dietz
Dept. of Medical Biometry
University of Tübingen
W-7400 Tübingen
Germany

Library of Congress Cataloging-in-Publication Data

AIDS epidemiology : methodological issues / edited by Nicholas P. Jewell, Klaus Dietz, Jr., Vernon T. Farewell.
p. cm.
Includes bibliographical references.
ISBN 0-8176-3632-3 (hard : alk. paper). -- ISBN 3-7643-3632-3 (hard : alk. paper)
1. AIDS (Disease)-- Epidemiology--Congresses. 2. Epidemiologic Methods. I. Jewell, Nicholas P., 1952- II. Dietz, Klaus 1940- . III. Farewell, Vernon T.
[DNLM: 1. Acquired Immunodeficiency Syndrome--epidemiology. WD 308 A28807]
RA644.A25A3616 1992 92-17877
614.5'993--dc20 CIP

Printed on acid-free paper

ISBN 0-8176-3632-3
ISBN 3-7643-3632-3

Camera-ready copy prepared by the Authors.
Printed and bound by Quinn-Woodbine, Woodbine, NJ.
Printed in the U.S.A.

9 8 7 6 5 4 3 2 1

TABLE OF CONTENTS

Foreword

In 1974, the Societal Institute of the Mathematical Sciences (SIMS) initiated a series of five-day Research Application Conferences (RAC's) at Alta, Utah, for the purpose of probing in depth societal fields in light of their receptivity to mathematical and statistical analysis. The first eleven conferences addressed ecosystems, epidemiology, energy, environmental health, time series and ecological processes, energy and health, energy conversion and fluid mechanics, environmental epidemiology: risk assessment, atomic bomb survival data: utilization and analysis, modern statistical methods in chronic disease epidemiology and scientific issues in quantitative cancer risk assessment.

These *Proceedings* are a result of the twelfth conference on Statistical Methodology for Study of the AIDS Epidemic which was held in 1991 at the Mathematical Sciences Research Institute, Berkeley, California. For five days, 45 speakers and observers contributed their expertise in the relevant biology and statistics. The presentations were timely and the discussion was both enlightening and at times spirited.

Members of the Program Committee for the Conference were Klaus Dietz (University of Tübingen, Germany), Vernon T. Farewell (University of Waterloo, Ontario), and Nicholas P. Jewell (University of California, Berkeley) (Chair).

The Conference was supported by a grant to SIMS from the National Institute of Drug Abuse.

D. L. Thomsen, Jr.
President, SIMS

Preface

In the United States there have been 202,730 reported cases of Acquired Immunodeficiency Syndrome (AIDS) as of January 31, 1992, resulting in 135,434 deaths by that date. These numbers rapidly grew throughout the 1980's, in part reflecting the epidemic of infections that occurred prior to behavioral changes and interventions. In many regards, our knowledge of the virology of the Human Immunodeficiency Virus (HIV), behavioral and therapeutic interventions, and the natural history of HIV disease have grown in a manner that matches the growth of the epidemic over this same period. Nevertheless, as might be expected, as the epidemic has entered its second decade, the focus of questions of interest has changed to respond to new demands and challenges. The twelfth Research Application Conference held under the auspices of the Societal Institute of the Mathematical Sciences brought together experts from around the world to discuss statistical and quantitative methodology which is designed to address issues surrounding ongoing study of the AIDS epidemic. The conference took place at the Mathematical Sciences Research Institute in October 1991.

Methods to reconstruct past HIV infection patterns and project AIDS incidence are primarily based on methods of backcalculation applied to AIDS incidence data using information on the incubation period distribution and models for the infection curve. The article by Gail and Rosenberg reviews the development of the backcalculation technique and considers the need to incorporate nonstationary effects into incubation assumptions due to the impact of treatment. Brookmeyer and Liao, Bacchetti *et al.*, and Becker and Watson all discuss smoothed non-parametric estimates of the infection curve. The article by Pagano illustrates application of backcalculation ideas to data for New York City.

The backcalculation approach is still hampered by the considerable uncertainty regarding the incubation distribution. Bacchetti *et al.* consider the effect of this uncertainty on backcalculation estimates and the ability to detect the impact of external nonstationary forces such as treatment. This paper also argues for a broadening of sensitivity analyses to truly characterize the uncertainty involved. Another source of variability in the prediction of AIDS incidence is highlighted in the article by Lawless and Sun, namely, the practice of treating counts of AIDS cases which have been adjusted for reporting delays as true counts.

Mathematical modeling of the AIDS epidemic can help in understanding the essential components of the epidemic, in the evaluation of control measures, and in the identification of needed data. Dietz and Tudor consider the role of the reproductive rate, the number of secondary cases per infective in a susceptible population, in characterization of the sustainability of the epidemic and discusses the extent to which information on such parameters can be acquired from simple summary measures. The article by Hadeler shows how comprehensive models can be reduced to a few simplified equations and comments on questions as to whether the reproductive rate always increases with infectivity rate and whether reproductive rate relationships are altered by variable infectivity over partnerships. Through models based on data arising in San Francisco and New York, Hethcote and Van Ark analyze the linkage between the epidemics in gay men and in IVDU's.

The evolution of immunological markers during the course of HIV disease and their relationship to the risk of onset of AIDS or death is an area of intense current interest. Not only are these concepts relevant to understanding natural history and for clinical monitoring but there is increasing pressure to utilize markers, especially CD4+ counts, as surrogate outcome variables in clinical trials. It is particularly important that statisticians involved in the analysis of AIDS clinical trials communicate the problems with the use of surrogate markers. With regard to HIV disease, only preliminary investigations have taken place with respect to the aspects of marker history, current values, rates of decline, changes in rate of decline, etc., which are in fact related to the disease process.

The article by Jewell and Kalbfleisch provides a mathematical framework for the consideration of marker models and considers some applications. Self and Pawitan, Tsiatis *et al.*, and DeGruttola and Tu all address various aspects of the joint distribution of the time to disease (or death) and the marker process. The article by Tsiatis *et al.* introduces methods to quantify the extent of the treatment effect due to zidovudine (AZT) which can be "explained" by changes in CD4+ count patterns. Robins and Rotnitzky outline methods which allow the effective use of marker data to enhance the information available from clinical endpoints when patients can be monitored longitudinally.

Lack of information on dates of infection, reliance on prevalent cohorts, and various kinds of truncated and censored sampling continue to pose fundamental problems inhibit accurate characterization of the natural history of AIDS. The article by Wang provides a framework for considering natural history analyses by defining restrictions on the information available about times of infection, AIDS diagnosis and death and noting a duality between retrospective and prospective studies. A particular problem of interest is estimation of the incubation distribution which is complicated by the lack of "pure data" of the kind provided by individuals under follow-up at the time of seroconversion. Parametric assumptions can help to make better use of incomplete data, and may be essential for time periods early in the epidemic, but nonparametric procedures are often preferable. Taylor and Chon examine a method for incubation estimation that makes minimal assumptions about the underlying distribution. The issue of partnership formation is addressed in the article by Castillo-Chavez *et al.* which presents methods for estimating the size of a population which might be in sexual contact with a defined subpopulation. On the clinical side, Berman and Dubin develop a simple model for the action of AZT on CD4+ counts which may provide guidance in scheduling the administration of AZT.

This conference made it evident that, while much has been accomplished in a short time span, the available data are often inadequate for describing the AIDS epidemic. Future methodologic work must further identify sources of uncertainty and help to direct resources to the collection of needed additional data. Further, the uncertainty present, and the requirements for informative data, must become more widely known.

The conference was marked by excellent presentations and lively discussion. This collection of papers provides a timely review of some of the key statistical and quantitative issues concerning the epidemiology of AIDS and will, we hope, stimulate further research as we face the challenges of the next decade.

Berkeley, California, USA — Nicholas P. Jewell
Tübingen, Germany — Klaus Dietz
Waterloo, Canada — Vernon T. Farewell

Contributors

Peter R. Bacchetti
Department of Epidemiology and Biostatistics, University of California, San Francisco, CA 94110

Niels Becker
Department of Statistics, La Trobe University, Bundoora VIC 3083, Australia

Simeon M. Berman
Courant Institute of Mathematical Sciences, New York University, New York, NY 10010

Ron Brookmeyer
Department of Biostatistics, Johns Hopkins University, Baltimore, MD 21205

Carlos Castillo-Chavez
Biometrics Unit, Cornell University, Ithaca, NY 14853-7801

Yun Chon
Division of Biostatistics, School of Public Health, University of California, Los Angeles, CA 90024

Urania Dafni
Department of Biostatistics, Harvard University, School of Public Health, Boston, MA 02115

Victor DeGruttola
Department of Biostatistics, Harvard University, School of Public Health, Boston, MA 02115

Klaus Dietz
Department of Medical Biometry, Eberhard-Karls-University D-7400 Tübingen 1, Germany

Neil Dubin
Department of Environmental Medicine, New York University Medical Center, New York, NY 10010

Mitchell H. Gail
National Cancer Institute, Epidemiologic Methods Section, Bethesda, MD 20892

Karl P. Hadeler
Lehrstuhl für Biomathematik, University of Tübingen, D-7400 Tübingen 1, Germany

Herbert Hethcote
Department of Mathematics, University of Iowa, Iowa City, IA 52242

Nicholas P. Jewell
Program in Biostatistics and Department of Statistics, University of California, Berkeley, CA 94720

John D. Kalbfleisch
Faculty of Mathematics, University of Waterloo, Waterloo, Ontario N2L 3G1, Canada

Jerald F. Lawless
Department of Statistics, University of Waterloo, Waterloo, Ontario N2L 3G1, Canada

Jiangang Liao
Department of Biostatistics, Johns Hopkins University, Baltimore, MD 21205

Samantha MaWhinney
Department of Biostatistics, Harvard University, School of Public Health, Boston, MA 02115

Marcello Pagano
Department of Biostatistics, Harvard University, School of Public Health, Boston, MA 02115

Yudi Pawitan
University of Washington, Seattle, WA 98195

Kathleen J. Propert
Department of Biostatistics, Harvard University, School of Public Health, Boston, MA 02115

James M. Robins
Department of Biostatistics, Harvard University, School of Public Health, Boston, MA 02115

Andrea Rotnitzky
Department of Biostatistics, Harvard University, School of Public Health, Boston, MA 02115

Philip S. Rosenberg
National Cancer Institute, Epidemiologic Methods Section, Bethesda, MD 20892

Gail Rubin
Biometrics Unit, Cornell University, Ithaca, NY 14853-7801

Mark R. Segal
Department of Epidemiology and Biostatistics, University of California, San Francisco, CA 94110

Steve G. Self
Biostatistics Department, Fred Hutchinson Cancer Research Center, 1124 Columbia Street, Seattle, WA 98104

Shwu-Fang Shyu
Biometrics Unit, Cornell University, Ithaca, NY 14853-7801

Robert L. Strawderman
Department of Biostatistics, Harvard University, School of Public Health, Boston, MA 02115

Jianguo Sun
Department of Statistics, University of Waterloo, Waterloo, Ontario N2L 3G1, Canada

Jeremy M. G. Taylor
Division of Biostatistics, School of Public Health, University of California, Los Angeles, CA 90024

Anastasios A. Tsiatis
Department of Biostatistics, Harvard University, School of Public Health, Boston, MA 02115

Xin Ming Tu
Department of Biostatistics, Harvard University, School of Public Health, Boston, MA 02115

David Tudor
Synthelabo Recherche, 31, avenue Paul Vaillant-Couturier, 92225 Bagneux CEDEX, France

David Umbach
National Institute of Environmental Health Sciences, P. O. Box 12233, Research Triangle Park, NC 27709

James W. Van Ark
Department of Mathematics, University of Iowa, Iowa City, IA 52242

Mei-Cheng Wang
Department of Biostatistics, School of Public Health, Johns Hopkins University, Baltimore, MD 21205

Lyndsey F. Watson
Department of Statistics, La Trobe University, Bundoora VIC 3083, Australia

Michael Wulfsohn
Department of Biostatistics, Harvard University, School of Public Health, Boston, MA 02115

Section 1
The Backcalculation Technique for Reconstruction of HIV Infection Patterns and AIDS Projections

Perspectives on Using Backcalculation to Estimate HIV Prevalence and Project AIDS Incidence

M.H. Gail and P.S. Rosenberg

Abstract

The method of backcalculation uses information on the AIDS incubation distribution to estimate the previous rates of HIV infection (the "infection curve") needed to account for the observed AIDS incidence series. Projections of future AIDS incidence are then obtained by distributing estimates of the numbers of previously infected people forward using the incubation distribution. We review the major sources of uncertainty for backcalculation procedures that were applicable to AIDS incidence data through mid-1987 and discuss estimates of cumulative HIV infections based on such data.

Beginning in mid-1987, projections of AIDS incidence derived from backcalculation exceeded observed AIDS counts in exposure groups with good access to zidovudine (AZT) (Gail, Rosenberg and Goedert, 1990; Rosenberg et al, 1991b). Such treatment can cause secular changes in the incubation distribution, and failure to take treatment into account can lead to sharp reductions in backcalculated estimates of cumulative HIV infections. The Stage model of Brookmeyer (1991) takes treatment into account, as does the "time-since-infection" (TSI) model of Rosenberg, Gail and Carroll (1991). The TSI model also allows for the broadened surveillance definition of AIDS that was adopted in 1987. Both models estimate a decreasing trend in the rate of HIV infection in the United States since the mid-1980s. Both models yield estimates of cumulative HIV infections through 1990 that are broadly consistent with estimates obtained by simpler backcalculation models applied to AIDS incidence data through mid-1987. However, estimates of numbers infected and projections of AIDS incidence are higher for the Stage model than for the TSI model, mainly because the parameters used with the Stage model imply that more treatment was in use and that treatment was more efficacious than in the TSI model. Both models predict continued high levels of AIDS incidence through 1994.

1 Introduction

Projecting AIDS incidence, estimating the number of people currently infected with HIV, and tracking trends in the rate of new HIV infections per unit time (the "infection curve") are central goals of public health efforts to monitor the AIDS epidemic. "Backcalculation" was originally proposed as a tool for projecting AIDS incidence and for determining the minimum number of people infected with HIV (Brookmeyer and Gail, 1986). However, as more reliable information became available on the incubation distribution, which governs the time from HIV infection to the onset of clinical AIDS, backcalculation was used as a method to estimate the infection curve (Brookmeyer and Gail, 1988; Taylor, 1989; Rosenberg et al, 1991a; Brookmeyer, 1991). Though subject to large uncertainties, such estimates complement entirely independent estimates of the number of persons infected based on serosurveys in selected populations (Centers for Disease Control (CDC), 1987a).

Backcalculation uses the incubation distribution and the observed AIDS incidence series to estimate the infection curve, $\nu(s)$, that is required to yield expected numbers of AIDS cases (see equation (1)) in good agreement with the observed AIDS incidence series. Letting $F(t|s)$ be the probability that a person infected at calendar time s will develop AIDS in the interval $[s, s+t)$, we calculate the expected number of AIDS cases, Y_j, in time interval $[T_{j-1}, T_j)$ as

$$E(Y_j) = \int_{-\infty}^{T_j} \nu(s)\{F(T_j - s|s) - F(T_{j-1} - s|s)\}ds. \tag{1}$$

The basic backcalculation strategy is to estimate $\nu(s)$ from data on Y_j by deconvolution and then to project incidence forward using (1) together with some assumptions on future values of $\nu(s)$. Expression (1) allows the incubation distribution to vary in calendar time in order to accommodate the effects of treatment and changes in the surveillance definition of AIDS. If one were to assume stationarity of the incubation distribution, as in the original formulation of Brookmeyer and Gail (1986), the quantities $F(T_j - s|s)$ and $F(T_{j-1} - s|s)$ would be expressed by the simpler terms $F(T_j - s)$ and $F(T_{j-1} - s)$.

Backcalculation was applied to AIDS incidence series through mid-1987 under the assumption of a stationary incubation distribution. We review the use of backcalculation for AIDS incidence data through mid-1987, including assessments of uncertainty for projections of AIDS incidence and for estimates of cumulative HIV infections (Section 2). This simple backcalculation model failed to predict the sudden improvements in AIDS incidence trends seen in mid-1987 in some exposure groups, such as gay men. Gail, Rosenberg and Goedert (1990) presented data suggesting that the introduction of zidovudine (AZT) and other treatments in mid-1987 could account for the improvements seen, and they pointed out that backcalculation methods that did not allow for secular changes in the incubation distribution beyond mid-1987 could lead to serious underestimates of cumulative HIV infections. In Section 3 we outline approaches used to model secular changes in the incubation distribution based on the effects of treatment and changes in the surveillance definition of AIDS. A summary and discussion is presented in Section 4. Several authors (Brookmeyer and Damiano, 1989; Gail and Brookmeyer, 1988, 1990) review many of these issues.

2 Backcalculation of AIDS Incidence Data Through Mid-1987

Even before mid-1987, when the AIDS incubation distribution could reasonably be assumed to be stationary, backcalculated estimates of the infection curve were subject to large uncertainties. AIDS incidence projections from backcalculation were much less uncertain, however. Systematic uncertainties include possible misspecification of $F(t)$, of the functional form of $\nu(s)$, and of methods used to correct the AIDS incidence series, $\{Y_j\}$, for reporting delays and other factors. Estimates are also subject to substantial random variation. We now discuss these sources of uncertainty.

2.1 The Incubation Distribution

Hessol et al (1989) estimated the incubation distribution from follow-up data on homosexual men who had participated in a study of vaccination against hepatitis B in San Francisco and whose approximate dates of seroconversion could be estimated from previously stored sera. Brookmeyer and Goedert (1989) used similar data to estimate the incubation distribution in people with hemophilia. A gay man infected in San Francisco in 1981, when many infections are thought to have occurred (Figure 3 in Bacchetti, 1990), might have received treatment six years later, in mid-1987, when AZT became available. Likewise, most people with hemophilia in the United States are believed to have been infected between 1981 and 1983 (Goedert et al, 1989), but it is thought that AZT treatment was introduced about six months later in this population than in homosexual men (Rosenberg et al, 1991b). Thus a person with hemophilia infected in 1982 might have received AZT after about six years of follow-up. Seroconverters in the Multicenter AIDS Cohort Study (MACS) provided only about 3 years of follow-up before mid-1987, though estimates of the incubation distribution beyond this interval have been obtained by imputing the dates of seroconversion for those who were already seropositive at entry into the MACS Cohort (Muñoz et al, 1989). Biggar et al (1990) estimated the incubation distribution from an international registry of seroconverters. "Backcalculated" estimates of the incubation distribution for homosexual men in San Francisco have been obtained by relating AIDS incidence to data on the infection curve (Bacchetti and Moss, 1989; Bacchetti, 1990). Several studies have shown that older men progress more rapidly to AIDS than younger men (Goedert et al, 1989; Darby et al, 1989; Biggar et al, 1990).

To evaluate the hazard of AIDS in the cohorts discussed by Hessol et al (1989), Brookmeyer and Goedert (1989), and Biggar et al (1990) and to eliminate the possible effects of treatment, we reanalyzed the data, using the earlier of the date last seen or 1 January, 1987 as the end of follow-up. Only people whose date of seroconversion could be determined to within an interval of less than two years were used, and the midpoint between the date of the last negative and first seropositive result was taken as the date of infection. To obtain smooth hazard estimates, the hazard function was modelled as a linear combination of B-splines with knots at selected quantiles of the empirical distribution of failure times (P. Rosenberg and R. Biggar, work in progress). To obtain non-negative hazard estimates, the hazard function was estimated by maximum likelihood under the constraints that coefficients of the B-splines be non-negative. These smoothed hazard estimates were extended to about the time of the last observed failure (Figure 1).

There is very little information about the hazard function beyond five years from these cohorts (Figure 1). However, the smoothed hazard estimate of Bacchetti (1990) extends to about ten years. Each of the curves shows a rapidly increasing hazard through year four or five, though the shapes of these spline estimates are not reliable near the ends of the curves. Little is known about the shape of the hazard beyond five years. However, the spline estimates continue to increase beyond five years among people with hemophilia age 18-30 at infection and among gay men in the hepatitis B vaccination trial (Hessol et al, 1989). Bacchetti (1990) finds a decrease in the rate of increase of the hazard function beyond six years, but he notes that treatment may play a role in this time period.

Short term projections of AIDS incidence before mid-1987 based on backcalculation were quite reliable (Brookmeyer and Damiano, 1989; Taylor, 1989), and backcalculated estimates of AIDS incidence fit observed incidence data well, as illustrated in Figure 2. These fits and projections were relatively insensitive to the choice of incubation distribution (Brookmeyer and Gail, 1988), because each of the estimated incubation distributions has an increasing hazard in the first few years following infection, and flexible models of the infection curve $\nu(s)$ can adapt to a particular incubation distribution to fit the AIDS incidence series.

In contrast, backcalculated estimates of cumulative HIV infections are very sensitive to the choice of $F(t)$ (Brookmeyer and Gail, 1986, 1988; Taylor, 1989; Rosenberg and Gail, 1990; Rosenberg et al, 1991a), because slow incubation distributions require large values of $\nu(s)$ to fit the AIDS incidence series and fast incubation distributions require small values of $\nu(s)$. Moreover, estimates of $\nu(s)$ corresponding to the last two or three years of the AIDS incidence series are very uncertain, because small variations in the initial hazard of $F(t)$ cause large variations in the late portion of the infection curve (Hyman and Stanley, 1988). Point estimates (Rosenberg and Gail, 1990) of the cumulative numbers infected to mid-1987 in the United States, adjusted for 15% underreporting, range from 765,000 to 1,312,000, depending on which incubation is chosen (Figure 3), and this uncertainty exceeds estimated uncertainty from random variation. Note that the range of variation is much smaller for estimates of cumulative incidence through January 1, 1985, because the portion of the infection curve between January 1, 1985 and July 1, 1987 is especially sensitive to the choice of $F(t)$.

2.2 Modelling the Infection Curve, $\nu(s)$

The choice of a particular parametric model for the infection curve can have a strong influence, particularly on estimates of the portion of the infection curve closest to the termination date of the AIDS incidence series (see CDC, 1987a; Day and Gore, 1989; Taylor, 1989; Isham, 1989). For example, a simple exponential model $\nu(s) = \alpha \exp(\beta s)$ will lead to estimates of α and β that fit the early portions of the AIDS incidence series well and will imply continued exponential growth of $\nu(s)$ later on, even if later AIDS incidence data would suggest less rapid later growth in the infection curve.

For this reason, Brookmeyer and Gail (1986, 1988) and Rosenberg et al (1991a) relied on weakly parametric step function models in which $\nu(s)$ is piecewise constant. These models, which usually contain four or five steps, are sufficiently flexible that later portions of the infection curve can vary quite independently of early values of $\hat{\nu}(s)$. An advantage of step function models is that estimates of $\hat{\nu}(s)$ constrained to be non-negative can be obtained by the expectation-maximization (EM) algorithm (Brookmeyer and Gail, 1988) or by examining the Kuhn-Tucker conditions and using iteratively reweighted least squares procedures (Rosenberg and Gail, 1991; Rosenberg et al, 1991b). The flexibility of step function models is increased by considering a set of such models with different locations and widths of steps and selecting the best fitting model from this set.

The performance of step function models has been studied (Rosenberg, Gail and Pee, 1991) by simulating data from infection curves of known form and with known incubation distributions. Procedures for estimating cumulative HIV infections through 1 January, 1985, based on selecting the best of several step function models, yielded percentage root mean square error (PRMSE) of less than 14% for each of 9 hypothetical epidemics, but the largest PRMSE increased to 33% for estimates of cumulative HIV infections through 1 July, 1987. Short term projections of AIDS incidence had a PRMSE always less than 18% in these studies. Simulations revealed that step function models with a long last step of about 4 years yielded a favorable tradeoff between bias and variance. Bias is less than 15% for estimating cumulative HIV infections through June 1, 1985, but the bias from using step function models to estimate cumulative HIV infections through mid-1987 can be as large as 30% in infection curves that are rapidly decreasing (overestimated cumulative incidence) or rapidly increasing (underestimated cumulative incidence) after January 1, 1985.

Some important functionals of the estimated infection curve

$\hat{\nu}(s)$, such as estimates of the cumulative HIV infections and projections of AIDS incidence are obtained from integrals involving $\hat{\nu}(s)$. For such functionals of $\hat{\nu}(s)$, the discontinuities in step function models of $\hat{\nu}(s)$ may not be a serious disadvantage. For other purposes, however, it may be desirable to have flexible models of $\nu(s)$ that are continuous and smooth. Rosenberg and Gail (1991) presented iteratively reweighted least squares methods for fitting spline models of $\nu(s)$. An alternative approach is to use many steps to approximate $\nu(s)$ and to impose smoothing constraints to insure that adjacent steps have similar values. Becker, Watson and Carlin (1991) smooth by taking running weighted averages over a "window" of adjacent steps, following each cycle of the EM algorithm. Brookmeyer (1991) smooths by minimizing a Poisson weighted residual sum of squares plus a penalty function. The penalty function is proportional to the sum of squared second differences in the step values (see Bacchetti, 1990) and is a discrete approximation to a penalty proportional to the integrated squared second derivative of $\nu(s)$. Estimation is obtained by iteratively reweighted least squares methods. These smoothed non-parametric or weakly parametric estimates of $\nu(s)$ are visually appealing and are more suggestive of trends in the infection curve than are step function models. However, recent simulation studies (Becker and Watson, 1991) and theoretical calculations (Brookmeyer and Liao, 1991) indicate that when sufficient smoothing is used to reduce variability in the infection curve, similar important biases arise as described for step function models with long last steps. Further work of this type would be useful for comparing the performance of these procedures and for determining which methods work best for choosing the appropriate degree of smoothing and for smoothing near the beginning and end of the parameter series.

2.3 The AIDS Incidence Series

Although the surveillance definition of AIDS was broadened slightly in 1985 (CDC, 1985) to include certain forms of non-Hodgkin's lymphoma, disseminated histoplasmosis, and certain other conditions in addition to the initial list of AIDS-defining opportunistic infections and malignancies (CDC, 1982), such changes in definition had minor effects on the AIDS incidence series through mid-1987. Of much greater consequence is the delay between the time AIDS is diagnosed and the time a report is received at the CDC. Failure to adjust for reporting delays can yield serious underestimates of numbers of incident cases and misleading extrapolations and backcalculations. Adjustments for reporting delay (Harris, 1987; Zeger, See and Diggle, 1989; Rosenberg, 1990; Brookmeyer and Damiano, 1989; Brookmeyer and Liao, 1990a) are usually made to the AIDS incidence series before separately applying backcalculation techniques, though Harris (1990) and Lawless and Sun (1991) have simultaneously corrected for reporting delays and performed backcalculation. Corrections for reporting delay can be substantial. For example, a typical adjustment for cases diagnosed 7 to 9 months before the date of the report is to increase the reported AIDS incidence by 22% (Brookmeyer and Damiano, 1989), and typical adjustments for cases diagnosed 16-24 months before the report amount to 6%.

Public health officials have estimated that 15% of AIDS cases are never reported; this phenomenon is termed "underreporting". To adjust for such underreporting, public health officials have inflated the entire delay-corrected AIDS incidence series by the factor 1/0.85=1.176 (CDC, 1990). Projections of the numbers of AIDS cases reported to the Centers for Disease Control (CDC) based on backcalculation are unaffected by the degree of underreporting, provided the degree of underreporting remains constant. However, secular trends in the degree of underreporting affect the shape of the AIDS incidence curve and can influence projections of the number of AIDS cases reported to CDC. Moreover, estimates of the level of underreporting are needed to convert projections of AIDS incidence as reported to the CDC into estimates of national AIDS incidence.

Rosenberg and Gail (1990) studied the sensitivity of backcalculated estimates of cumulative HIV infections through mid-1987 to perturbations in the AIDS incidence series, such as might arise from changes in the degree of underreporting or from variability in delay adjustments. Various perturbations decreased estimates of cumulative HIV infections by as much as 16% or increased such estimates by as much as 1.5%. Though not negligible, these changes are much smaller than those associated with varying the incubation distribution (Figure 3).

2.4 Stochastic Error and the Construction of Plausible Ranges for Cumulative HIV Infections Based on AIDS Incidence Data Through Mid-1987

The uncertainty in estimates of the cumulative HIV infections through mid-1987 derives both from possible systematic model misspecification, as described in Sections 2.1-2.3, and from random error. Taylor (1989) suggested Bayesian methods to incorporate both sources of error by assigning prior probabilities to members of a set of possible models for $F(t)$ and $\nu(s)$. The approach used by Rosenberg et al (1991a) is to carry out sensitivity analyses to cover major systematic uncertainties and then to broaden the intervals defined by extreme or near extreme point estimates from the sensitivity analyses by taking random variation in to account.

Brookmeyer and Gail (1988) regarded the AIDS incidence series $\{Y_j\}$ having a multinomial distribution with unknown index $N = \int_{-\infty}^{T} \nu(s)ds$, where T is the end of the AIDS reporting series. Under multinomial sampling, Rosenberg and Gail (1991) showed that standard likelihood and quasi-likelihood methods for generalized linear models could be used to estimate infection curves of the form $\nu(s) = \sum_{i=1}^{I} \beta_i g_i(s)$, where $g_i(s)$ are known positive functions, and to provide variance estimates for quantities like estimated future AIDS incidence and estimated cumulative HIV infections. The class of models defined by various choices of $g_i(s)$ includes step function models and spline models. The suggested variance estimates are valid provided the model for $\nu(s)$ is specified in advance and provided no non-negativity constraints are imposed on $\{\beta_i\}$. In the case of step function models, it has been useful to impose the non-negativity constraints $\hat{\beta}_i \geq 0$ (Section 2.2), and if some $\hat{\beta}_i$ is thereby constrained to be zero, standard variance estimates are no longer valid (Chernoff, 1954). Rosenberg et al (1991a) did not choose a particular step function model for $\nu(s)$ in advance, but selected the model that provided the best non-negative estimate of $\nu(s)$ from a set of such models (Section 2.2). For these reasons, a bootstrap procedure was used to estimate the variance of functionals of $\hat{\nu}(s)$. Multinomial bootstrap samples were generated from the best fitting non-negative model for $\nu(s)$, and, for each bootstrap sample, the entire procedure of model selection with constrained estimation was carried out. The covariances of functionals of $\hat{\nu}(s)$ were calculated from these bootstrap replicates, and confidence ellipsoids based on normal theory were calculated from such covariance estimates (Figure 3).

To produce a "plausible range", 1.96 estimated bootstrap standard deviations were added to the largest plausible point estimate found in the sensitivity analyses, and 1.96 bootstrap standard deviations were subtracted from the smallest such point estimate.

Using such techniques, Rosenberg et al (1991a) estimated that between 411,000 and 756,000 persons had been infected in the United States by January 1, 1985, and that between 707,000 and 1,376,000 had been infected by July 1, 1987. If an adjustment for underreporting of 15% is used, instead of 10% as in Rosenberg et al (1991a), these ranges are increased by the factor 0.90/0.85=1.059 (Table 1).

3 Backcalculation After Mid-1987

3.1 Treatment, Changes in the Surveillance Definition, and Other Complications

Backcalculation had yielded good fits to the observed AIDS incidence series before mid-1987 and reasonably accurate short term projections. Thus it was surprising when previously successful backcalculation models were unable to fit the abrupt improvements in AIDS incidence trends noted among gay men in the United States for the year beginning in mid-1987, as indicated in Figure 2 of Gail, Rosenberg and Goedert (GRG) (1990). This failure of backcalculation to fit the data from mid-1987 to mid-1988 was especially noticeable if one studied a "consistently defined" AIDS incidence series. The "consistent" series included cases defined under the surveillance definition in use since 1985 but allowed for presumptive as well as pathologically proven AIDS-defining conditions in HIV antibody-positive people. The surveillance definition of AIDS was broadened in the fall of 1987 to include wasting syndrome, dementia, extrapulmonary tuberculosis and certain other conditions in addition to conditions in the "consistently defined" AIDS series (CDC, 1987b). This expanded definition increased AIDS counts (Selik et al, 1990) and tended to obscure the dramatic improvements seen in incidence trends for consistently defined AIDS. Nonetheless, improvements were noted in gay men beginning in mid-1987 (CDC, 1990), even when one analyzed all AIDS cases under the broadened definition (Figure 2).

GRG argued that the abrupt improvement in AIDS incidence for the one year period beginning in mid-1987 could not be completely explained by a previous slow-down in the infection curve because even abrupt changes in $\nu(s)$ tend to be smoothed out by the convolution equation (1) and cannot result in abrupt changes in AIDS incidence. For example, using the incubation distribution of Brookmeyer and Goedert (1989), they found that constrained models of $\nu(s)$ that allowed no new infections among gay men in the United States after mid-1985 could account for less than one third of the improvement seen (Figure 2).

GRG concluded that only factors that suddenly altered the incubation distribution or that affected reporting delays could cause such an abrupt bend in the AIDS incidence curve. They reviewed evidence for the hypothesis that newly introduced treatments, such as AZT and pentamidine, caused the abrupt improvements in AIDS incidence seen beginning in mid-1987. They cited clinical trial evidence that AZT, in combination with pentamidine, had the potential to reduce the hazard of progression to AIDS by a factor of θ=0.5 to θ=.25 among AIDS-free persons with severe immunodeficiency (Fischl et al, 1987; Golden et al, 1989; Leoung et al, 1990) and in persons with somewhat less severe immunodeficiency (Fischl et al, 1990; Volberding et al, 1990). Based on data on AZT use among gay men in the San Francisco Men's Health Study, GRG calculated that enough AZT was being given to AIDS-free gay men with severe immunodeficiency to account for the observed improvements in AIDS incidence for the one year period beginning in mid-1987, through perhaps not for the last half of 1988.

The argument that treatment had had a favorable impact on AIDS incidence was further supported by correlations between AIDS incidence trends and AZT usage showing that gay men and people with hemophilia, who had received substantial amounts of AZT before AIDS developed, had experienced abrupt improvements in AIDS incidence trends, whereas intravenous drug abusers and persons infected by heterosexual contact, who had received very little AZT while still AIDS-free, had not shown improvements in AIDS incidence trends (Rosenberg et al, 1991b). Improvements in AIDS incidence trends were also more pronounced among whites than non-whites and in urban rather than non-urban locations, as one might expect if access to treatment were an important factor in reducing

AIDS incidence (Rosenberg et al, 1991b).

GRG were unable to account for sudden improvements in AIDS incidence among gay men by using different incubation distributions in the backcalculation model. However, Bacchetti, Segal and Jewell (1991) showed that the sudden improvement in AIDS incidence could be explained, at least in part, if both the infection curve decreased sharply beginning in 1981 and if the "natural history" hazard of the incubation distribution leveled off at about 6 years. Thus, the precise quantitative contribution of AZT and other treatments to improvements in AIDS incidence seen from mid-1987 to mid-1988 remains uncertain.

Backcalculation methods must deal with the following complexities and uncertainties that affect AIDS incidence data after mid-1987:

1. The incubation distribution must be allowed to change in calendar time to reflect the introduction of effective therapies. Models that incorporate treatment are uncertain because it is not known precisely how effective treatments are, how long the beneficial effects of treatment last, and exactly over what time period and at what intensity treatments are being used in selected populations.

2. Models must accommodate the broadening of the surveillance definition of AIDS in the fall of 1987 (CDC, 1987b). There were about 8% more delay-corrected AIDS cases under the broadened definition than under the delay-corrected "consistent" definition for gay men in the third quarter of 1987 and about 22% more for intravenous drug users.

3. Little is known about the incubation distribution of untreated patients beyond five years (Section 2.1). This limitation had little impact on projections of AIDS incidence through mid-1987. However, available models to incorporate treatment (Brookmeyer and Liao, 1990; Brookmeyer, 1991; Solomon and Wil-

son, 1990; Rosenberg, Gail and Carroll, 1991) do so by altering the natural history incubation distribution. Since many people infected in the early 1980's are expected to develop AIDS in the 1990's, one must assume knowledge of the natural history incubation distribution beyond 10 years. Sensitivity analyses on the long term features of this natural history incubation distribution are essential not only for estimating cumulative HIV infections, as was the case before for estimates derived from AIDS incidence data through mid-1987, but also for projecting AIDS incidence in the 1990's.

We now review two approaches that attempt to extend backcalculation models to allow for treatment, Stage models (Section 3.2) and "time-since-infection" (TSI) models (Section 3.3).

3.2 Stage Models of Treatment Effect

If one assumes that HIV infection is a progressive disease, that all persons who develop AIDS must first pass through a state of severe immunodeficiency defined by T helper lymphocyte (CD4) levels $\leq$200 cells/mm^3, and that the time from entry into that state to AIDS is independent of the period between infection with HIV and arriving at the state of severe immunodeficiency, one is led to a semi-Markov model for the natural history incubation distribution. For example, Brookmeyer (1991) assumes that the sojourn time T_{12}, from infection (state 1) to severe immunodeficiency (state 2) has a Weibull distribution, $1 - \exp(-.0141t^{2.08})$ with median 6.5 years, and the sojourn time T_{23}, from state 2 to AIDS (state 3) has an exponential distribution with median 2.5 years. The corresponding natural history distribution of the incubation time from infection to AIDS, $T_{12}+T_{23}$, has a median of 10 years. Earlier workers had used a Stage model of this type with somewhat different parameters (Brookmeyer and Liao, 1990b) or with multiple stages defined by clinical criteria (Longini et al, 1989) or by multiple CD4 levels (Longini, 1990; Longini et al, 1990).

An attractive feature of the Stage model used by Brookmeyer (1991), is that one can assume that only those AIDS-free people, in state 2 receive AZT, which reflects the early patterns of AZT use in 1987. From the progressive nature of the model, it is clear that treating only the relatively small numbers of patients with severe immunodeficiency can have an important impact on the population incubation distribution.

Brookmeyer (1991) makes two assumptions to incorporate treatment into the model:

1. The hazard that a person in state 2 receives treatment is 0.2 per person-year beginning from the later of the date at which the person enters state 2 and mid-1987. Eventually all persons in state 2 will receive pre-AIDS treatment or develop AIDS, whichever comes first.

2. The effect of treatment is to reduce the hazard of the transition from state 2 to AIDS from .277/person-year to 0.277θ, where $\theta=0.35$ is a measure of treatment efficacy. Brookmeyer (1991) explores a range of treatment efficacies from $\theta=0.25$ to $\theta=1$.

Brookmeyer (1991) used delay-adjusted AIDS incidence data through 1 April 1990, based on the broadened case definition of August 1987 (CDC, 1987b). A correction of 10% was added to account for underreporting. Brookmeyer (1991) does not explicitly model the effect of the change in the surveillance definition of AIDS, but he notes that when the consistently defined AIDS series is analyzed, estimates of cumulative numbers infected decrease by 16%.

Using step functions with yearly intervals, except for the initial period from 1977.0 to 1979.0 and the final period from 1989.0 to 1990.25, Brookmeyer (1991) applied a penalty, as described in Section 2.2, to obtain smoothed estimates of the infection curve. He concluded that the HIV infection curve in the United States peaked in the mid-1980's (about 1984) both for all exposure categories combined and for homosexual and bisexual men. He estimated that between 850,000 and 1,205,000 people had been infected through 1 April 1990, and gave a point estimate of 1,050,000. This range was based on a sensitivity analysis covering three incubation distributions, each with median 10 years, and on an analysis of stochastic error. The incubation distributions used in the sensitivity analysis had median sojourn times T_{23} of 1.5, 2.5 or 3.5 years. Higher values of θ corresponding to less effective treatment produced lower point estimates of cumulative HIV infections, and if treatment was assumed to be ineffective (θ=1.0), the point estimate dropped to 715,000. To compare Brookmeyer's estimates with results from the time since infection model (Section 3.3 and 3.4), we multiplied his plausible range of 850,000 to 1,205,000 by the factor (1/0.85)/1.10 =1.069, so that the same correction for underreporting, (1/.85), is applied in each calculation (Table 1). This adjustment results in the plausible range 909,000 to 1,289,000. Projections of AIDS incidence increased from 65,000 cases in 1991 to 73,200 cases in 1994. These estimates also include an adjustment for underreporting of 1/0.85=1.176, whereas Brookmeyer (1991) used 1.10. Professor Brookmeyer kindly provided the uncorrected counts used to produce Table 2.

3.3 The Time Since Infection TSI Model

Rosenberg, Gail and Carroll (RGC) (1991) incorporated both the effects of treatment and the effects of changes in the surveillance definition through the hazard model

$$\begin{aligned} h(t|s,\tau) &= h_0(t)\{\theta(t)I(t+s \geq \tau) + I(t+s < \tau)\} \\ &\times \{\delta I(t+s \geq \Delta) + I(t+s < \Delta)\}. \end{aligned} \tag{2}$$

Here $h(t|s,\tau)$ is the hazard of AIDS at t years after infection for a person infected at calendar date s and given treatment at calendar time τ, $h_0(t)$ is the "natural history" hazard for an untreated patient under the "consistently defined" surveillance definition in use until the fall of 1987, the quantity δ reflects the increase in the AIDS hazard from broadening the AIDS definition at Δ=1 October, 1987, and $\theta(t)$ is an "efficacy function" that reflects treatment. The function $\theta(t)$ equals 1.0 for t near zero but decreases beginning in year 4 to an asymptotic value of $\theta_{\text{min}}=0.5$ by about year 7. Note that even people who are receiving "treatment" do not have a reduced hazard, under this model, until some time has elapsed since infection, because it was common practice during the period 1987-1990 to withhold the use of powerful agents like AZT and pentamidine until advanced immunodeficiency developed. Model (2) is called a "time-since-infection" (TSI) model because the efficacy function varies with time since infection.

A typical pattern for the multiplier of $h_0(t)$ in equation (2) is shown in Figure 4. Although treatment begins two years after infection in October 1984 in this example, no effect is seen on the natural history hazard until the definition of AIDS is broadened in October, 1987, when the hazard increased by the factor $\delta \geq 1$. Only in October, 1989, five years after infection does the beneficial effect of treatment become apparent.

Equation (2) induces an incubation distribution $F(t|s,\tau)$ for a person infected at calendar time s and first brought into treatment at time τ. In order to obtain the conditional incubation distribution $F(t|s)$ needed in equation (1), we must average over the distribution $P(\tau|s)$ of times of treatment onset for persons infected at calendar time s. Indeed,

$$F(t|s) = \int F(t|s,\tau)dP(\tau|s). \tag{3}$$

Data from the San Francisco Men's Health Study (Rosenberg et al, 1991b; Lang et al, 1991), and from the multicenter AIDS Cohort Study (Graham et al, 1991) indicate that the proportion of AIDS-free gay men with severe immunodeficiency who were receiving AZT began increasing in mid-1987 and then reached a final proportion in treatment, p, between 0.35 and 0.55 after two or three years. A similar pattern was seen for intravenous drug users (Rosenberg et al, 1991b), but AZT use began later and stabilized at only about p = 0.10. Data of this type were used to define the treatment onset distribution $P(\tau|s)$ for various exposure groups (RGC). We use the notation 1987.25 to denote 1 April, 1987 and a similar notation for other calendar quarters. For $s \leq 1987.25$, RGC assumed for gay men that $P(\tau|s)$ increased linearly from $p = 0$ to $p = .4$ on [1987.25, 1990.25] and remained constant at $p = 0.4$ thereafter. For $1987.25 < s \leq 1990.25$, they assumed $P(\tau|s)$ had point mass, $p = .4$, at $\tau = 1990.25$, and for $s > 1990.25$, they assumed $P(\tau|s)$ had point mass, $p = 0.4$, at $\tau = s$. The same distribution was used for gay intravenous drug users except $p = 0.3$. For other intravenous drug users and for persons infected by heterosexual contact, $p = 0.1$, and the three year phase-in of treatment began in 1988.25.

The surveillance change parameter δ in equation (2) was estimated as the average ratio of the number of delay-corrected AIDS cases under the broadened 1987 definition to the number of consistently defined AIDS cases in each of six successive quarters beginning on 1 October, 1987. Persons who were prevalent on 1 October, 1987 with a new AIDS defining condition like wasting syndrome were not included in these calculations. For gay men, $\hat{\delta}$=1.10, whereas estimates $\hat{\delta}$=1.25, 1.17 and 1.17 were found respectively for intravenous drug users (IVDUs), gay IVDUs, and people infected by heterosexual contact.

To estimate the infection curve and project AIDS incidence for the entire United States, RGC analyzed the four major exposure groups, (gay men, IVDUs, gay IVDUs and people infected by heterosexual contact) separately, added these results, and multiplied by 1/0.94 to account for other exposure groups and people with no identified risk. Backcalculation was applied to delay-corrected consistently defined AIDS counts (including presumptive diagnoses) through 30 September, 1987, and thereafter to all newly incident delay-corrected AIDS counts through 31 December, 1990.

The choice of "natural history" incubation distribution had a major impact on estimates of cumulative numbers infected. Therefore four incubation distributions, whose hazards are depicted in Figure 5, were used in sensitivity analyses. In addition to a "Standard" and "Fast" Weibull distribution, RGC modified these distributions to have a slowly increasing ("levelling") hazard after 8.0 years, as described in the footnote to Figure 5. Note that the natural history hazard implicit in the model of Brookmeyer (1991) falls among these other hazard functions (Figure 5).

A single step function model was used with knots at 1977.0, 1980.0, 1984.0, 1986.0, and 1991.0.

On the basis of extensive sensitivity analyses, RGC defined a plausible lower limit as the 2.5^{th} percentile obtained from bootstrap replications based on a Fast Weibull distribution with levelling hazard and with $\theta_{\min}=0.5$. The upper limit of the plausible range was defined as the 97.5^{th} percentile of bootstrap replications based on the Standard Weibull distribution with $\theta_{\min}=0.35$. To account for overdispersion in AIDS incidence counts compared to Poisson variation (see Brookmeyer and Liao, 1990; Lawless and Sun, 1991), RGC bootstrapped from a normal approximation to a negative binomial distribution with mean $\hat{E}(Y_j)$ and variance $\tilde{\sigma}^2\hat{E}(Y_j)$, where $\hat{E}(Y_j)$ is obtained from equation (1) with $\hat{\nu}(s)$ in place of $\nu(s)$, and where $\tilde{\sigma}^2$ is the ratio of the observed Poisson deviance to the degrees of freedom.

To test these methods, RGC used AIDS incidence data through 31 December, 1989 to project AIDS incidence in 1990 and then compared projections with observed data in 1990. For example, for gay men, projections based on the Fast Weibull incubation distribution with $\theta_{\min}=0.5$ yielded a good fit to the data in 1990 (see the solid circles in Figure 6). The step function estimate of the infection curve decreases after 1984, and the estimated infection curve is zero beyond 1985. However, the HIV infection rate is very uncertain after 1985, as indicated by the bootstrap confidence interval, and this uncertainty reflects itself in the large upside uncertainty in projections of AIDS incidence. This model predicts fairly constant high levels of AIDS incidence from 1990 to 1995.

Using AIDS incidence data through 31 December, 1990, RGC constructed plausible ranges for estimated cumulative numbers infected for various time periods (Table 1) and for projections of AIDS incidence (Table 2).

3.4 Comparison of Classical Backcalculation with the Time-Since-Infection Model

Based on classical backcalculation and consistently defined AIDS incidence data through 1 July, 1987, Rosenberg et al (1991a) estimated that between 435,000 and 800,000 people had been infected by 1 January, 1985 and between 749,000 and 1,457,000 by 1 July, 1987 (Table 1). These figures are based on an assumption of 15% underreporting, rather than the 10% used originally, and are therefore higher by a factor of 0.90/0.85=1.059 than in Rosenberg et al (1991a). Taylor (1989) obtained similar results based on incidence data through mid-1987. After correction for 15% underreporting, his estimates for the numbers infected through April 1987 ranged from 630,000 to 1,306,000. If one bases the upper limit of the plausible range on the Standard Weibull distribution, which was used in the TSI model, rather than the Slow incubation distribution that was used originally by Rosenberg et al (1991a), then from Table 2 in Rosenberg and Gail (1990) one obtains an upper limit of the plausible range of 587,000 infected by 1 January, 1985 and 1,103,000 infected by 1 July, 1987 (Table 1).

These estimates based on classical backcalculation agree well with estimates from the TSI model through 1 January, 1985, but the classical backcalculation estimates exceed those from the TSI model after 1985. It is likely that classical backcalculation with a long last step yielded a positively biased estimate of the cumulative HIV infections to July, 1987 if the infection curve decreased rapidly between 1983 and 1987 (Section 2.2).

3.5 Comparisons Between the TSI and Stage Models

The lower limit of the plausible range for the estimated HIV infections through early 1990 is 30% lower for the TSI model than for the Stage model, and the upper limit is 23% lower (Table 1). Despite these differences, there is overlap between the two plausible ranges. Likewise, limits of the plausible ranges for projections of AIDS incidence are between 13% and 22% lower for the TSI model than for the Stage model (Table 2), but there is broad overlap in the plausible ranges. Both models suggest a decrease in the infection curve since the mid-1980s (compare Figures 2 and 3 in Brookmeyer, 1991 with Figure 6).

One reason the Stage model tends to produce higher estimates of HIV infections is that more treatment is assumed to be in use and the effect of treatment is assumed to be stronger (θ=0.35). In particular, by 1 January, 1989, it is assumed that about 25% of persons with advanced immunodeficiency in the United States are in treatment (see Figure 4 in Brookmeyer, 1991). The TSI model assumes a smaller proportion in treatment. From parameters used to define the distributions of times of treatment onset for gays, gay IVDUs, IVDUs and people infected by heterosexual contact (Section 3.3), and from estimates of numbers infected in these exposure groups in RGC, we calculate that 15.7% of infected people were in treatment as of 1 January, 1989, compared to 25% for the Stage model. Moreover, not every person "in treatment" in the TSI model is receiving agents like AZT or pentamidine, because some would have been infected only a short time before. Even ignoring this feature of the TSI model, the sensitivity analyses in Figure 4 of Brookmeyer (1991) suggest that the assumptions that only 15.7% are in treatment on 1 January, 1989 and that $\theta_{\text{min}}=0.5$, compared to $\theta=0.35$ in the Stage model, account for a 24% reduction in the estimated numbers infected by the TSI model, compared to the Stage model.

Other differences help to explain the higher estimates from the Stage model. The Stage model was fitted to all incident AIDS cases, and no attempt was made to model the effect of the change in the surveillance definition. In fact, the expansion of the surveillance definition in 1987 tends to shorten the incubation distribution, partially offsetting the effects of treatment. Thus, ignoring the surveillance change has the effect of increasing estimates of the numbers infected in the Stage model. If the consistently defined AIDS incidence series is analyzed by the Stage model, the estimated numbers infected are reduced by 16% (see footnote 24 in Brookmeyer, 1991).

The TSI model was fitted to AIDS incidence data through 31 December 1990, whereas Brookmeyer (1991) used data through 1 April, 1990. The additional incidence data beyond 1 April, 1990 tends to decrease estimates of numbers infected by the Stage model slightly. For example, applying the Stage model to AIDS incidence data through 1 October, 1990 reduced the point estimate of cumulative HIV infections from 1,125,000 to 1,112,000, a 1% decrease. The effects on projections of AIDS incidence are slightly greater and lead to reductions of 3.9%, 3.8%, 3.5% and 3.0% respectively in the point estimates for 1991, 1992, 1992 and 1994 (personal communication from Professor Brookmeyer).

The natural history incubation distribution implicit in the Stage model is similar to incubation distributions used with the TSI model (Figure 5), and the hazard functions for the three incubations distributions used by Brookmeyer (1991) in sensitivity analyses also fall within the hazard plots used for the TSI model in Figure 5 (loci not shown). Thus, we do not believe that differences seen in Table 1 and 2 result mainly from differences in the choice of incubation distribution.

4 Discussion

Models that fail to take treatment into account after mid-1987 yield substantially smaller estimates of the numbers infected than models that account for treatment. For example, Brookmeyer's (1991) point estimate of the numbers infected (recalculated for 15% underreporting) decreases from 1,123,000 to 765,000 if treatment is removed (θ=1.0).

Models that take treatment and surveillance changes into account are necessarily more complex than the simpler models that apply to data before mid-1987. It is therefore encouraging that the Stage model and TSI model yield similar trends in the infection curve and that corresponding ranges of estimates of cumulative HIV infections and projected AIDS counts overlap. The higher estimates of numbers infected obtained by the Stage model seem mainly to reflect higher assessments of the extent of treatment in use and efficacy of treatment. Likewise, it is reassuring that estimates of cumulative infections from the TSI model agree reasonably well with estimates obtained by classical backcalculation applied to AIDS incidence data through mid-1987 (Table 1).

It would be helpful to have additional information on the "natural history" hazard beyond five years, because such data could help determine the quantitative impact of treatment on AIDS incidence (see Bacchetti, Segal and Jewell, 1991 and Section 3.1). Helper lymphocyte (CD4) marker data that extend beyond mid-1987 may be useful for estimating the "natural history" hazard beyond five years, because treatments such as AZT and pentamidine were usually administered after CD4 counts had fallen to low levels.

Table 1: Estimated plausible ranges for cumulative HIV infections (in thousands) in the United States based on backcalculation*

Method	Through 1 January, 1985	Through 1 July, 1987	Through Early 1990
Classical backcalculation†			
Data to 1 July, 1987			
	435-800	749-1,457	
	435-587	749-1,103	
Time-since-infection model			
Data to 1 January, 1991			
	444-599	590-791	628-988 (to 1 January, 1990)
Stage model			
Data to 1 April, 1990			909-1,289 (to 1 April, 1990)

* All calculations are multiplied by 1/0.85 to account for 15% underreporting. Estimates previously based on 10% underreporting are revised accordingly. Methods for constructing the plausible ranges for the Stage model and the time-since-infection model are outlined in Sections 3.2 and 3.3.

† The lower limit of the plausible range was based on the Fast Weibull incubation distribution (see legend to Figure 3) and the upper limit was based either on the Slow incubation distribution (See Rosenberg et al, 1991a), which yielded the highest estimates, or on the Standard Weibull distribution (see Table 2 of Rosenberg and Gail, 1990) which yielded lower estimates of the upper limit. The Standard Weibull distribution is defined with Figure 3.

Table 2: Projections of AIDS incidence for the broadened surveillance definition adopted in 1987 (in thousands)*

	Stage model		Time-since-infection model	
Year	Point Estimate	Plausible Range	Point Estimate†	Plausible Range
1991	65.0	59.0-69.6	54.7	51.4-58.8
1992	70.0	59.8-77.6	55.9	50.3-64.2
1993	72.6	58.0-84.2	54.8	47.0-68.1
1994	73.2	54.1-89.5	51.6	42.3-70.7

* All counts are based on a correction of 1/0.85 to account for 15% underreporting.

† Based on a Fast Weibull incubation distribution (see legend to Figure 3).

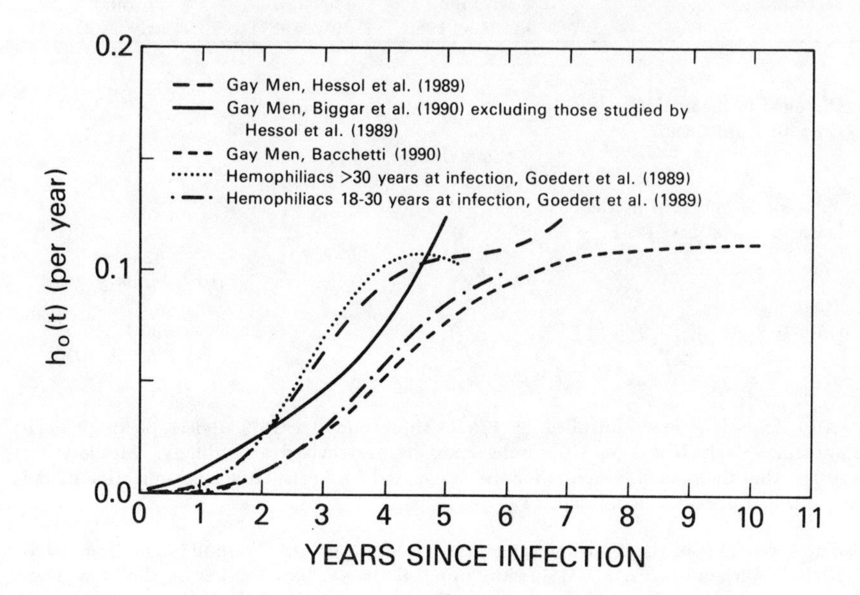

Figure 1. Smoothed estimates of the hazard of AIDS. Spline models using AIDS incidence data through 1 January, 1987 are presented for gay men studied by Hessol et al (1989), gay men studied by Biggar et al (1990) who were not in the cohort studied by Hessol et al, and hemophiliacs studied by Goedert et al (1989) and stratified by age group. The numbers of AIDS events in these groups were respectively 27, 19, 7 (for hemophiliacs infected when >30 years old) and 11 (for hemophiliacs infected when 18-30 years old). The hazard estimated by Bacchetti (1990) was obtained by backcalculation using seroconversion and AIDS incidence data in San Francisco through 31 December, 1988.

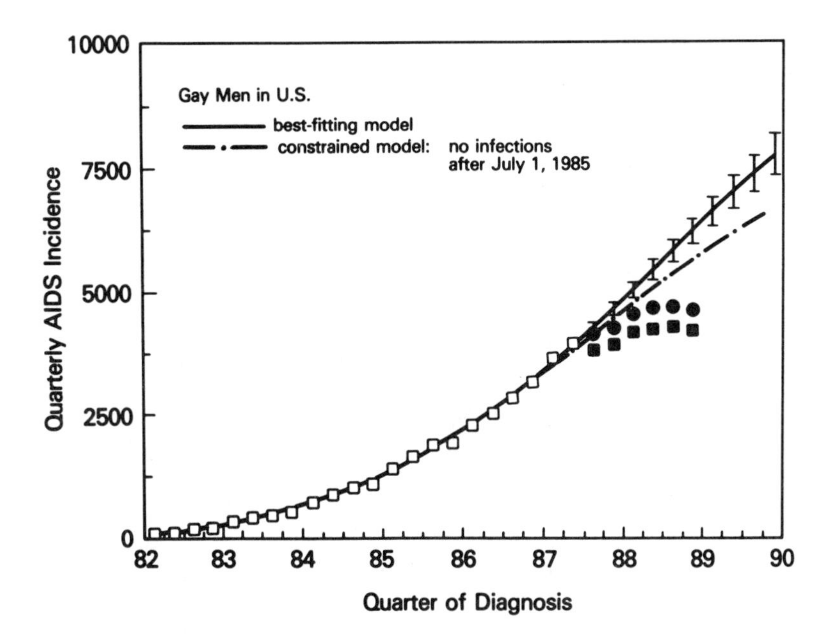

Figure 2. Consistently defined AIDS (squares) and all AIDS (circles) among U.S. gay men. The best fitting backcalculation projection (solid line) based on AIDS incidence data through June, 1987 and the backcalculated projection constrained to have no infections after July 1, 1985 (dot-dash line) exceed observed AIDS incidence beginning in mid-1987. Further details are in Gail, Rosenberg and Goedert (1990).

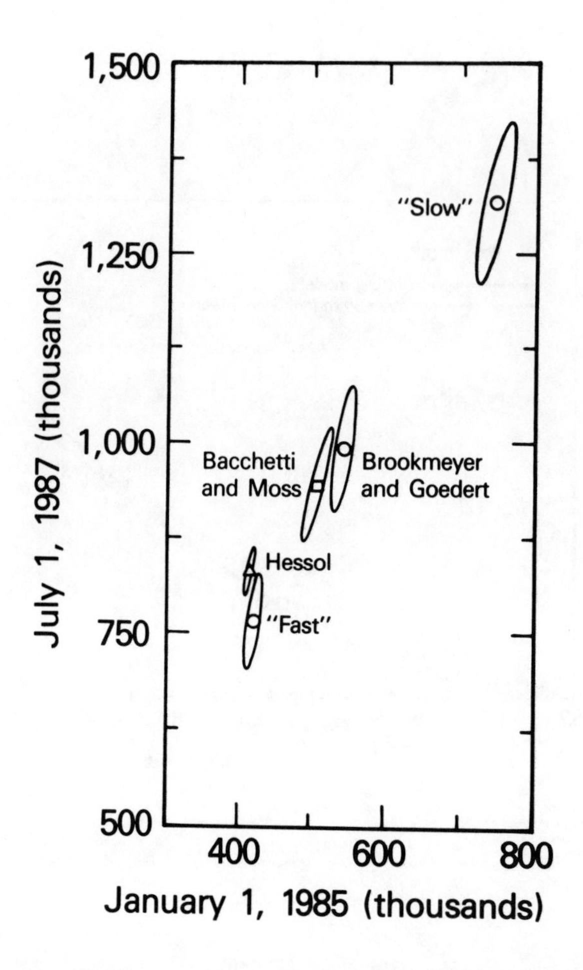

Figure 3. Sensitivity to the choice of incubation distribution of backcalculated estimates of cumulative HIV infections, based on consistently defined AIDS incidence data through 30 June, 1987 (taken from Rosenberg and Gail, 1990). Ninety-nine percent confidence ellipsoids are based on normal theory and bootstrap estimates of covariances. The incubation distribution of Brookmeyer and Goedert (1989), which we call the "Standard Weibull" distribution, is 1-exp(-.0021$t^{2.516}$). The incubation distribution estimated by Bacchetti and Moss (1989) has median 9.8 years, and that of Hessol et al (1989) about 10 years (see Rosenberg and Gail, 1991). The "Slow" model is given in Figure 1 of Rosenberg and Gail (1990) and has median 11.6 years, whereas the "Fast Weibull" distribution, which is approximately 1-exp(-.0021$t^{2.650}$), has median 9.0 years. The estimates shown are adjusted for 10% underreporting.

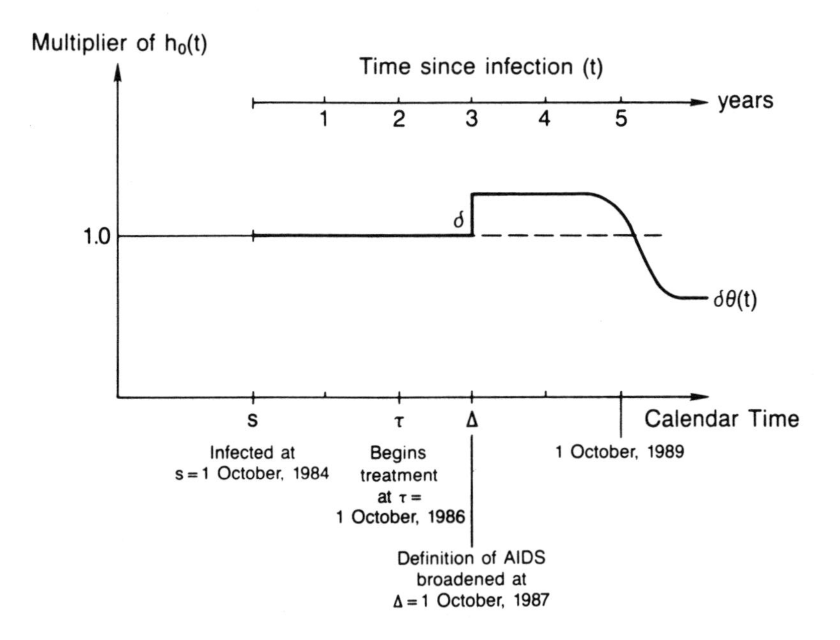

Figure 4. Multiplier of the natural history hazard function, $h_0(t)$, for the time-since-infection model. This example illustrates the multiplier for a person infected at s=1 October, 1984 who came under good medical care at τ=1 October, 1986. The multiplier δ takes effect on Δ=1 October, 1987 when the definition of AIDS is broadened, and the beneficial effects of treatment are first seen about 5 years after infection.

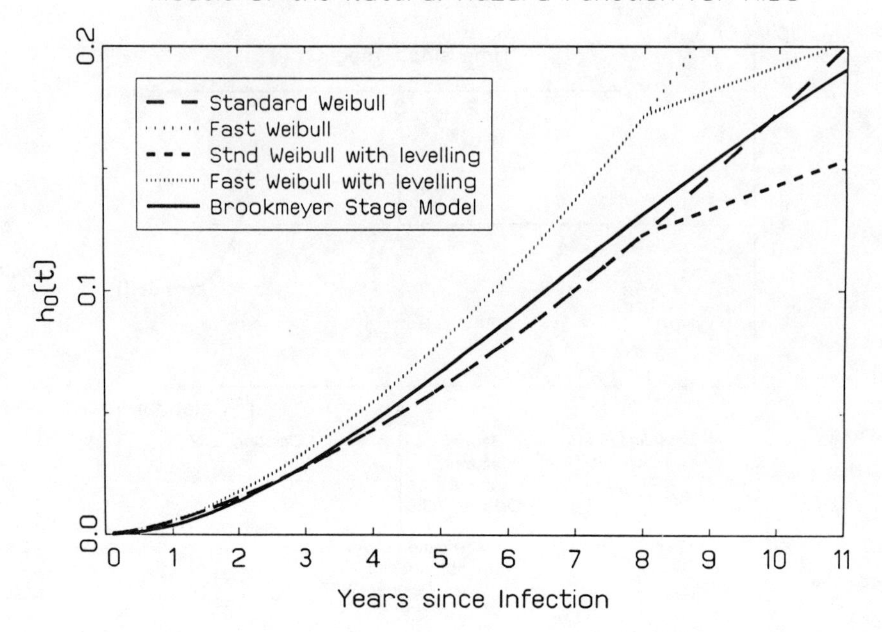

Figure 5. Hazard functions used in sensitivity analyses for the natural history incubation distribution. The "Standard" and "Fast Weibull" distributions are defined in the legend to Figure 3. Standard and Fast Weibull hazards with "levelling" are obtained by replacing the hazard functions by a straight line with slope 0.01 per year beginning at year 8. The solid locus corresponds to the natural history incubation used in the Stage model of Brookmeyer (1991).

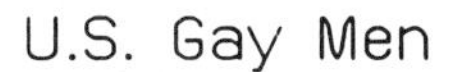

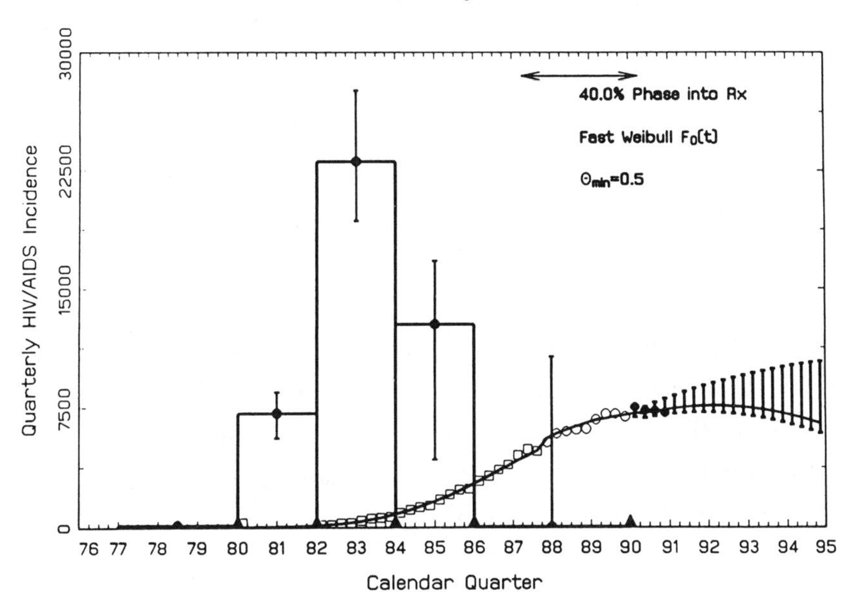

Figure 6. Estimates of the infection curve (rectangles) and projections of quarterly AIDS incidence (solid line) for gay men in the U.S. based on a Fast Weibull natural history incubation distribution. AIDS incidence data through 1989 were used to fit the backcalculation model, and treatment was phased in from 1 April, 1987 to 1 April, 1990. Eventually 40% receive treatment and the efficacy reaches θ_{min}=0.5. Vertical bars indicate 95% confidence based on percentiles of the bootstrap distribution, which takes overdispersion into account. Taken from Rosenberg, Gail and Carroll (1991).

Given the uncertainties in backcalculation, it is important to try to confirm the results of such analyses using other sources. In the rare event that unbiased information on the infection curve is available from serosurveys, such data may be formally combined with backcalculation by weighted least squares (Brookmeyer and Liao, 1990b). Data on HIV incidence trends in selected cohorts (CDC, 1987a) may also be very useful for checking trends estimated by backcalculation.

Acknowledgements

We thank Dr. Ronald Brookmeyer for helpful comments and for unpublished data on estimates of numbers infected and projections of AIDS incidence from the Stage model (Brookmeyer, 1991) and Dr. Robert Biggar for data on the incubation distribution. We also thank Mrs. Jennifer Donaldson for typing the manuscript.

References

Bacchetti, P. (1990). Estimating the incubation period of AIDS by comparing population infection and diagnosis patterns. *Journal of the American Statistical Association* **85**, 1002-1008.

Bacchetti, P. and Moss, A. R. (1989). Incubation period for AIDS in San Francisco. *Nature* **338**, 251-253.

Bacchetti, P., Segal, M. and Jewell, N. P. (1991). Uncertainty about the incubation period of AIDS and its impact on backcalculation. In AIDS Epidemiology: Methodological Issues, N. Jewell, K. Dietz and V. Farewell (eds). Boston: Birkhäuser-Boston.

Becker, N. G., Watson, L. F. and Carlin, J. B. (1991). A method of nonparametric back-projection and its application to AIDS data. *Statistics in Medicine*, in press.

Becker, N. G. and Watson, L. F. (1991). Use of empirical transformations in nonparametric back-projection of AIDS incidence data. In AIDS Epidemiology: Methodological Issues, N. Jewell, K. Dietz and V. Farewell (eds.). Boston: Birkhäuser-Boston.

Biggar, R. J. and the International Registry of Seroconverters (1990). AIDS incubation distribution in 1891 HIV seroconverters from different exposure groups. *AIDS* **4**, 1059-1066.

Brookmeyer, R. (1991). Reconstruction and future trends of the AIDS epidemic in the United States. *Science* **253**, 37-42.

Brookmeyer, R. and Damiano, A. (1990). Statistical methods for short-term projections of AIDS incidence. *Statistics in Medicine* **8**, 23-24 .

Brookmeyer, R. and Gail, M. H. (1986). Minimum size of the acquired immunodeficiency syndrome (AIDS) epidemic in the United States. *Lancet* **2**, 1320-1322.

Brookmeyer, R. and Gail, M. H. (1988). A method for obtaining short term projections and lower bounds on the size of the AIDS epidemic. *Journal of the American Statistical Association* **83**, 301-308.

Brookmeyer, R. and Goedert, J. J. (1989). Censoring in an epidemic with application to hemophilia-associated AIDS. *Biometrics* **45**, 325-335.

Brookmeyer, R. and Liao, J. (1990a). The analysis of delays in disease reporting: Methods and results for the acquired immunodeficiency syndrome. *American Journal of Epidemiology* **132**, 355-365.

Brookmeyer, R. and Liao, J. (1990b). Statistical modelling of the AIDS epidemic for forecasting health care needs. *Biometrics* **46**, 1151-1163.

Brookmeyer, R. and Liao, J. (1991). Statistical methods for reconstructing infection curves. In AIDS Epidemiology: Methodological Issues, N. Jewell, K. Dietz and V. Farewell (eds.). Boston: Birkhäuser-Boston.

Centers for Disease Control (1982). Update on acquired immune deficiency syndrome (AIDS) - United States. *Morbidity and Mortality Weekly Reports*, **31** 507-508.

Centers for Disease Control (1985). Revision of the case definition of acquired immunodeficiency syndrome for national reporting - United States. *Morbidity and Mortality Weekly Reports*, **34** 373-375.

Centers for Disease Control (1987a). Human immunodeficiency virus infection in the United States: A review of current knowledge. *Morbidity and Mortality Weekly Reports* **36**, 1-48.

Centers for Disease Control (1987b). Revision of the CDC surveillance case definition for acquired immunodeficiency syndrome. *Morbidity and Mortality Weekly Reports* **36**, 3S-15S.

Centers for Disease Control (1990). Estimates of HIV prevalence and projected AIDS cases: Summary of a workshop, October 31-November 1, 1989. *Morbidity and Mortality Weekly Reports* **39**, 110-119.

Chernoff, H. (1954). On the distribution of the likelihood ratio. *Annals of Mathematical Statistics* **25**, 573-578.

Darby, S. C., Rizza, C. R., Doll, R., Spooner, R. J. D., et al. (1989). Incidence of AIDS and excess of mortality associated with HIV in haemophiliacs in the United Kingdom: Report on behalf of the directors of hemophilia centers in the United Kingdom. *British Medical Journal* **298**, 1064-1068.

Day, N. E. and Gore, S. M. (1989). Prediction of the number of new AIDS cases and the number of new persons infected with HIV up to 1992: The results of 'back projection methods', Short-term Prediction of HIV Infections and AIDS in England and Wales, London: HMSO.

DeGruttola, V. and Lagakos, S. W. (1989). The value of AIDS incidence data in assessing the spread of HIV infection. *Statistics in Medicine* **8**, 35-43.

Fischl, M. A., Richman, D. D., Grieco, M. H., Gottlieb, M. S., et al. (1987). The efficacy of azidothymidine (AZT) in the treatment of patients with AIDS and AIDS-related complex. *New England Journal of Medicine* **317**, 185-191.

Fischl, M. A., Richman, D. D., Hansen, N., Collier, A. C., et al. (1990). The safety and efficacy of zidovudine (AZT) in the treatment of patients with mildly symptomatic HIV infection: A double blind placebo-controlled trial. *Annals of Internal Medicine* **112**, 727-737.

Gail, M. H. and Brookmeyer, R. (1988). Methods for projecting course of Acquired Immunodeficiency Syndrome epidemic. *Journal of the National Cancer Institute* **80**, 900-911.

Gail, M. H. and Brookmeyer, R. (1990). Modeling the AIDS epidemic. *AIDS Update* **3**, 1-8.

Gail, M. H., Rosenberg, P. S. and Goedert, J. J. (1990a). Therapy may explain recent deficits in AIDS incidence. *Journal of Acquired Immune Deficiency Syndromes* **3**, 296-306.

Goedert, J. J., Kessler, C. M., Aledort, L. M., Biggar, R. J., et al. (1989). A prospective study of human immunodeficiency virus type 1 infection and the development of AIDS in subjects with hemophilia. *New England Journal of Medicine* **321**, 1141-1148.

Golden, J. A., Chernoff, D., Hollander, H. and Conte, J. E. (1989). Prevention of pneumocystis carinii pneumonia by inhaled pentamidine. *Lancet* **1**, 654-657.

Graham, N. M., Zeger, S. L., Kuo, V., Jacobson, L. P., et al. (1991). Zidovudine use in AIDS-free HIV-1-seropositive homosexual men in the multicenter AIDS cohort study (MACS), 1987-1989. *Journal of Acquired Immune Deficiency Syndromes* **4**, 267-276.

Harris, J. E. (1987). Delay in reporting acquired immunodeficiency syndrome (AIDS). Working paper No. 2278. National Bureau of Economic Research.

Harris, J. E. (1990). Reporting delays and the incidence of AIDS. *Journal of the American Statistical Association* **85**, 915-924.

Hessol, N. A., Lifson, A. R., O'Malley, P. M., Doll, L. S., et al. (1989). Prevalence, incidence, and progression of human immunodeficiency virus infection in homosexual and bisexual men in hepatitis B vaccine trials, 1978-1988. *American Journal of Epidemiology* **130**, 1167-1175.

Hymen, J. M. and Stanley, E. A. (1988). Using mathematical models to understand the AIDS epidemic. *Mathematical Biosciences* **90**, 415.

Isham, V. (1989). Estimation of the incidence of HIV infection - the back projection method. Short-term Prediction of HIV Infections and AIDS in England and Wales, London: HMSO.

Lang, W., Osmond, D., Samuel, M., Moss, A., et al. (1991). Population-based estimates of zidovudine and aerosol pentamidine use in San Francisco: 1987-1989. *Journal of Acquired Immune Deficiency Syndromes* **4**, 713-716.

Lawless, J. and Sun, J. (1991). A comprehensive back-calculation framework for the estimation and prediction of AIDS cases. In AIDS Epidemiology: Methodological Issues, N. Jewell, K. Dietz and V. Farewell (eds.). Boston: Birkhäuser-Boston.

Leoung, G. S., Feigal, D. W., Jr., Montgomery, A. B., Corkery, K., et al. (1990). Aerosolized pentamidine for prophylaxis against pneumocystis carinii pneumonia: The San Francisco Community Prophylaxis Trial. *New England Journal of Medicine* **323**, 769-775.

Longini, I. M., Jr. (1990). Modeling the decline of CD4+ T-lymphocyte counts in HIV-infected individuals. *Journal of Acquired Immune Deficiency Syndromes* **3**, 930-931.

Longini, I. M., Byers, R. H., Horsburgh, C. R. and Hessol, N. A. (1990). Estimation of the stage-specific incidence and prevalence of HIV infection using a Markov model and back-calculation. Abstract F.C. 212. Presented at the Sixth International Conference on AIDS. San Francisco.

Longini, I. M., Clark, W. S., Byers, R. H., Ward, J. W., et al. (1989). Statistical analysis of the stages of HIV infection using a Markov model. *Statistics in Medicine* **8**, 831-843.

Muñoz, A., Wang, M-C., Bass, S., Taylor, J. M. G., et al.(1989). Acquired immunodeficiency syndrome (AIDS)-free time after human immunodeficiency virus type I (HIV-1) seroconversion in homosexual men. *American Journal of Epidemiology* **130**, 530-539.

Rosenberg, P. (1990). A simple correction of AIDS surveillance data for reporting delays. *Journal of Acquired Immune Deficiency Syndromes* **3**, 49-54.

Rosenberg, P., Biggar, R. J., Goedert, J. J. and Gail, M. H. (1991a). Backcalculation of the number with human immunodeficiency virus infection in the United States. *American Journal of Epidemiology* **133**, 276-285.

Rosenberg, P. S. and Gail, M. H. (1990). Uncertainty in estimates of HIV prevalence derived by backcalculation. *Annals of Epidemiology* **1**, 105-115.

Rosenberg, P. S. and Gail, M. H. (1991). Backcalculation of flexible linear models of the human immunodeficiency virus infection curve. *Applied Statistics* **40**, 269-282.

Rosenberg, P. S., Gail, M. H. and Carroll, R. J. (1991). Estimating HIV prevalence and projecting AIDS incidence in the United States: A model that accounts for therapy and changes in the surveillance definition of AIDS. (Submitted).

Rosenberg, P. S., Gail, M. H. and Pee, D. (1991). Mean square error of estimates of HIV prevalence and short-term AIDS projections derived by backcalculation. *Statistics in Medicine* **10**, 1167-1180.

Rosenberg, P. S., Gail, M. H., Schrager, L., Vermund, S. H., et al. (1991b). National AIDS incidence trends and the extent of zidovudine therapy in selected demographic and transmission groups. *Journal of Acquired Immune Deficiency Syndromes* **4**, 392-401.

Selik, R. M., Buehler, J. W., Karon, J. M., Chamberland, M. E., et al. (1990). Impact of the 1987 revision of the case definition of acquired immune deficiency syndrome in the United States. *Journal of Acquired Immune Deficiency Syndromes* **3**, 73-82.

Solomon, P. J. and Wilson, S. R. (1990). Accommodating change due to treatment in the method of back projection for estimating HIV infection incidence. *Biometrics* **46**, 1165-1170.

Taylor, J. M. G. (1989). Models for the HIV infection and AIDS epidemic in the United States. *Statistics in Medicine* **8**, 45-58.

Volberding, P. A., Lagakos, S. W., Koch, M.A., Pettinelli, C., et al. (1990). Zidovudine in asymptomatic human immunodeficiency virus infection: A controlled trial in persons with fewer than 500 CD4-positive cells per cubic millimeter. *New England Journal of Medicine* **322**, 941-949.

Zeger, S. L., See, L-C. and Diggle, P.J. (1989). Statistical methods for monitoring the AIDS epidemic. *Statistics in Medicine* **8**, 3-21.

Mitchell H. Gail and Philip S. Rosenberg, National Cancer Institute, Epidemiologic Methods Section, 6130 Executive Blvd., EPN/403, Rockville, Maryland 20892

STATISTICAL METHODS FOR RECONSTRUCTING INFECTION CURVES

Ron Brookmeyer and Jiangang Liao

Abstract: The objective of this paper is to consider statistical issues for reconstructing infection curves. We investigate the method of back-calculation using a nonstationary incubation period distribution to account for recent treatment advances. A spline methodology based on a penalized likelihood is used for estimating historical infection rates. Estimates can be obtained through iteratively reweighted least squares. Some theoretical calculations to investigate mean square error are presented. There is tradeoff between bias and variance when choosing the smoothing parameter. An approach for choosing a range of sensible smoothing parameters is suggested. Some of the methods are illustrated with the U.S. AIDS epidemic.

1. Introduction

The method of back-calculation (Brookmeyer and Gail, 1986; 1988) involves using disease (AIDS) incidence data and the incubation period distribution to reconstruct historical infection rates. These rates are then propagated forward according to the incubation period distribution to obtain short-term projections of disease (AIDS) incidence. The fundamental equation underlying the back-calculation method is given by the convolution equation

$$a(t) = \int_0^t I(s)F(t-s)ds \tag{1}$$

where $a(t)$ is the expected cumulative number of AIDS cases diagnosed by year t, $I(s)$ is the infection rate at time s, and $F(t)$ is the incubation period distribution which is the probability of developing AIDS within t years of infection. The basic idea of back-calculation is to use AIDS incidence data, $a(t)$, together with an estimate of the incubation period distribution, $F(t)$, to glean information about past HIV infection rates, $I(s)$, from equation (1). The main sources of uncertainty from this approach arise from uncertainties in the incubation distribution, the shape of the infection curve, and the AIDS incidence data (Rosenberg and Gail, 1990). Furthermore, estimates of recent infection rates are very imprecise because recent infections are not yet reflected in AIDS incidence data due to the long incubation period.

Beginning in 1987, therapies such as AZT and aerosolized pentamidine were introduced for HIV infected individuals who do not yet have AIDS. These therapies could potentially lengthen the incubation period (Gail, Rosenberg and Goedert, 1990). Accordingly, back-calculation methods were generalized to account for secular changes in the incubation period distribution (Brookmeyer and Liao, 1990). The generalization of equation (1) is

$$a(t) = \int_0^t I(s) \cdot F(t-s|s)ds \qquad (2)$$

where $F(t|s)$ is the incubation period distribution for an individual infected at calendar time s; that is, $F(t|s)$ is the probability of developing AIDS within t years of infection for an individual who was infected at calendar time s. The objective of this paper is to consider statistical issues and methods for the deconvolution of AIDS incidence data to produce smoothed reconstructions of infection rates by solving equation (2). Integral equations such as equation (2) arise in many different applications (O'Sullivan, 1986) and have been called Fredholm integral equations of the first kind (Wahba, 1985).

An important question in the statistical solution of equation (2) is how to parameterize the infection curve $I(s)$. If $I(s)$ is parameterized very weakly, the estimates of $I(s)$ can exhibit implausible oscillations and sensitivity to small perturbation in the data. Some previous attempts to overcome these problems have used strongly parametric models (e.g., log-logistic, or exponential growth models; see for example: Brookmeyer and Damiano (1989); Taylor (1989); Day and

Gore (1989); and DeGruttola and Lagakos (1989)). However, this approach can produce severely biased infection rates, especially in the most recent past, if the assumptions are incorrect. Another approach is to use parametric models such as flexible step functions with relatively few parameters. This was the original approach used by Brookmeyer and Gail (1986) in the first attempts at back-calculation of AIDS incidence data. Simulation studies suggested that step-function models for the infection curve yield satisfactory estimates of HIV prevalence and AIDS incidence as measured by mean square error (Rosenberg, Gail and Pee, 1991). A disadvantage of step-function models is it produces unsmoothed estimates of the infection curve.

An alternative approach, based on splines, uses Phillips-Tikhonov regularization (Phillips, 1962; Tikhonov, 1963). Bacchetti (1990) employed this approach to estimate the incubation period distribution ($F(t)$) by solving equation (1) using AIDS incidence data, $a(t)$ and infection rates, $I(s)$, obtained from HIV seroprevalence surveys in San Francisco. In this paper, we use a methodology similar to the Bacchetti approach in order to estimate infection rates from knowledge of $F(t|s)$ and $a(t)$. The methods allow for secular changes in the incubation distribution.

2. Models for Secular Changes in the Incubation Period Distribution

In order to use equation (2) we need an external estimate of $F(t|s)$. We have used a staging model for the natural history of HIV infection to induce secular changes in the incubation period distribution due to therapeutic advances. It is assumed individuals progress from infection (stage 1) to an advanced stage of HIV disease without an AIDS diagnosis (stage 2) to AIDS (stage 3). Advanced stage HIV disease (stage 2) could be defined in terms of CD4 cells or clinical signs and symptoms.

The main assumptions of our model for evaluating the effects of treatment on the incubation distribution are as follows: Individuals in advanced stage HIV disease (stage 2) may be treated but individuals with early stage HIV disease are not treated. An individual who entered stage 2 at calendar time s has a hazard, $h(u|s)$, of receiving treatments u time units after entry into stage 2 and the effect of treatment is to reduce the hazard of progression to AIDS by the factor θ (the treatment relative risk). A schematic illustration of this four-state competing risk model is shown in Figure 1. In the absence

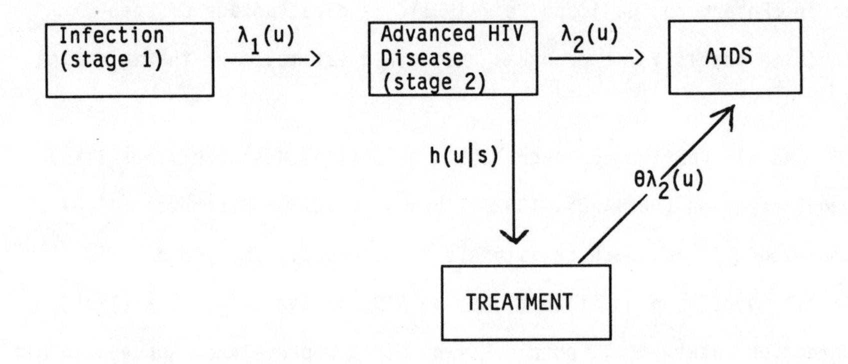

Figure 1. Four State (staging) Model to Incorporate Secular Changes in Incubation Period Due to Treatment

of treatment, the hazard of progression from stage i to stage i+1 after u time units in stage i is called $\lambda_i(u)$. In our previous work (Brookmeyer and Liao, 1990; Brookmeyer, 1991) we assumed $\lambda_1(u)$ was Weibull ($\lambda_1(u) = .029u\ 1.08$, median = 6.5 years), and $\lambda_2(u)$ was exponential ($\lambda_2 = .277$, median = 2.5 years). Treatment was assumed to be phased in at a constant rate beginning July 1, 1987, that is $h(u|s) = 0$ for $u + s \leq 1987.5$ and $h(u|s) = \lambda_3 = .20$ for $u + s >$ 1987.5. The expression for the resulting distribution of the time in advanced stage HIV disease (stage 2) as a function of calendar time of entry into stage 2 is given by equation 9 of Brookmeyer and Liao (1990). An important advantage of modelling treatment effects by a staging model is that treatment decisions are typically based on CD4 count and other clinical symptoms. Furthermore, empirical estimates of $h(u|s)$ can be obtained from surveys and cohort studies of HIV infected populations.

3. A Spline Methodology

The data consist of the numbers of AIDS cases diagnosed in intervals of calendar time. Let y_i represent the number of cases diagnosed in calendar interval $[T_{i-1}, T_i)$, $i = 1,\ldots,N$. Our statistical model specifies the mean and variance of y_i. The mean is

$$E(y_i) = \int_0^{T_i} I(s)\ \{F(T_i-s|s)-F(T_{i-1}-s|s)\}ds \qquad (3)$$

where $F(t|s)$ is defined to be 0 for $t < 0$. The variance of y_i is taken to be proportional to the mean

$$Var(y_i) = \sigma^2 E(y_i) \qquad (4)$$

where σ^2 is the overdispersion parameter to account for extra-Poisson variation.

The infection curve $I(s)$ will be approximated by a step function with a large number, p, of short steps. That is,

$$I(s) = \beta_j \quad \text{for } c_{j-1} < s < c_j \qquad j = 1,\ldots,p$$

where the calendar times, $\{c_j\}$, are the knots (jump points) for the step function. Under this model for $I(s)$, $E(Y_i)$ is linear in the unknown parameters (Rosenberg and Gail, 1991):

$$E(Y_i) = \sum_{j=1}^{p} \beta_j X_{ij}$$

where

$$X_{ij} = \int_{c_{j-1}}^{c_j} \{F(T_i - s|s) - F(T_{i-1} - s|s)\}ds \qquad (5)$$

In matrix notation,

$$E(\underset{\sim}{Y}) = X\underset{\sim}{\beta}$$

Without additional structure on the shape of the infection curve, the estimates of I(s) can exhibit implausible oscillation and high sensitivity to small perturbation in the data especially if the widths of the steps, $w_j = (c_j - c_{j-1})$, are small. Following Bacchetti (1990), our approach to deal with this problem is Phillips-Tikhonov regularization. This involves maximizing a penalized log-likelihood:

$$\log L - \frac{\lambda}{2} J \tag{6}$$

where log L is the log-likelihood function, J measures the roughness of the infection curve, and λ is the smoothing parameter which calibrates the desired degree of smoothness of the estimated function I(s). Our measure of roughness, J, is a discretized approximation to the integrated squared second derivative of the infection curve, $\int_0^{T_N} [I''(s)]^2 \, ds$. This is given by

$$J = \sum_{k=1}^{p-2} \frac{4}{w_{k+1}} \left\{ \frac{\beta_{k+2} - \beta_{k+1}}{w_{k+2} + w_{k+1}} - \frac{\beta_{k+1} - \beta_k}{w_{k+1} + w_k} \right\}^2$$

where $w_k = c_k - c_{k-1}$ is the width of the kth step. For intervals of equal width this reduces to

$$J = \frac{1}{w^3} \sum_{k=1}^{p-2} (\beta_{k+2} - 2\,\beta_{k+1} + \beta_k)^2$$

The roughness penalty J can be expressed as a quadratic form

$$\underset{\sim}{\beta}' K \underset{\sim}{\beta}$$

where the p×p matrix K is $K = Q'Q$ where the elements of the (p-2)×p matrix Q are

$$Q_{j,j} = \frac{2}{(w_{k+1} + w_k)\sqrt{w_{k+1}}}$$

$$Q_{j,j+2} = \frac{2}{(w_{k+1} + w_{k+2})\sqrt{w_{k+1}}}$$

$$Q_{j,j+1} = - Q_{j,j} + Q_{j,j+2}$$

for $j = 1,\ldots,p-2$. All other elements of Q are 0. O'Sullivan, Yandell and Raynor (1986) note that maximizing (6), for a Poisson likelihood, is equivalent to minimizing

$$(\underset{\sim}{Y} - X\underset{\sim}{\beta})'W(\underset{\sim}{Y} - X\underset{\sim}{\beta}) + \lambda\underset{\sim}{\beta}'K\underset{\sim}{\beta} \tag{7}$$

where the weight matrix, W, is an N×N diagonal matrix with diagonal entries $(X\underset{\sim}{\beta})^{-1}$. Differentiating (6) with respect to $\underset{\sim}{\beta}$ where L is the Poisson likelihood, it can be shown that $\hat{\underset{\sim}{\beta}}$ satisfies

$$\hat{\underset{\sim}{\beta}} = (X'\hat{W}X + \lambda K)^{-1}X'\hat{W}\underset{\sim}{Y} \tag{8}$$

where $\hat{W}$ is the N×N diagonal matrix with diagnonal entries $(X\hat{\underset{\sim}{\beta}})^{-1}$. Thus, $\hat{\underset{\sim}{\beta}}$ can be obtained by an iteratively reweighted least squares procedures: equation (8) is used to update the estimate $\hat{\underset{\sim}{\beta}}$ where the weight matrix W is updated at each iteration by using the current estimate of β.

The asymptotic distribution of the estimator $\hat{\beta}$ can be derived under the following conditions. Consider a sequence of Poisson models defined by (3) where $I_n(s) = nI_0(s) \to \infty$ as $n \to \infty$, and where N (the dimension of $\underset{\sim}{Y}$) and p (the dimension of $\underset{\sim}{\beta}$) are held fixed. If $I_n(s) \to \infty$ then $E(\sum_{i=1}^{N} y_i) \sum_{i=1}^{n} \mu_{in} = \mu_{\cdot n} \to \infty$. We also assume $\lambda_n \to 0$ fast enough so that $\lambda_n\mu_{\cdot n} \to c$ for some constant $c < \infty$. We consider the limiting distribution of $(\hat{\beta}_n - \beta_n)/\sqrt{\mu_{\cdot n}}$ where $\hat{\underset{\sim}{\beta}}_n$ satisfies (8) and $\underset{\sim}{\beta}_n$ satisfies

$$\underset{\sim}{\beta}_n = (X'W_nX + \lambda K)^{-1} \; X'W_nE(\underset{\sim}{Y}) \tag{9}$$

where $E(\underset{\sim}{Y})$ is given by expression (3) with $I_n(s)$ substituted for $I(s)$, and W_n is a diagonal matrix with entries $(X\underset{\sim}{\beta}_n)^{-1}$. Expression (8) together with the fact that $W_n^{1/2}(\underset{\sim}{Y}_n - \underset{\sim}{\mu}_n)$ converges to a multivariate normal distribution with mean 0, and a covariance matrix given by the identity matrix, under suitable regularity conditions, establish that $(\hat{\beta}_n - \underset{\sim}{\beta}_n)/\sqrt{\underset{\sim}{\mu}_{\cdot n}}$ converges to a multivariate normal distribution with mean 0 and asymptotic variance-covariance matrix, Σ, given by

$$\Sigma = \lim_{n\to\infty} \mu_{\cdot n}^{-1} \left[X'W_nX+\lambda_nK\right]^{-1} X'W_nW_{on}^{-1}W_nX\left[(X'W_nX+\lambda_nK)^{-1}\right]' \tag{10}$$

where W_n is an $N\times N$ diagonal matrix with entries $(X\underset{\sim}{\beta}_n)^{-1}$ and W_{on} is an $N\times N$ diagonal matrix with entries $[E(\underset{\sim}{Y})]^{-1}$.

A heuristic derivation of this asymptotic result is obtained directly from expression (8) by writing $\hat{\underset{\sim}{\beta}} = C\underset{\sim}{Y}$. If we consider C as a fixed matrix, and $\underset{\sim}{Y}$ as approximately normal then $E(\hat{\beta}) \approx CE(\underset{\sim}{Y})$ and $Var(\hat{\underset{\sim}{\beta}}) \approx CV(\underset{\sim}{Y})C'$. This yields equations (9) and (10).

One estimate of the overdispersion parameter, σ^2, is

$$\hat{\sigma}^2 = \frac{\sum_{i=1}^{N} (y_i - \hat{y}_i)^2/\hat{y}}{N-\text{Trace}(H)} \tag{11}$$

where H is the smoothing spline hat matrix, that is

$$\hat{Y} = HY$$
$$H = X(X'\hat{W}X + \lambda K)^{-1}X'\hat{W} \; .$$

Intuitively, the denominator of (11) is an adjusted degrees of freedom. Trace (H) which is never greater than p, represents the effective number of parameters which are being estimated (because of the roughness penalty we in fact are not estimating p independent parameters). A fuller discussion of the estimator $\hat{\sigma}^2$ is given in

Wahba (1990) and Nychka (1988). Some simulation studies suggest $\hat{\sigma}^2$ is a good estimate of σ^2 (Wahba, 1983; Silverman, 1985).

The main question with smoothing splines is how to choose the smoothing parameter, λ. One approach is to perform a sensitivity analysis of the estimated infection curve, $\hat{I}(s)$, to different choices for λ. At the end of section 5, we outline a strategy for choosing a range of values of the smoothing parameter for such a sensitivity analysis. An alternative approach is to use automatic smoothing procedures such as the generalized cross-validation score GCV(λ), to guide the degree of smoothing. The generalized cross-validation score is

$$GCV(\lambda) = \frac{\hat{\sigma}^2}{N - \text{Trace}(H)} \quad .$$

Some theoretical and simulation work suggests that the λ which minimizes the generalized cross-validation score will minimize a weighted mean squared error criterion, for the AIDS incidence curve (O'Sullivan, Yandell and Raynor, 1986). Although for our purpose it should be noted that a more relevant criterion might be a mean square error criterion for the infection curve rather than the AIDS incidence curve.

4. Computational Notes

It is useful to note that existing computer algorithms which fit step function models for I(s) by iteratively reweighted least squares can be easily adapted to incorporate the smoothing methodology described in Section 2. To see this note that $\lambda \underset{\sim}{\beta}' K \underset{\sim}{\beta}$ in (7) can be thought of as sum of squares for a weighted regression analysis where the data vector is a column of zeros, the expected value of the data is $\underset{\sim}{\beta}$, and the weight matrix is K. To implement the spline methodology on existing iteratively least squares computer programs, one would augment "pseudo-data" to the $\underset{\sim}{Y}$ data vector which would consist of a vector, $\underset{\sim}{D}$, of p-2 zeros. Computing algorithms for fitting step functions for I(s) could be used for fitting smoothing splines by defining the data vector $\underset{\sim}{Y}^*$, design matrix X^* and weight matrix W^* as follows:

$$\underset{\sim}{Y}^* = \begin{pmatrix} \underset{\sim}{Y} \\ D_{p\times 1} \end{pmatrix} \quad X^* = \begin{pmatrix} X \\ -I \end{pmatrix}$$

$$W^*_{(N+p)\times(N+p)} = \begin{bmatrix} W_{N\times N} & D_{N\times p} \\ D_{p\times N} & \lambda K_{p\times p} \end{bmatrix}$$

where I is the (p×p) identity matrix and $D_{m\times n}$ represents an m×n matrix all of who's entries are zero.

5. Mean Square Error and the Trade-off Between Bias and Variance

In general, strongly parametric models for I(s) yield smaller variances of the estimated infection rates than do weakly parametric models. However, there could be considerable bias in the estimated infection rate if the assumed parametric model is incorrect (Brookmeyer and Damiano (1989); De Gruttola and Lagakos (1989); Taylor (1989); Day and Gore (1989)). There is a tradeoff between bias and variance. In this section, we calculate the bias and variance of estimated infection rates based on the smoothing spline procedure (Section 2) for arbitrary infection curves, I(s).

The procedures and asymptotic results described above refer to unconstrained estimation. However, constrained optimization should be used to insure that $\hat{\underset{\sim}{\beta}}$ is non-negative. A simple ad-hoc, alternative to fully constrained optimization is to, first, perform unconstrained optimization, and then, redefine any negative estimates of $\hat{\underset{\sim}{\beta}}$ to be 0. The sampling distribution of this "constrained estimator", $\hat{\beta}_c$, is a truncated normal with asymptotic mean

$$\beta_c = \int_0^\infty u f(u) du \tag{12}$$

and variance

$$\text{Var}(\hat{\beta}_c) = \int_0^\infty u^2 f(u) du - \beta_c^2 \tag{13}$$

where f is a normal density with mean β given by expression (9) variance obtained from expression (10). Of course, $\hat{\beta}_c$ is not the fully constrained estimator. Below we report theoretical calculations to evaluate the mean square error of $\hat{\beta}_c$. Alternatively, a simulation study could be undertaken to evaluate the performance of the fully constrained estimator. One would expect the fully constrained estimator would perform better than $\hat{\beta}_c$, and thus our mean square error results for $\hat{\beta}_c$ should be upper bounds on the mean square error for the fully constrained estimator.

We computed the bias, variance, and mean square error of estimated infection rates from $\hat{\beta}_c$ based on smoothing splines from equation (12) and (13) for a range of the smoothing parameter and for several hypothetical infection curves using the theoretical results of this section. For our theoretical calculations, we considered three hypothetical infection curves which were scaled to produce 150,000 AIDS cases by April 1, 1991. The infection curves A, B, and C are illustrated in Figure 2 and correspond to situations 5, 9, and 7 respectively in Figure 1 of Rosenberg, Gail and Pee (1991). Rosenberg, Gail and Pee (1991) estimated mean square error of cumulative HIV infections and AIDS projections from a simulation study based on an assumed step function model for I(s) (without smoothing). For our calculations, the knots for the step function $\{c_j\}$, were chosen so that the step widths were yearly except for the first and last intervals which were 2.0 and 1.25 years respectively (i.e., the c_j were 1977.0, 1979.0, 1980.0, 1981.0, 1988.0, 1989.0, 1990.25).

The results for infection curve A (increasing then falling infection rates) are given in Table 1. Table 1 gives the standard deviation (SD) of the estimated infection rate at several different points in calendar time and the percent root mean square (PRMS) for a range of smoothing parameters ($-11.0 \leq \log \lambda \leq -3.0$). The percent root mean square (see footnote to Table 1) was also used by Rosenberg, Gail and Pee (1991) to assess the performance of the estimators. The table shows that the standard error decreases as the smoothing parameter increases. Generally, it is also true that standard errors are considerably larger for infection rates in the recent

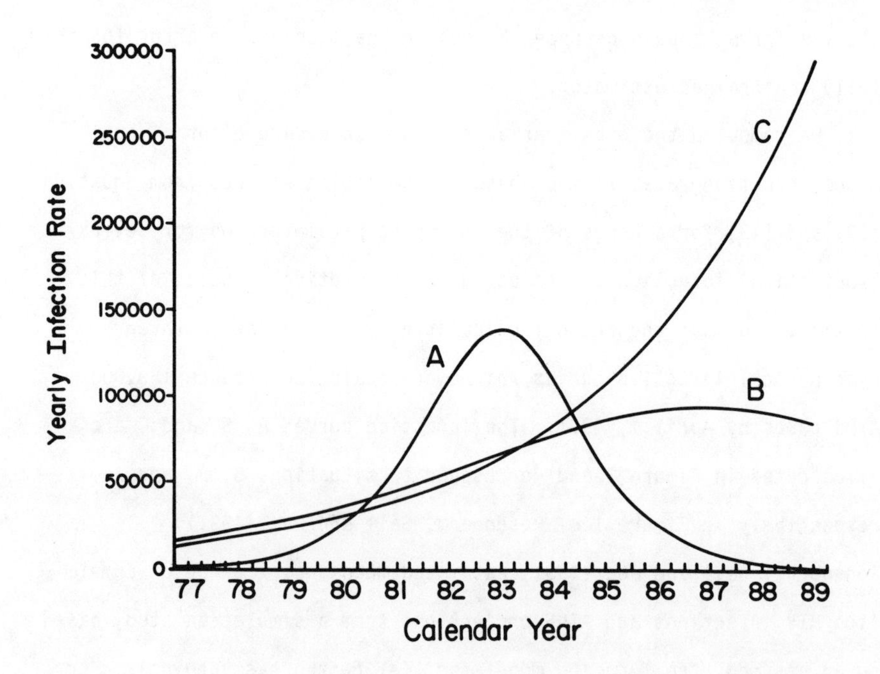

Figure 2. Three Hypothetical Infection Curves. Infection Curves are proportional to $I(s) = e^{\sigma_1+\sigma_3 s}/(1 + e^{\sigma_2+\sigma_3 s})^2$ where proportionality constant is chosen to yield 150,000 expected cumulative AIDS cases by 1990.25 using incubation distribution, $F(t|s)$, described in Figure 1: Curve A: $\sigma_1=1$, $\sigma_2=6$, $\sigma_3=1$; Curve B: $\sigma_1=1$, $\sigma_2=-3$, $\sigma_3=0.3$; Curve C: $\sigma_1=1$, $\sigma_2=-20.0$, $\sigma_3=0.25$.

past than the distant past. The PRMS tends to be higher both for small values of log λ (because of large standard errors) and for large values of log λ (because of large bias), which illustrates the trade-off between bias and variance. The lower values of PRMS are obtained when log λ is in the range of -8.0 to -6.0.

Similar calculations for infection curve B (increasing then plateauing infection rates) are given in Table 2. Again, standard errors are markedly reduced with increased smoothing. The PRMS decreases as log λ increases, and then approximately stablizes for log $\lambda \geq -7.0$. Choosing log $\lambda = -7.0$ gives good values for the PRMS for the infection rates at all the considered calendar time points. Table 3 gives he results for infection curve C (increasing infection rates). The PRMS first decreases and then increases as log λ increases. Again, log λ near -7.0 produces good values for the PRMS at all considered calendar time points.

Tables 1-3 suggest a strategy for choosing the smoothing parameter. One would consider several plausible infection curves which are scaled to produce the observed number of AIDS cases. The PMSE (or an alternative measure of performance) could be computed for various values of log λ. The range of log λ would be identified which gave good (lower) values for the PRMS for the considered infection curves. Sensitivity analyses of the estimated infection rates to this range of log λ would be performed. The results in Tables 1-3 suggest that with 150,000 cumulative AIDS cases, a value of log λ in the neighborhood of -7.0 would give low values of PRMS for the range of true infection curves illustrated in Figure 2.

The optimum choice of the smoothing parameter (i.e. λ which minimizes the PRMS) depends on the sample size (the expected cumulative number of cases, $E(\Sigma Y_i)$). Generally the optimum λ gets smaller with increasing sample sizes. Table 4 gives the optimum value of log λ for epidemics of different sizes (cumulative cases between 25,000 and 250,000). This table can be used, as a starting point, for choosing a smoothing parameter for epidemics of different sizes.

6. Application to the U.S. AIDS Epidemic

The methods outlined in sections 2 and 3 were applied to the U.S. AIDS epidemic. A more complete description of the substantive findings is in Brookmeyer (1991). Quarterly AIDS incidence data based on cases diagnosed before April 1, 1990 and reported by September 1, 1990, and adjusted for reporting delays was obtained from the Centers for Disease Control. The knots for the step function, $\{c_j\}$, were the same as described in section 5 for our mean square error calculation. The nonstationary incubation period distribution described in section (2) was used. Figure 3 shows the estimated infection curves for different choices of the smoothing parameter, λ. The estimates before 1987 are not nearly as sensitive to the smoothing parameter compared to estimates after 1987.

Further insight into the smoothing spline procedures can be obtained by reexpressing the estimated smoothed infection rates, $\hat{\beta}_\lambda$, based on smoothing parameter λ, in terms of estimated unsmoothed infection rates, $\hat{\beta}_0$, based on the smoothing parameter $\lambda = 0$:

$$\hat{\underset{\sim}{\beta}}_\lambda = (X'\hat{W}_\lambda X + \lambda k)^{-1}(X'\hat{W}_0 X)\hat{\underset{\sim}{\beta}}_0$$

$$= A \cdot \hat{\underset{\sim}{\beta}}_0$$

where $\hat{W}_\lambda$ is a diagonal matrix with entries $[X\hat{\underset{\sim}{\beta}}_\lambda]^{-1}$. Technically, this is not a linear decomposition of the smoothed rates into unsmoothed rates, because A depends (somewhat) on the unsmoothed rates through $\hat{W}_\lambda$. Nevertheless the averaging matrix, A, provides some insight into how the unsmoothed infection rates, $\hat{\underset{\sim}{\beta}}_0$, are weighted to produce smoothed infection rates, $\hat{\beta}_\lambda$. For example, Table

5 gives the averaging matrix A corresponding to one of the smoothed infection curves shown in Figure 3. Inspection of the matrix A shows that generally, the diagonal elements are large suggesting that the unsmoothed infection rate is given considerable weight in determining the smoothed rate. The smoothed infection rate is approximately equal to the unsmoothed infection rates for the period 1977-1979. For later periods in calendar time, the smoothed infection rate is a weighted average of the neighboring unsmoothed infection rates. For example, the smoothed infection rate for 1983.0-1984.0 is a linear combination principally of unsmoothed infection rates for the period 1981.0-1986.0

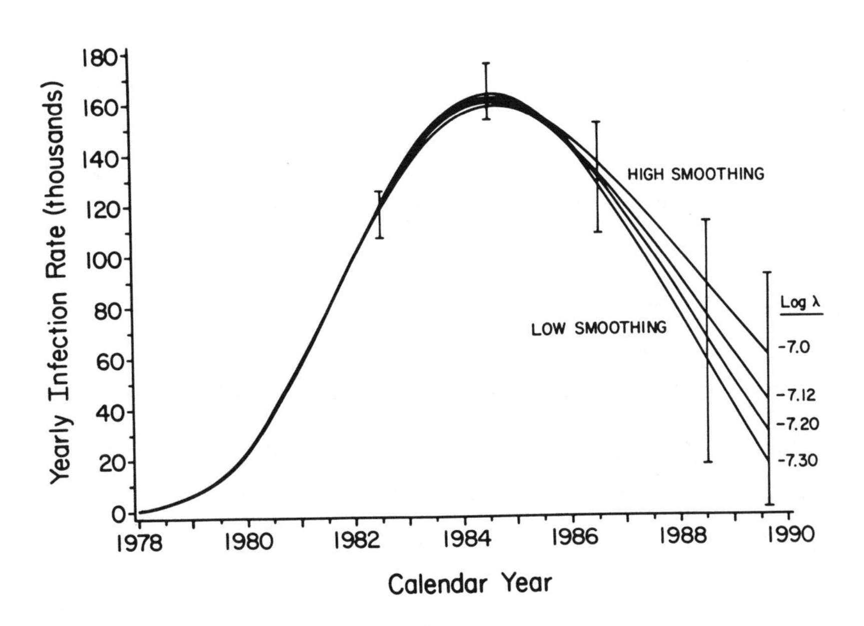

Figure 3. Sensitivity Analysis of Reconstructed Infection Rate to Smoothing Parameter.

with most weight given to the period 1982.0-1984.0. In the most recent calendar period, the smoothed infection rate is a linear combination of all previous unsmoothed rates with no obvious pattern to the weights. Negligible weight is given to the unsmoothed rate for period 1989-1990.25 when determining any of the smoothed rates.

These observations about the averaging matrix A suggest an alternative smoothing approach: Smoothed estimates could be obtained by simply taking a weighted average of the unsmoothed infection rates. The weights given by the averaging matrix A (the kernel) would be chosen by the data analyst (e.g. weight neighboring points 1/3, 1/3, 1/3). Questions arise concerning how to choose the weights (the kernel). A comparison of various smoothing procedures including the EMS procedure of Becker et al. (1991) is an important area of inquiry. An interesting additional question is whether there are advantages to using different amounts of smoothing for different parts of the infection curve. Since there is more information in the data about the early infection rates one might want to use increasingly more smoothing for I(s) with increasing calendar time s. One would redefine the roughness penalty giving more weight to roughness that occurs in the recent past.

The most appreciable improvements in our ability to reconstruct recent infection rates may come, not from alternative smoothing algorithms, but rather from obtaining empirical data on recent infection rates. Incorporating external information about recent infection rates, along the lines suggested in Brookmeyer and Liao (1990), may drastically improve our ability to reconstruct infection rates.

7. References

Bacchetti, P. (1990). Estimating the Incubation Period of AIDS by Comparing Population Infection and Diagnosis Patterns. Journal of the American Statistical Association 88,1002-1008.

Becker, N. G., Watson, L. F. and Carlin, J. B. (1991). A Method of Nonparametric Back-projection and its Application to AIDS Data. Statistics in Medicine 10, 1527-1542.

Brookmeyer, R. (1991). Reconstruction and Future Trends of the AIDS Epidemic in the United States. Science 253,37-42.

Brookmeyer, R., Damiano, A. (1989). Statistical Methods for Short-Term Projections of the AIDS Incidence. Statistics in Medicine 8,23-34.

Brookmeyer, R., Liao, J. (1990). Statistical Modelling of the AIDS Epidemic for Forecasting Health Care Needs. Biometrics 46,1151-1163.

Brookmeyer, R., Gail, M. H. (1986). Minimum Size of the Acquired Immunodeficiency Syndrome (AIDS) Epidemic in the United States. Lancet 2,1320.

Brookmeyer, R., Gail, M. H. A Method for Obtaining Short-Term Projections and Lower Bounds on the Size of the AIDS Epidemic (1988). Journal of the American Statistical Association 83,301-308.

Day, N. E., Gore, S. M. (1989). Prediction of the Number of New AIDS Cases and the Number of New Persons Infected with HIV up to 1992: The Results of "Back Projection" Methods. In: Short-term Prediction of HIV Infections and AIDS in England and Wales. London: Her Majesty's Stationary Office.

DeGruttolla, V., Lagakos, S. W. (1989). The Value of AIDS Incidence in Assessing the Spread of HIV Infection. Statistics in Medicine 8,35-44.

Gail, M. H., Brookmeyer, R. (1988). Methods for Projecting the Course of the Acquired Immunodeficiency Syndrome Epidemic. Journal of the National Cancer Institute 80,900-911.

Gail, M. H., Rosenberg, P. S., Goedert, J. J. (1990). Therapy May Explain Recent Deficits in AIDS Incidence. Journal of AIDS 3,296-306.

Nychka, D. (1988). Confidence Intervals for Smoothing Splines. Journal of the American Statistical Association 83,1134-1143.

O'Sullivan, F., Yandell, B., Raynor, W. (1986). Automatic Smoothing of Regression Functions in Generalized Linear Models. Journal of the American Statistical Association 81,96-103.

Rosenberg, P. S. and Gail, M. H. (1990). Uncertainty in Estimates of HIV Prevalence Derived by Backcalculation. Annals of Epidemiology 1,105-115.

Rosenberg, P. S., Gail, M. H. (1991). Back-calculation of Flexible Linear Models of the HIV Infection Curve. Applied Statistics 40,269-282.

Rosenberg, P. S., Gail, M. H. and Pee, D. (1991). Mean Square Error of Estimates of HIV Prevalence and Short-Term AIDS Projections Derived by Back-calculation. Statistics in Medicine 10,1167-1180.

Silverman, B. (1985). Some Aspects of the Spline Smoothing Approach to Non-parametric Regression Curve Fitting. Journal of the Royal Statistical Society B 47,1-52.

Taylor, J. M. G. (1989). Model for the HIV Infection and AIDS Epidemic in the United States. Statistics in Medicine 8,45-58.

Wahba, G. (1983). A Comparison of GCV and GML for Choosing the Smoothing Parameter in the Generalized Spline Smoothing Problem. Technical Report 712, Department of Statistics, University of Wisconsin.

Wahba, G. (1990). Spline Models for Observational Data. Society for Industrial and Applied Mathematics, Philadelphia.

Department of Biostatistics
Johns Hopkins University
School of Hygiene and Public Health
Baltimore, Maryland 21205

Table 1. Standard Deviation (SD) and Per-Cent Root Mean Square (PRMS)[1] of Infection Rates as a Function of Smoothing Parameter for Infection Curve A in Figure 2.

Interval midpt[2]	1982.5			1984.5			1986.5			1988.5		
Infections/year[3]	129,330			83,810			16,480			2,360		
log λ	Bias	SD	PRMS	Bias	SD	PRMS	Bias	SD	PRMS	Bias	SD	PRMS
-11.0	4,080	48,000	37	1,090	51,100	61	16,100	40,400	264	27,600	42,600	2.151
-10.0	4,300	18,700	15	1,170	20,770	25	1,940	18,900	115	18,700	29,400	1,476
- 9.0	1,280	10,200	8	4,220	9,640	13	-3,040	10,310	65	11,010	19,240	938
- 8.0	-6,200	6,980	7	9,200	6,210	13	1,060	4,540	28	-1,920	2,320	127
- 7.0	-14,790	6,130	12	15,530	5,503	20	8,590	3,270	56	-2,360	1	100
- 6.0	-29,350	5,250	23	13,400	5,120	17	35,150	3,410	214	-2,160	818	98
- 5.0	-43,890	4,362	34	10,530	4,950	14	73,560	4,880	447	79,930	4,820	3,390
- 4.0	-50,080	4,140	39	20,300	5,430	25	109,570	6,580	666	144,940	7,750	6,140
- 3.0	-52,180	4,030	40	24,580	5,650	30	122,820	7,260	747	167,770	8,880	7,113

[1] The Per-cent Root Mean Square (PRMS) is defined as $100 \cdot (\text{bias}^2 + (SD)^2)^{1/2}/\beta^*$ where β^* is the true average infection rate in the interval, bias = $\beta - \beta^*$ where β is computed from expression 12 and SD is the standard deviation of the estimated infection rate computed from expression 13. The overdispersion parameter σ^2 was assumed to be 1.0.

[2] The intervals refer to (c_{j-1}, c_j).

[3] The infections per year cited is the true average number of infections in the interval, $\beta^* = \left[\int_{c_{j-1}}^{c_j} I(s)ds \right] / (c_j - c_{j-1})$.

Table 2. Standard Deviation (SD) and Per Cent Root Mean Square (PRMS) of Infection Rates as a Function of Smoothing Parameter for Infection Curve B in Figure 2.

Interval midpt	1982.5			1984.5			1986.5			1988.5		
Infections/year	62,370			82,020			94,660			90,550		
log λ	Bias	SD	PRMS	Bias	SD	PRMS	Bias	SD	PRMS	Bias	SD	PRMS
-11.0	4,160	45,800	74	3,430	59,800	72	-36	47,680	50	7,120	78,410	87
-10.0	1,360	19,840	32	-643	21,300	26	623	25,110	27	-880	47,660	53
- 9.0	-590	8,340	13	590	9,490	11	-620	12,660	13	900	32,740	36
- 8.0	-1,370	4,400	07	690	5,990	07	-940	6,590	07	3,740	18,950	21
- 7.0	-290	3,560	06	-1,600	4,610	06	-350	5,790	06	12,450	10,750	18
- 6.0	-211	3,320	05	-3,160	4,240	06	930	5,410	06	19,810	7,240	23
- 5.0	-560	3,230	05	-3,570	4,180	07	2,040	5,220	06	23,250	6,370	27
- 4.0	-750	3,220	05	-3,470	4,170	07	2,770	5,120	06	24,750	6,090	28
- 3.0	-850	3,270	05	-3,500	4,160	07	2,860	5,160	06	24,980	6,040	28

Table 3. Standard Deviation (SD) and Per-Cent Root Mean Square (PRMS) of Infection Rates as a Function of Smoothing Parameter for Infection Curve C in Figure 2.

Interval midpt	1982.5			1984.5			1986.5			1988.5		
Infections/year	59,290			97,750			161,160			265,760		
log λ	Bias	SD	PRMS	Bias	SD	PRMS	Bias	SD	PRMS	Bias	SD	PRMS
-11.0	3,860	44,980	76	741	55,640	57	-2,140	58,400	36	-2,100	75,580	28
-10.0	780	19,340	33	-1,114	21,160	22	-990	26,450	16	-4,580	52,350	20
- 9.0	-390	8,100	14	-1,140	9,790	10	139	14,340	09	-7,940	35,830	14
- 8.0	-1,760	4,220	08	-730	6,490	07	2,180	9,600	06	-17,280	22,740	11
- 7.0	-2,250	3,330	07	890	5,460	06	1,610	9,040	06	-29,580	15,530	13
- 6.0	230	3,170	05	3,390	5,320	06	-5,260	8,400	06	-50,930	12,070	20
- 5.0	3,870	3,310	09	2,220	5,240	06	-18,670	7,550	12	-79,250	10,000	20
- 4.0	7,670	3,500	14	-3,120	4,960	06	-37,470	6,470	24	-112,620	8,040	40
- 3.0	8,790	3,560	16	-5,040	4,850	07	-43,650	6,140	27	-123,340	7,480	47

Table 4. Optimal[1] Log λ as a Function of Sample Size, $E(Y_{\bullet}) = \sum_{i=1}^{N} E(Y_i)$.

Cumulative[2] cases (thousands)	1982.5 Infection curve A	B	C	1984.5 Infection curve A	B	C	1986.5 Infection curve A	B	C	1988.5 Infection curve A	B	C
25	-7.2	-3.2	-5.2	-7.4	-5.2	-5.8	-6.8	-3.2	-5.6	-5.6	-5.2	-6.2
50	-7.8	-3.8	-5.6	-7.8	-6.0	-6.2	-7.2	-4.0	-6.0	-6.8	-6.2	-6.8
75	-8.0	-4.2	-5.8	-8.2	-6.4	-6.6	-7.6	-4.6	-6.2	-7.0	-6.8	-7.1
100	-8.2	-4.4	-5.8	-8.4	-6.6	-6.8	-7.6	-5.6	-6.4	-7.4	-7.0	-7.6
150	-8.4	-5.4	-6.0	-8.6	-7.0	-7.0	-8.0	-6.0	-6.6	-7.6	-7.4	-8.0
200	-8.6	-5.8	-6.2	-8.8	-7.2	-7.2	-8.0	-6.2	-6.6	-7.8	-7.6	-8.2
250	-8.8	-5.8	-6.2	-9.0	-7.4	-7.4	-8.2	-6.4	-6.8	-8.0	-7.8	-8.4

[1] Optimal log λ was defined as the value which minimized the PRMS.

[2] Expected cumulative cases, in thousands, by April 1, 1990. Infection curves (A,B,C) scaled to produce expected cumulative cases.

Table 5. Example[1] of Averaging Matrix A Which Decomposes the Smoothed Infection Rates Into Linear Combination of Unsmoothed Infection Rates.

$$(\hat{\beta}_{\lambda} = A\hat{\beta}_{o})$$

79.0[2]	80.0	81.0	82.0	83.0	84.0	85.0	86.0	87.0	88.0	89.0	90.25
.99	.07	-.04	-.02	.00	.01	.00	.00	.00	.00	.00	.00
.07	.57	.31	.05	-.03	-.03	-.01	.00	.00	.00	.00	.00
-.05	.47	.39	.21	.07	.00	-.02	-.01	.00	.00	.00	.00
-.04	.14	.31	.33	.22	.10	.02	-.01	-.01	.00	.00	.00
.00	-.11	.15	.33	.33	.22	.10	.01	-.01	-.02	.00	.00
.03	-.19	.00	.22	.32	.29	.17	.09	.02	-.01	-.01	.00
.03	-.13	-.07	.08	.23	.29	.26	.17	.08	.03	.00	.00
.02	-.02	-.09	-.05	.09	.22	.28	.25	.17	.09	.03	.00
.00	.11	-.07	-.16	-.07	.11	.26	.32	.28	.17	.06	.01
-.03	.24	-.03	-.24	-.23	-.03	.22	.37	.38	.26	.11	.01
-.06	.26	.02	-.32	-.37	-.17	.17	.42	.49	.36	.16	.01
-.11	.63	.08	-.52	-.70	-.40	.14	.60	.75	.58	.26	.03

[1] Averaging matrix A corresponds to infection curve with log λ = -7.20 in Figure 3.

[2] Endpoint of step function interval, (c_{j-1}, c_j).

UNCERTAINTY ABOUT THE INCUBATION PERIOD OF AIDS AND ITS IMPACT ON BACKCALCULATION

Peter R. Bacchetti, Mark R. Segal and Nicholas P. Jewell

ABSTRACT: We analyze three sets of doubly-censored cohort data on incubation times, estimating incubation distributions using semiparametric methods and assessing the comparability of the estimates. Weibull models appear to be inappropriate for at least one of the cohorts, and the estimates for the different cohorts are substantially different. We use these estimates as inputs for backcalculation, using a nonparametric method based on maximum penalized likelihood. The different incubations all produce fits to the reported AIDS counts that are as good as the fit from a nonstationary incubation distribution that models treatment effects, but the estimated infection curves are very different. We also develop a method for estimating nonstationarity as part of the backcalculation procedure and find that such estimates also depend very heavily on the assumed incubation distribution. We conclude that incubation distributions are so uncertain that meaningful error bounds are difficult to place on backcalculated estimates and that backcalculation may be too unreliable to be used without being supplemented by other sources of information on HIV prevalence and incidence.

1. INTRODUCTION

Backcalculation is the main method used to reconstruct the past pattern of HIV infections in the USA, and it is also widely used to predict future numbers of AIDS cases (Centers for Disease Control 1990). The method is known to be sensitive to the incubation period used (Brookmeyer and Gail 1988), but recent backcalculation articles have given optimistic assessments of the state of knowledge about the distribution of the incubation period of AIDS (Brookmeyer 1991; Rosenberg, *et al*. 1991), claiming that there is close agreement among estimates that use different data and different methods. We argue here that in fact very little is known about the incubation distribution and that it is likely to be quite different in different populations. In section 2, we use well-known cohort data to produce several different incubation estimates, and we assess the comparability of the estimates. We explore the impact of differing incubations estimates on backcalculations in section 3, showing that enough error can result to make any interpretation of the estimated infection rates questionable.

2. INCUBATION ESTIMATES

2.1. Methods. The ideal data for estimating the AIDS incubation distribution would be a large number of observed incubation times from representative individuals. Available cohort data on the natural history of AIDS fall short of this ideal in three respects: incubation times are observed inexactly due to interval-censoring of seroconversion times and right-censoring of AIDS diagnosis times, there may be truncation effects due to selection of only AIDS-free subjects, and the cohorts may not be representative of the populations that we would like to extrapolate to.

The first problem, interval-censored data, is easily handled by using an appropriate statistical method (DeGruttola and Lagakos 1989). This method is easily modified to account for truncation, as described by Bacchetti and Jewell (1991) for a similar situation. Here, we discretize the data into months and estimate the seroconversion pattern by maximum penalized likelihood (Bacchetti 1990). We estimate the incubation distribution using two different parametric models. One specifies that the logit of the hazard is a linear function of log time and is just a discrete analog of the widely-used Weibull distribution. (We use logits here instead of logs for mathematical convenience and to prevent the possibility of hazards greater than one.) The other allows the logit hazard to be quadratic in log time. This three-parameter model overcomes an important limitation of the Weibull distribution—the fact that the hazard must increase as a fixed exponent of time. Because this includes the Weibull as a special case, the likelihoods from the two models can be compared to test whether the Weibull assumption is appropriate.

If different populations share a common incubation distribution, then who a cohort represents is not an issue. If this were the case, then it would be very desirable to combine data from different sources to obtain a more accurate meta-estimate. This can be accomplished by modelling two or more cohorts as having distinct seroconversion patterns but a common incubation. In addition, the combinability of the cohorts can be assessed by comparing the likelihood to the sum of the likelihoods from modelling the cohorts as completely separate. If the cohorts do not appear to be combinable, then there may be systematic differences in different populations as well, and the question of which populations are accurately represented by which cohorts becomes important.

2.2. Data. Public use data sets from hemophiliacs (Goedert *et al*. 1989) and from gay men screened for the Hepatitis B Vaccine Trial in San Francisco (Hessol *et al*. 1989) provide doubly-censored data on times from HIV seroconversion to AIDS diagnosis. Because of previously documented heterogeneity in the infection patterns and incubation periods of the hemophiliacs (Brookmeyer and Goedert 1989), we use only those with severe type A hemophilia who were over age 19 at their estimated seroconversion times. We divided the San Francisco cohort into two groups, those in the Hepatitis B Vaccine Trial, and those who were ineligible for the Trial because of previous HBV exposure but who were later part of a random sample chosen for HIV followup. To eliminate the influence of treatment on development of AIDS, we censored all the San Francisco subjects at June 1987 if they did not have AIDS by that time. Only one of the hemophiliacs was reported to have been treated prior to development of AIDS, so the censoring date of November 1988 provided in the data set was not changed. Thus, we have three groups: hemophiliacs, with 56 diagnosed and 229 censored individuals; Hepatitis B Vaccine Trial participants, with 33 diagnosed and 114 censored; and the random sample from San Francisco, with 51 diagnosed and 364 censored.

2.3. Results. The value of the smoothing parameter for the maximum penalized likelihood estimation of the seroconversion patterns had little influence on the incubation estimates. The comparison of two- and three-parameter models showed significant evidence against the Weibull assumption for the hemophiliacs ($p=0.007$) and some evidence against it for the Hepatitis B Vaccine Trial participants ($p=0.16$). The strength of the evidence against the Weibull for the hemophiliacs is due to their later censoring date—if they are censored at June 1987, then the evidence is not as strong ($p=0.07$). The three-parameter estimate, however, changes very little as the censoring date is pushed back, while the Weibull estimate does vary with the censoring date. Thus, the Weibull appears to be a poor fit. Figure 1 compares the CDFs for the Weibull and three-parameter estimates.

Figure 2 shows the estimated CDFs for the three-parameter model on each of the three groups. (The fourth curve is shown for later reference to illustrate another incubation distribution that will be used in section 3.) The three groups show substantial differences, which appear to preclude creation of a meta-estimate. Table 1 shows the results of formal tests of whether any

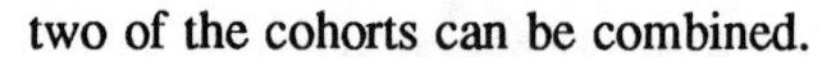

two of the cohorts can be combined.

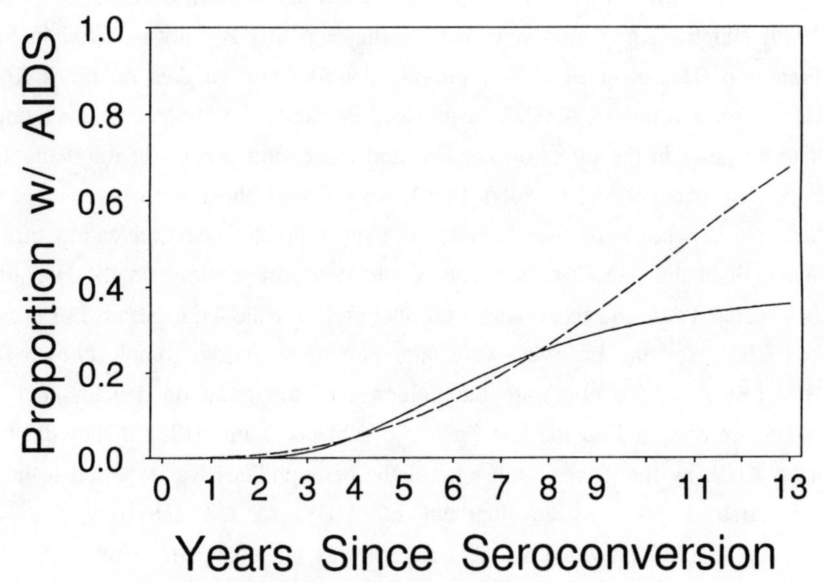

Figure 1. Estimated cumulative distribution functions for the AIDS incubation period in the hemophiliac cohort. Dashed line: Weibull model. Solid line: three-parameter generalization of Weibull.

3. BACKCALCULATION

3.1. Estimation Method. In addition to knowledge of the incubation distribution, we will make use of the observed numbers of AIDS diagnoses up to month n that are reported by some time $n^* \geq n$. Assume that the number of new infections in month i is Poisson with parameter θ_i and that given $\boldsymbol{\theta}$ the numbers of infections in different months are independent. We observe

$$y_{jk} = \#\text{ diagnosed month } j \text{ and reported month } k\,,\quad j \leq n\,,\quad j \leq k \leq n^*$$

and we wish to estimate $\boldsymbol{\theta}$ using knowledge of

$$a_{ijk} = Pr\{\text{ diagnosed at } j \;\&\; \text{reported at } k \mid \text{infected at } i\;\}\,.$$

Letting $y_j = \sum_{k=j}^{n^*} y_{jk}$, we write the likelihood of $\boldsymbol{\theta}$ given $\mathbf{a}$ as $L(\boldsymbol{\theta}|\mathbf{a}) = L_c \times L_m$ where L_c is the likelihood of the y_{jk} conditional on the y_j and L_m is the marginal likelihood of the y_j. We have

$$L_c \propto \prod_{j=0}^{n} \prod_{k=j}^{n^*} A_{jk}^{y_{jk}}\,,\quad \text{where } A_{jk} = \frac{\sum_{i=0}^{j} a_{ijk}\theta_i}{\sum_{r=j}^{n^*} \sum_{i=0}^{j} a_{ijr}\theta_i}\,, \tag{1}$$

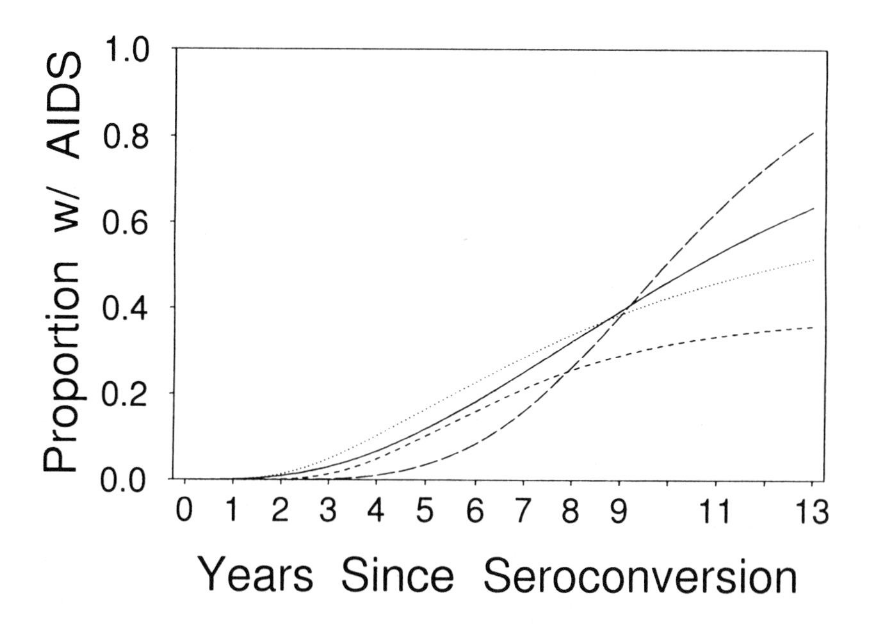

Figure 2. Comparison of cumulative distribution functions for the AIDS incubation period from different sources. Solid line: Brookmeyer's (1991) nonstationary model, for a person infected in January 1982. Dotted line: three-parameter model from the Hepatitis B Vaccine Trial cohort (N=147, 33 diagnosed). Long-dashed line: three-parameter model from the Random Sample cohort (N=415, 51 diagnosed). Short-dashed line: three-parameter model from the hemophiliac cohort (N=285, 56 diagnosed).

Table 1. P-values from tests of whether cohorts share a common incubation distribution. Tests are based on fitting common and separate three-parameter models for the incubation and comparing twice the difference in the log-likelihoods to the chi-squared distribution with 3 degrees of freedom.

	Hepatitis B Vaccine Trial	Random Sample
Hemophiliacs	.084	.0095
Hepatitis B Vaccine Trial	--	<.0001

and

$$L_m \propto \prod_{j=0}^{n} \left[\sum_{k=j}^{n^*} \sum_{i=0}^{j} a_{ijk} \theta_i \right]^{y_j} \exp\left[-\sum_{k=j}^{n^*} \sum_{i=0}^{j} a_{ijk} \theta_i \right] .$$

To simplify this likelihood, we make the assumption that $a_{ijk} = I_{ij} R_{jk}$, where I_{ij} is the probability of diagnosis at j given infection at i and R_{jk} is the probability of reporting at k given diagnosis at j. Then we have

$$A_{jk} = \frac{R_{jk}}{\sum_{m=j}^{n^*} R_{jm}} ,$$

so that L_c does not depend on $\boldsymbol{\theta}$. We can therefore estimate $\boldsymbol{\theta}$ using the log-likelihood

$$\log(L_m) = \sum_{j=0}^{n} \left[y_j \log\left(\sum_{i=0}^{j} R_j I_{ij} \theta_i \right) - \sum_{i=0}^{j} R_j I_{ij} \theta_i \right] , \tag{2}$$

where $R_j = \sum_{k=j}^{n^*} R_{jk}$, the probability that a case diagnosed at time j is reported by time n^*. A minor complication is the fact that confidentiality concerns may prevent release of exact diagnosis and reporting times of early cases, say those diagnosed up to time g. (For example, the CDC does not release month of diagnosis for cases diagnosed before 1982.) In this case, we observe only $y^* = \sum_{j=0}^{g} y_j$, and we have

$$\log(L_m) = y^* \log\left(\sum_{j=0}^{g} \sum_{i=0}^{j} R_j I_{ij} \theta_i \right) - \sum_{j=0}^{g} \sum_{i=0}^{j} R_j I_{ij} \theta_i + \sum_{j=g+1}^{n} \left[y_j \log\left(\sum_{i=0}^{j} R_j I_{ij} \theta_i \right) - \sum_{i=0}^{j} R_j I_{ij} \theta_i \right] . \tag{2a}$$

The penalized likelihood criterion that we optimize is

$$\log(L_m) - \frac{\lambda_\theta}{2} \sum_{i=0}^{n-2} \left(\log(\theta_i) - 2\log(\theta_{i+1}) + \log(\theta_{i+2}) \right)^2 . \tag{3}$$

This penalty forces $\theta_i > 0$ for any $\lambda_\theta > 0$, so that constrained optimization is not needed. The criterion (3) can be optimized by an EM algorithm, or directly by the Newton-Raphson method. Further details will be provided in a future manuscript.

Goodness of fit for various estimates of $\boldsymbol{\theta}$ is measured by the deviance

$$-2\left(\log(L_m) - \sum_{j=0}^{n}[y_j \log(y_j) - y_j]\right). \tag{4}$$

This depends on the estimates used for the I_{ij} and the R_j in addition to the resulting estimate of $\boldsymbol{\theta}$.

3.2. Modelling Nonstationarity. The above formulation allows for incubation and reporting delay distributions that are nonstationary over chronological time. Nevertheless, if good estimates of any nonstationarity are not available, then it may be of interest to allow for estimation of nonstationarity in the backcalculation itself. This is accomplished by by replacing the terms $R_j I_{ij}$ in (2) by $R_j I_{ij} e^{\beta_j}$, with $\boldsymbol{\beta}$ estimated along with θ by maximum penalized likelihood. The vector $\boldsymbol{\beta}$ captures the effect of chronological time on the chance of being diagnosed and subsequently reported by time n^*, beyond the effects that are reflected in the R_j and I_{ij}. Note that β_j can be thought of as modifying either or both of R_j and the I_{ij}, because these terms only appear multiplied together in (2).

The roughness penalty used for $\boldsymbol{\beta}$ is the sum of squared second differences, so the criterion optimized is

$$\log(L_m) - \frac{\lambda_\theta}{2}\sum_{i=0}^{n-2}\left(\log(\theta_i) - 2\log(\theta_{i+1}) + \log(\theta_{i+2})\right)^2$$
$$- \frac{\lambda_\beta}{2}\sum_{j=0}^{n-2}(\beta_j - 2\beta_{j+1} + \beta_{j+2})^2 .$$

We set β_j equal to zero for j before January 1987, noting that the penalty includes terms to ensure that the β_j's diverge from zero gradually after that date. The joint optimization in $\boldsymbol{\theta}$ and $\boldsymbol{\beta}$ is accomplished by the Newton-Raphson method, with a starting value determined by optimizing θ with β set to zero.

3.3. Diagnosis Counts, Incubation, and Reporting Delay. We examine a large subgroup of the cases on the CDC's AIDS Public Information Data Set for cases reported through December 1990. We restrict attention to homosexual and bisexual men from the Northeast area who did not use intravenous drugs and who were over age 19 at the time of their diagnoses. The epidemic is probably as old in this group as in any other, and recent infection rates are thought to have been low, so backcalculation should perform about as well as possible when applied to this group. We include diagnoses through September 1990, so that with $i=1$ set to January 1975 we have $n=189$ and $n^*=192$. A total of 16,561 cases meet these criteria.

We use values of the I_{ij} corresponding to the stationary distributions estimated in section 2, along with a nonstationary model proposed by Brookmeyer (1991). This nonstationary model allows for treatment effects that slow progression to AIDS beginning in mid-1987. The CDF for this model for someone infected at the beginning of 1982 is shown in Figure 2. Persons infected earlier would have higher CDFs and those infected later would have lower CDFs.

The reporting delay factors R_j used here are from the model estimated for Northeast homosexual/bisexual men by Brookmeyer and Liao (1990, Table 4), which has reporting delays lengthening for later calendar years of diagnosis. This model was fitted on only pre-1987 definition cases, so we assume that cases who met only the 1987 definition were being reported with similar delays by the end of 1990, although they may have initially had longer delays due to retrospective reporting shortly after the expansion of the definition. We also assume that all cases who will be reported at all will be reported by 48 months following diagnosis, because the model is conditional on reporting by 48 months. We set underreporting (cases never reported) at 10 percent before 1987 and increase it linearly from 10 to 15 percent from January 1987 to December 1990. Because we focus on a specific risk group, a few cases who have no identified risk will eventually be added to the group studied here, but we make no attempt to adjust for these classification delays by changing the R_j's.

3.4. Choosing the Amount of Smoothness and Estimating Confidence Intervals. The estimate of θ depends on the value used for λ_{θ}. The choice of λ_{θ} can be based on a method for testing $\lambda_{\theta}=\lambda_0$ versus $\lambda_{\theta}=\lambda_1$, with $\lambda_1<\lambda_0$. The method creates simulated values of y^* and the y_j's based on the estimate of θ that results from setting $\lambda_{\theta}=\lambda_0$. These simulated epidemics are then used to estimate θ with both $\lambda_{\theta}=\lambda_0$ and $\lambda_{\theta}=\lambda_1$, and the improvement in the deviance from using λ_1 instead of λ_0 is calculated. This improvement is due to the greater flexibility allowed with a smaller λ_{θ} even though the "true" underlying model (the one used to create the simulated data) is based on λ_0. This improvement is compared to the improvement actually observed for the real y^* and $\{y_j\}$. The simulation procedure is repeated a number of times, and the frequency with which the simulated improvements exceed the observed improvement is tabulated.

To select a value for λ_θ, we begin with a value that is clearly too large and test it against an alternative whose log is 0.5 smaller. The logs of the test values λ_0 are decreased by 0.5 until one is found where 1000 simulations produce more than 100 simulated improvements that are larger than the observed improvement. This procedure is applied using the nonstationary treatment model, and the same value of λ_θ is used for the other incubation models to facilitate comparisons. Although a similar procedure could be used to find a suitable value for λ_β, such a procedure would be quite vulnerable to overdispersion of the y_j's because β_j influences the fitted value of y_j directly. For this reason, we choose λ_β subjectively by examining the estimates resulting from a range of reasonable values.

Simulations as described above are used to produce pointwise confidence intervals using the bias-corrected percentile method (Efron 1985). Confidence intervals are also produced by using the inverse of the observed information matrix and assuming normality.

3.5. Results. Table 2 shows the results of the simulations used to choose a value of λ_θ, using the nonstationary treatment model for the incubation distribution.

Table 2. Results of simulations used to choose λ_θ as described in section 3.4.

	λ_0=exp(12) versus λ_1=exp(11.5)	λ_0=exp(11.5) versus λ_1=exp(11)	λ_0=exp(11) versus λ_1=exp(10.5)	λ_0=exp(10.5) versus λ_1=exp(10)	λ_0=exp(10) versus λ_1=exp(9.5)
Proportion of 1000 Simulated Improvements Exceeding Observed	.000	.020	.093	.218	.333

Based on these results we choose $\lambda_\theta = 10.5$, and we use this for all the other incubation distributions, as well. A plot of the deviance versus λ_θ (Figure 3) confirms that smaller values do not meaningfully improve the fit. In addition, Figure 4 shows that the choice of λ_θ has fairly little influence on the estimate of θ. For λ_β, we choose exp(15) because it is the smallest value that does

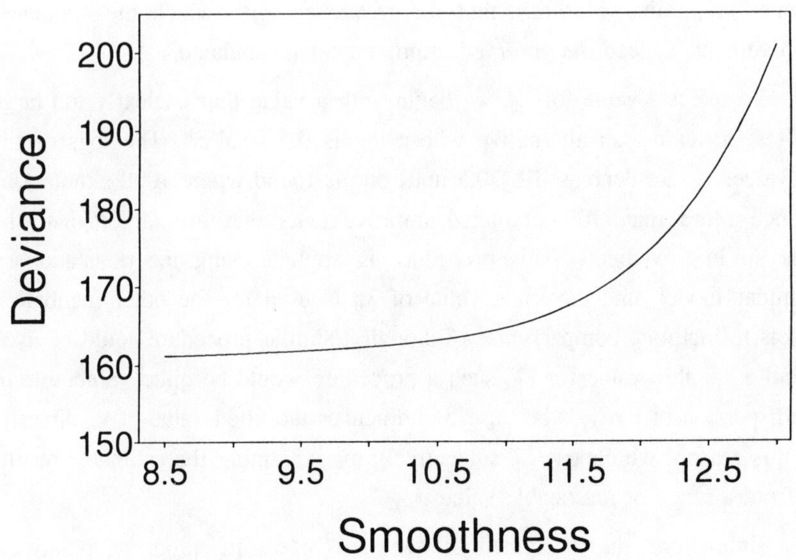

Figure 3. Deviance of backcalculation estimates of infection rates as a function of the smoothness parameter used for the estimates, with the incubation distribution assumed to follow the nonstationary treatment model. The smoothness axis corresponds to values of $\log(\lambda_\theta)$.

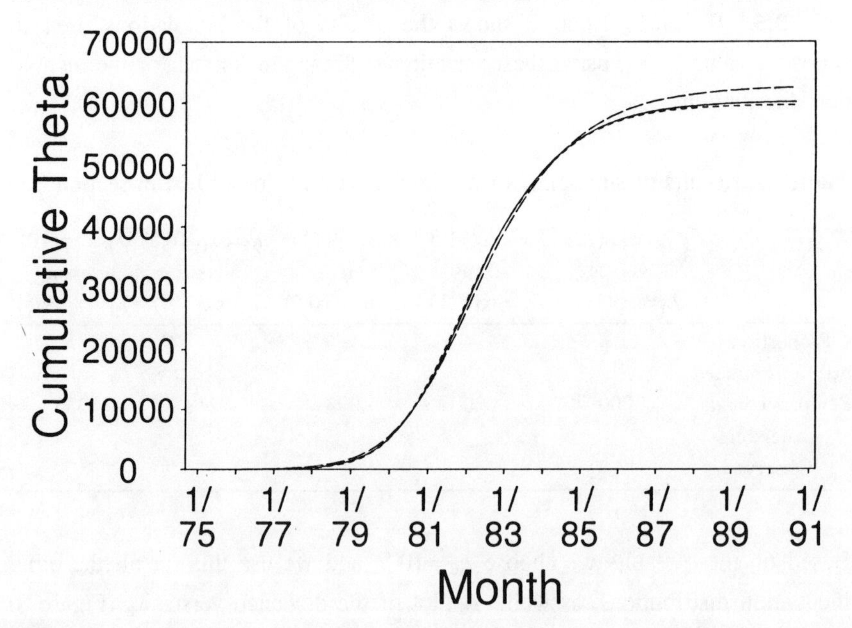

Figure 4. Cumulative infections estimated using different values of λ_θ in backcalculations, with the incubation distribution assumed to follow the nonstationary treatment model. Short-dashed line: $\lambda_\theta = \exp(9)$. Solid line: $\lambda_\theta = \exp(10.5)$. Long-dashed line: $\lambda_\theta = \exp(12)$.

not allow the estimated β_j's to change direction. The choice of λ_β has a similarly small influence on the estimate of $\boldsymbol{\theta}$ (not shown).

Table 3 summarizes the goodness of fit for models fitted using I_{ij}'s corresponding to the nonstationary treatment model and all of the models fitted in section 2. Only the two-parameter models from section 2 fit poorly.

Table 3. Goodness of fit as measured by the deviance (4) for models fitted with $\lambda_\theta = \exp(10.5)$ and $\lambda_\beta = \exp(15)$, with all β_j constrained to equal zero and with β_j after 1986 allowed to be nonzero.

Incubation Model	Deviance	Deviance with Nonzero $\boldsymbol{\beta}$	Deviance Reduction from Nonzero $\boldsymbol{\beta}$
Non-Stationary Treatment Model	163.2	161.1	2.1
Hepatitis B Vaccine Trial Three-Parameter	158.9	158.1	0.8
Random Sample Three-Parameter	161.0	161.2	-0.2*
Hemophiliac Cohort Three-Parameter	158.5	158.2	0.3
Hepatitis B Vaccine Trial Two-Parameter	186.4	157.8	28.6
Random Sample Two-Parameter	196.1	190.1	6.0
Hemophiliac Cohort Two-Parameter	248.7	162.0	86.7

*Allowing nonzero $\boldsymbol{\beta}$ here alters the trade-off between the deviance and the roughness of $\boldsymbol{\theta}$, so that a slightly worse deviance results in a large improvement in the penalty term for $\boldsymbol{\theta}$. The overall criterion (3) is necessarily better when $\boldsymbol{\beta}$ is allowed to be nonzero.

Figure 5 shows the estimates of $\boldsymbol{\theta}$ from the first four models in Table 3, and Figures 6a and 6b show the fit to the data for the nonstationary model and the three-parameter model from the hemophiliacs. The fits for the other three-parameter models are very close to that for the hemophiliac-based incubation estimate. The kink in the fit from the nonstationary model is due to the introduction of a treatment effect beginning in June 1987, and the minor

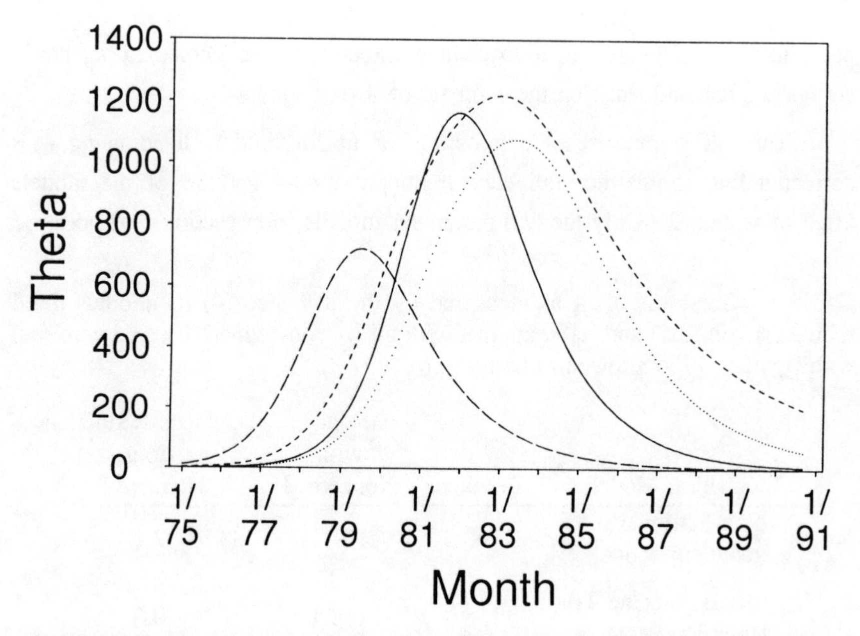

Figure 5. Infection rates estimated by performing backcalculation using four different incubation distributions, with $\lambda_{\theta}=\exp(10.5)$. Solid line: nonstationary treatment model. Dotted line: three-parameter model from the Hepatitis B Vaccine Trial cohort. Long-dashed line: three-parameter model from the Random Sample cohort. Short-dashed line: three-parameter model from the hemophiliac cohort.

wiggliness in all the later fits in Figure 6a is due to some wiggliness in the R_j's for the last 47 months. Despite the very comparable deviances and fits to the data, the estimates of $\boldsymbol{\theta}$ are quite different.

Table 4 summarizes some properties of the curves shown in Figure 5. In contrast to the wide range in the Table, 95% confidence intervals for the nonstationary model (based on 1000 simulations) are 52,700 to 55,200 at 12/84, 56,000 to 61,000 at 6/87, and 56,300 to 62,900 at 9/90. We note, however, that in addition to ignoring uncertainty due to the incubation distribution, these intervals also do not reflect uncertainty in the R_j's and the choice of λ_{θ}.

Two of the poorly-fitting models in Table 3 can be repaired by fitting additional nonstationarity as part of the backcalculation, i.e., by allowing nonzero β. Figure 7 shows the fit from backcalculations based on the two-parameter incubation model from the hemophiliac data with and without the estimation of additional nonstationarity. Without nonstationarity beyond what is reflected in the R_j's, the model produces lack of fit similar to that used to deduce the existence of "AIDS deficits" (Gail *et al*. 1990). With nonzero β, the fit is very close to that produced by the three-parameter incubation models. If we knew that the two-parameter model were correct, then we would be able to deduce the presence of significant additional nonstationarity, as shown in Figure 8a. The use of the more appropriate three-parameter model, however, leads to no evidence for additional nonstationarity, as shown by Figure 8b.

4. DISCUSSION

Backcalculation requires a fairly large amount of certainty about the AIDS incubation distribution in order to be useful. As can be seen from the convolution relationship, multiplying an incubation subdensity by a constant will divide the resulting estimate of θ by the same constant, and reducing or extending an initial period with essentially zero probability of diagnosis will shift the resulting estimate of θ to the right or left by the same amount. Beyond the location and scale of the incubation distribution, its shape has a more complex influence on estimates of θ. In addition, the possibility of nonstationarity adds another layer of complexity. Thus, an exhaustive sensitivity analysis can be extremely difficult to formulate.

We show here how four different plausible incubation distributions lead to very different reconstructions of the infection distribution for a large population for which AIDS diagnosis counts are available. These four distributions certainly do not constitute an exhaustive sensitivity analysis, but they nevertheless produce widely varying estimates of θ. The uncertainty demonstrated in Figure 5 and Table 4 results only from uncertainty about which of four incubation distributions to use—other sources of uncertainty are ignored. Accounting for other sources of uncertainty would lead to an even larger range. Three of the distributions are estimated from cohorts that have been heavily relied on for information about the AIDS incubation period. These estimates are very different when used for backcalculation. Furthermore, the incubation distribution for each cohort appears to differ systematically from the others, as described in section 2. This is not surprising, because one would expect the well-known individual variability in incubations to lead to systematic differences between different cohorts and between different populations. Thus, uncertainty about the incubation stems not only from the limitations of available data, but also from what data one assumes can be

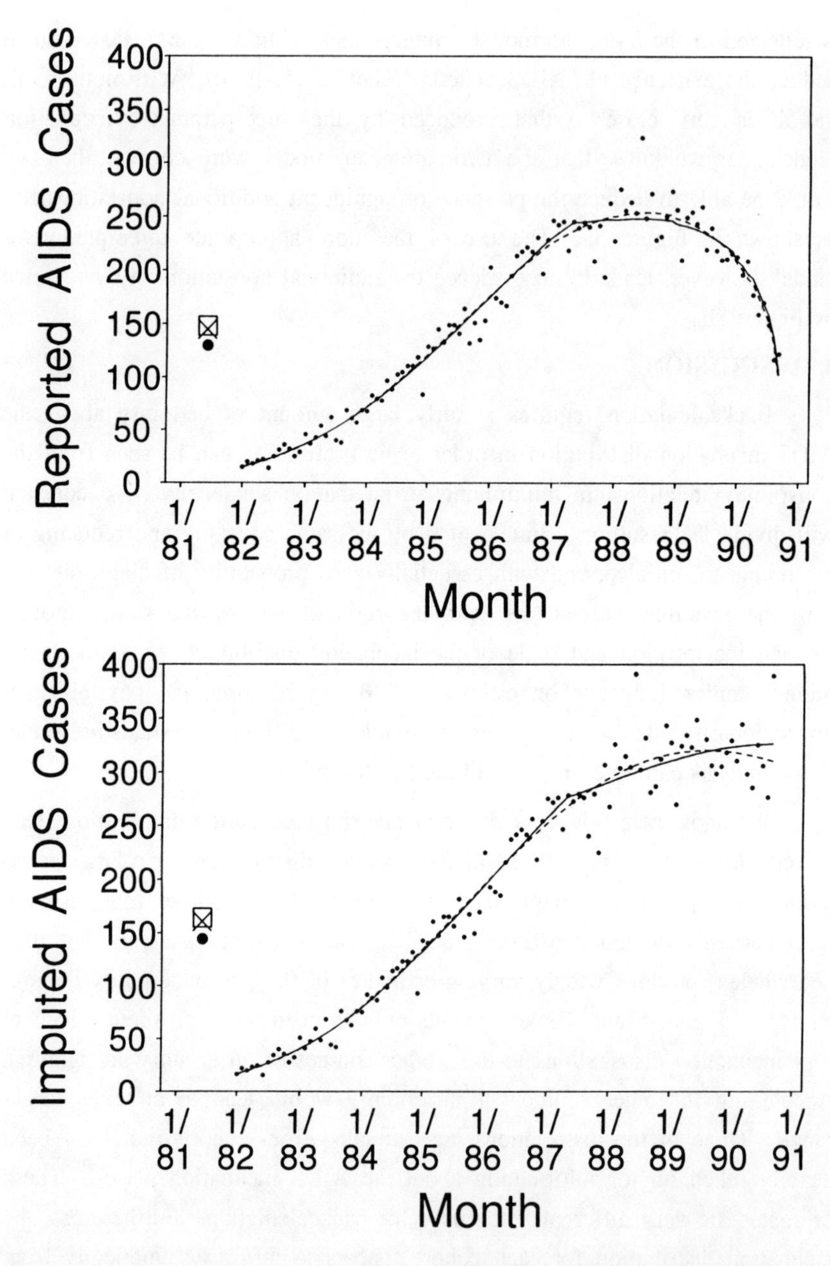

Figure 6. Fitted numbers of AIDS cases from backcalculations using two different incubation distributions, both with $\lambda_0 = \exp(10.5)$. Filled circles: reported cases, y^* and $\{y_j\}$. X and solid line: nonstationary treatment model. Square and dashed line: three-parameter model from the hemophiliac cohort. (a) Fit to reported cases. (b) Fit to estimated actual numbers of cases. Same as (a) but with all values divided by R_j.

Table 4. Summary measures for the estimates of θ shown in Figure 5.

Incubation Model	Month of Peak in Infections	Cumulative Infections by 12/84	Cumulative Infections by 6/87	Cumulative Infections by 9/90
Non-Stationary Treatment Model	12/81	54,100	59,100	60,200
Hepatitis B Vaccine Trial Three-Parameter	5/83	53,900	69,900	75,300
Random Sample Three-Parameter	7/79	35,200	35,900	36,000
Hemophiliac Cohort Three-Parameter	12/82	71,900	92,600	101,900

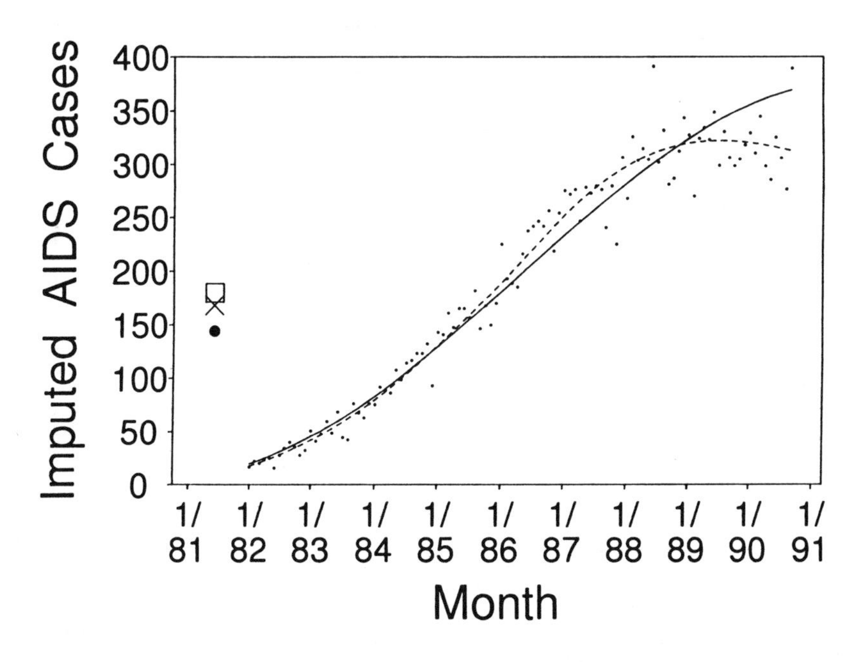

Figure 7. Fitted actual AIDS counts from backcalculations using the two-parameter model of incubation from the hemophiliac cohort, with and without the estimation of nonstationarity factors $\{\beta_j\}$ as described in section 3.2, with $\lambda_\theta = \exp(10.5)$ and $\lambda_\beta = \exp(15)$. Filled circles: imputed cases, y_j/R_j. X and solid line: without nonstationarity factors ($\beta = 0$). Square and dashed line: with nonstationarity factors (nonzero β).

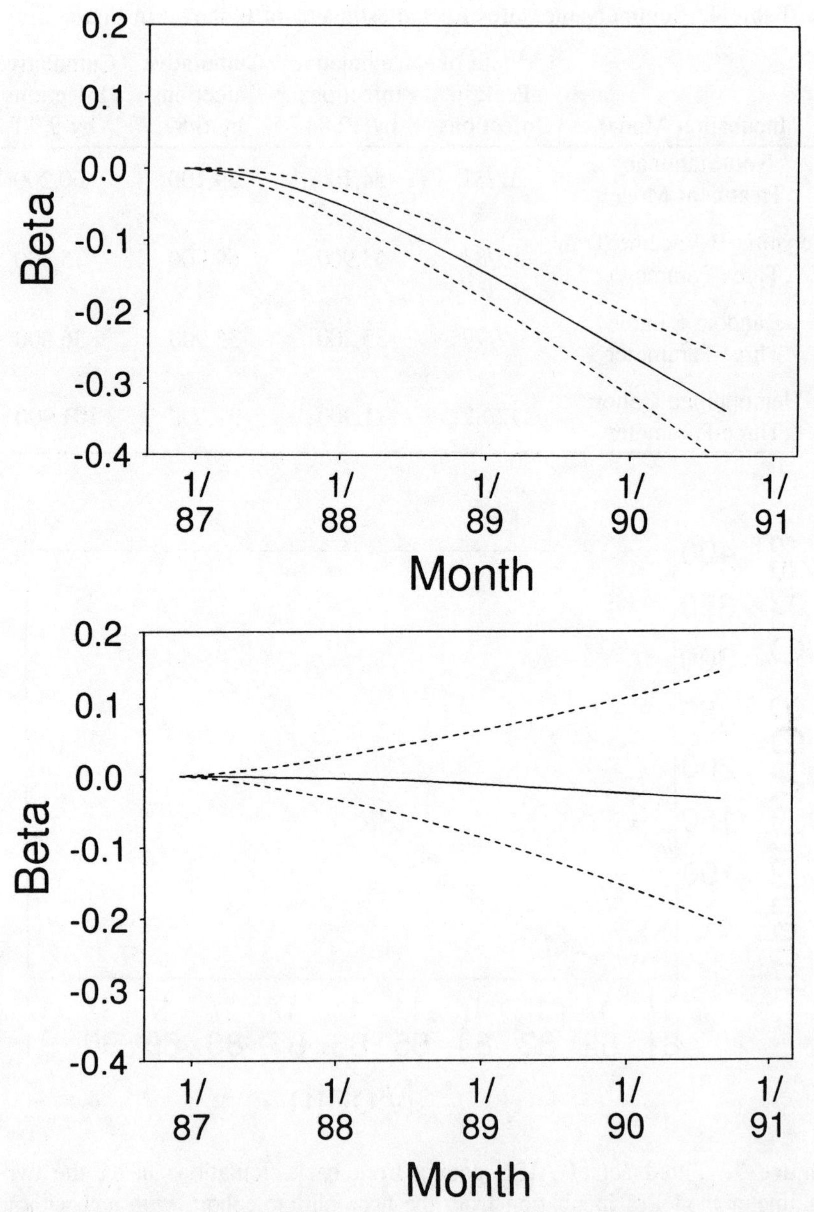

Figure 8. Nonstationarity factors $\{\beta_j\}$ estimated as described in section 3.2 using two different models of the incubation distribution, with $\lambda_\theta = \exp(10.5)$ and $\lambda_\beta = \exp(15)$. Solid lines are the estimates and the dashed lines are pointwise 95% confidence intervals calculated using the inverse of the observed information matrix.

(a) Two-parameter incubation model from the hemophiliac cohort.

(b) Three-parameter incubation model from the hemophiliac cohort.

extrapolated to the population one wishes to perform backcalculation on. This problem is particularly acute for populations such as intravenous drug users and heterosexuals, whose incubation distributions have not been extensively studied.

Methods could be developed to produce confidence intervals that account for most of the sources of uncertainty in estimates of θ. If we leave aside the issue of which incubation data can be extrapolated to which populations, then we can envision capturing the uncertainty in the incubation by generating replicates of our incubation estimate using simulated or resampled incubation data. This would produce estimates representing the range of plausible possibilities for the incubation distribution. These estimates could then be used in backcalculations that simultaneously estimate $\boldsymbol{\theta}$ and the R_{jk}'s, thereby accounting for some of the uncertainty in the R_j's, as well. (Uncertainty about underreporting also contributes to uncertainty about the R_j's.) Uncertainty due to model selection could be addressed by using flexible nonparametric methods for all the estimates, possibly using automatic smoothness selection methods that could be incorporated into replications of the estimation procedure on simulated or resampled data. Recent backcalculation efforts have adopted similar approaches that attempt to account for a variety of sources of uncertainty (Brookmeyer 1991; Rosenberg *et al*. 1991). It is possible that confidence intervals constructed by such an elaborate scheme would be much wider and more compatible with the amount of variability shown in Figure 5 and Table 4. Nevertheless, it seems likely that sensitivity analysis would still be necessary to address extrapolation of incubation data to the target population, and possibly to address underreporting.

Considerable attention has been focused on how to model the infection curve when performing backcalculation (Rosenberg, Gail, and Pee 1991; Segal and Bacchetti 1990; Taylor 1989). The method used here is appealing because it avoids parametric assumptions, requiring only that the infection curve be smooth. Furthermore, choosing an appropriate amount of smoothness appears to be quite easy, at least for the situation considered here.

We introduce in section 3.2 a method for estimating nonstationarity that may be present in the incubation or reporting delay distributions. This method is limited to detecting the influence of calendar time on the product $R_j I_{ij}$ beyond any influence that may already be reflected in the reporting and incubation distributions used. Figures 8a and 8b show that the estimate of such influence depends heavily on the incubation distribution used, even if attention is restricted to stationary distributions. A stationary incubation distribution is not implausible, because the influence of treatment could be countered by earlier diagnoses due to the expanding case definition and changes in clinical practice.

Although we have not incorporated estimation of the reporting delay into our backcalculations, estimation of the nonstationarity factors β_j does provide a check on the adequacy of the assumed distribution. Badly misspecified R_j's could be corrected by the β_j's, so the small improvements from nonzero β in Table 3 suggest that the R_j's used here are adequate. Simultaneous estimation of θ and the R_{jk} could be accomplished by including a term corresponding to L_c (1) in the criterion to be optimized (Harris 1990). Even in this case, however, the influence of the nonstationarity factors β_j from section 3.2 cannot be identified as applying either to the R_j's or the I_{ij}'s. This is because multiplying R_{jk} by a factor of e^{β_j} for each k leaves the conditional likelihood L_c unchanged. Thus, the factors still only appear when R_j and I_{ij} appear together, as described in section 3.2. This implies that it does not matter for estimation of θ whether nonstationarity is present in the incubation distribution versus the reporting delay distribution. Where the nonstationarity lies, however, is of great importance for making projections of future AIDS cases, so it is essential that the amount of nonstationarity in the incubation distribution be accurately estimated using external data.

The presence of systematic differences between incubation estimates based on different cohorts has serious implications for backcalculation. Uncertainty concerning what incubation data to use when performing backcalculation on a population can lead to substantial uncertainty in the resulting estimates of infection rates. For some populations there is little or no population-specific information about the incubation distribution. It is not clear how different such a population's incubation distribution might be from the distributions estimated from available data on other groups. It is not even clear how to specify a number of possibilities that would span a plausible range. Thus, applying backcalculation to populations of intravenous drug users or heterosexuals is very difficult, and methods for gauging the uncertainty of the resulting estimates are unavailable. For such populations (arguably for any population), methods for supplementing backcalculation with relevant survey and cohort data on seroprevalence and seroconversion rates are essential.

5. REFERENCES

Bacchetti, P. (1990). Estimating the Incubation Period of AIDS by Comparing Population Infection and Diagnosis Patterns. *Journal of the American Statistical Association* **85**: 1002-1008.

Bacchetti, P. and Jewell, N.P. (1991). Nonparametric Estimation of the Incubation Period of AIDS Based on a Prevalent Cohort with Unknown Infection Times. *Biometrics* **47**: 947-960.

Brookmeyer, R. (1991). Reconstruction and Future Trends of the AIDS Epidemic in the United States. *Science* **253**: 37-42.

Brookmeyer, R. and Gail, M.H. (1988). A Method for Obtaining Short-term Projections and Lower Bounds on the Size of the AIDS Epidemic. *Journal of the American Statistical Association* **83**: 301-308.

Brookmeyer, R. and Goedert, J.J. (1989). Censoring in an Epidemic with an Application to Hemophilia-Associated AIDS. *Biometrics* **45**: 325-335.

Brookmeyer, R. and Liao, J. (1990). The Analysis of Delays in Disease Reporting: Methods and Results for the Acquired Immunodeficiency Syndrome. *American Journal of Epidemiology* **132**: 355-365.

Centers for Disease Control (1990). HIV Prevalence Estimates and AIDS Case Projections for the United States: Report Based on a Workshop. *Morbidity and Mortality Weekly Report* **39(RR-16)**: 1-31.

DeGruttola, V. and Lagakos, S.W. (1989). Analysis of Doubly-Censored Survival Data, with Application to AIDS. *Biometrics* **45**: 1-11.

Efron, B. (1985). Bootstrap Confidence Intervals for a Class of Parametric Problems. *Biometrika* **72**: 45-58.

Gail, M.H., Rosenberg, P.S. and Goedert, J.J.(1990). Therapy May Explain Recent Deficits in AIDS Incidence. *Journal of Acquired Immune Deficiency Syndromes* **3**: 296-306.

Goedert, J.J., Kessler, C.M., Aledort, L.M., *et al*. (1989). A Prospective Study of Human Immunodeficiency Virus Type 1 Infections and the Development of AIDS in Subjects with Hemophilia. *New England Journal of Medicine* **321**: 1141-1148.

Harris, J.E. (1990). Reporting Delays and the Incidence of AIDS. *Journal of the American Statistical Association* **85**: 915-924.

Hessol, N.A., Lifson, A.R., O'Malley, P.M., Doll, L.S., Jaffe, H.W. and Rutherford, G.W. (1989). Prevalence, Incidence, and Progression of Human Immunodeficiency Virus Infection in Homosexual and Bisexual Men in Hepatitis B Vaccine Trials, 1978-1988. *American Journal of Epidemiology* **130**: 1167-1175.

Rosenberg, P.S., Biggar, R.J., Goedert, J.J. and Gail, M.H. (1991). Backcalculation of the Number with Human Immunodeficiency Virus Infection in the United States. *American Journal of Epidemiology* **133**: 276-285.

Rosenberg, P.S., Gail, M.H. and Pee, D. (1991). Mean Square Error of Estimates of HIV Prevalence and Short Term AIDS Projections Derived by Backcalculation. To appear.

Segal, M. and Bacchetti, P. (1990). Deficits in AIDS Incidence. *Journal of Acquired Immune Deficiency Syndromes* **3**: 832-833.

Taylor, J.M.G. (1989). Models for the HIV Infection and AIDS Epidemic in the United States. *Statistics in Medicine* **8**: 45-58.

Peter Bacchetti and Mark R. Segal
Department of Epidemiology and Biostatistics
University of California
San Francisco, California 94110

Nicholas P. Jewell
Group in Biostatistics
University of California
Berkeley, California 94720

A Comprehensive Back-Calculation Framework for the Estimation and Prediction of AIDS Cases

Jerry Lawless and Jiangue Sun

Abstract

We discuss a model for the occurrence of AIDS cases that incorporates uncertainty due to the HIV infection process, incubation times, and delays in the reporting of AIDS cases. The analysis is based on AIDS cases diagnosed and reported by a given time, and provides standard errors for estimates and predictions that recognize the different sources of uncertainty. The approach is illustrated on U.S. AIDS cases reported to the end of 1989.

1 Introduction and Notation

The analysis of AIDS incidence and prediction of future cases in a population has been studied by many authors, including several in this volume. The most appealing and flexible current methods assume a process of human immunodeficiency virus (HIV) infections in the population and an incubation distribution for the time from HIV infection to clinical AIDS. These so-called "back-calculation" methods (Brookmeyer and Gail, 1988) have been extensively used (e.g. see Becker, Watson and Carlin, 1991, Brookmeyer and Damiano 1989, Day et al. 1989, Brookmeyer and Liao 1990a, 1992, Brookmeyer 1991, Gail and Rosenberg 1992, Pagano et al. 1992, and Rosenberg and Gail 1991) to estimate HIV and AIDS incidence. Jewell (1990, section 3) discusses and compares several approaches.

Models are generally fitted using AIDS incidence data. There are several sources of uncertainty in the fitted models and estimates based on them, including uncertainty about the form of the HIV infection curves and AIDS incubation distributions, uncertainty about the numbers of AIDS cases diagnosed due to substantial delays in the reporting of cases and the non-reporting of many cases, inherent random variation in the HIV infection and disease processes, and sampling variation in estimates. The effect of the choice of models for the infection density and incubation distribution is usually investigated by fitting a variety of models. Other sources of uncertainty should be reflected in the standard errors of estimates or predictions. The purpose of this paper is to discuss a flexible model for AIDS case analysis and projection and to present realistic standard errors. The approach is a unification and extension of those of Harris (1990), Brookmeyer and Liao (1990a) and others. It is not our objective to give a critical analysis of the information available in the U.S. or elsewhere about incubation distributions, AIDS incidence, AIDS reporting and the like. Bacchetti, Segal and Jewell (1991), Gail and Rosenberg (1992) and others address these exceedingly important issues.

Ideal incidence data would consist of the numbers of AIDS cases diagnosed in different time intervals but as noted, the time lag between when a case is diagnosed and when it is reported to the surveillance agency responsible for collecting the data can be substantial (see e.g. Brookmeyer and Damiano 1989, Brookmeyer and Liao 1990b, Harris 1990). Most current methods therefore use adjusted numbers of AIDS cases, the adjustments being based on estimated reporting delay probabilities (e.g. Harris 1990). The uncertainty related to the use of estimated (adjusted) counts is usually ignored. We start here with counts for AIDS cases diagnosed in discrete time periods $i = 1, 2, \ldots$ and reported in time periods $j \geq i$. Estimation of reporting delay probabilities and other model parameters are considered jointly. We define

n_{ij} = number of AIDS cases diagnosed in period i and reported in period j ($j \geq i$; $i = 1, 2, \ldots$)

$N_i(T) = \sum_{j=i}^{T} n_{ij}$ = number of AIDS cases diagnosed in period i and reported by period T ($T \geq i$).

$N_i = N_i(\infty)$ = number of cases diagnosed in period i and eventually reported.

We suppose further that HIV infections, AIDS cases and reports of those cases are generated by a random process and in connection with that we define

$$\mu_{ij} = E(n_{ij}),\ \mu_i(T) = E\left(N_i(T)\right),\ \mu_i = E(N_i). \tag{1.1}$$

We assume further that

$$\mu_{ij} = \mu_i g_i(j-i) \tag{1.2}$$

$$\mu_i = \sum_{t \leq i} \lambda(t) f_t(i-t) \tag{1.3}$$

where

$g_i(r)$ = probability a case diagnosed in period i is reported in period $i+r$ $(r \geq 0)$

$\lambda(t)$ = expected number of HIV infections occurring in period t

$f_t(s)$ = probability an HIV infection in period t leads to a diagnosis of AIDS in period $t+s$ $(s \geq 0)$.

The structure of (1.3) is that used in the back-calculation method (e.g. Brookmeyer and Gail 1988, Becker et al. 1991, Rosenberg and Gail 1991). The $f_t(s)$'s are often called incubation probabilities but it is preferable here to refer to them as "progression" probabilities that represent, for the population under discussion, the expected proportion of persons infected in period t who will be diagnosed with AIDS in period $t+s$. Most authors have taken $f_t(s)$ to be independent of t; recent exceptions are Brookmeyer and Liao (1990a), Brookmeyer (1991), Gail and Rosenberg (1992) and Solomon and Wilson (1990) who allow $f_t(s)$ to reflect the introduction of treatments such as zidovudine (AZT).

It is not possible to estimate all of the $g_i(r)$'s, $\lambda(t)$'s and $f_t(s)$'s from observed counts n_{ij} and we take the common approach of assuming the $f_t(s)$'s are known; we discuss uncertainty due to this later. Aside from a truncation factor (see section 3) reporting delay probabilities are readily estimated and it is both flexible and convenient to treat them nonparametrically. On the other hand, nonparametric estimation of the $\lambda(t)$'s is more difficult, and we consider parametric models $\lambda(t;\boldsymbol{\theta})$, where $\boldsymbol{\theta}$ is a $p \times 1$ vector of parameters. Concurrently, we write $\mu_i = \mu_i(\boldsymbol{\theta})$ in (1.3). We comment on the choice between parametric and nonparametric representations of $\lambda(t)$ in section 6.

If we assume that the n_{ij}'s are independent Poisson random variables, as is often done, then maximum likelihood procedures follow easily. Jewell (1990, section 3) surveys this area. Since extra-Poisson variation is present, however, we use generalized least squares (quasi-likelihood) estimation of $\boldsymbol{\theta}$ jointly with nonparametric estimation of the $g_i(r)$'s. For convenience and to facilitate comparison with other approaches we discuss estimation of $\boldsymbol{\theta}$ and the $g_i(r)$'s separately in sections 2 and 3, and then in section 4 we give prediction limits for AIDS cases that reflect the uncertainty in both $\boldsymbol{\theta}$ and the $g_i(r)$'s. Section 5 provides examples based on U.S. data and section 6 makes a few concluding remarks.

2 Estimation of $\lambda(t;\ \boldsymbol{\theta})$

We assume that the data consist of AIDS case counts n_{ij} reported up to period T, i.e. with $1 \le i \le j \le T$. We estimate $\boldsymbol{\theta}$ by assuming that the $N_i(T)$'s ($N_i(T)$ = the number of cases diagnosed in period i and reported by period T) are independent ($i = 1, \ldots, T$) with

$$E\left\{N_i(T)\right\} = \mu_i(T;\boldsymbol{\theta}), \quad Var\left\{N_i(T)\right\} = V\left[\mu_i(T;\boldsymbol{\theta}), \alpha\right]$$

where α is a scalar parameter designed to allow extra-Poisson variation. We remark that the strict independence of the $N_i(T)$'s may be questioned, but assuming independence does not seem likely to bias results much.

We assume for now that the $g_i(r)$'s are known, and consider the quasi-likelihood estimating equations for $\boldsymbol{\theta}$ (e.g. McCullagh and Nelder 1989, ch. 9),

$$\sum_{i=1}^{T} \left\{ \frac{N_i(T) - \mu_i(T;\boldsymbol{\theta})}{V\left[\mu_i(T;\boldsymbol{\theta}), \alpha\right]} \right\} \frac{\partial \mu_i(T;\boldsymbol{\theta})}{\partial \boldsymbol{\theta}} = \mathbf{0}. \tag{2.1}$$

It should be noted that

$$\mu_i(T;\boldsymbol{\theta}) = \mu_i(\boldsymbol{\theta}) G_i(T-i) \tag{2.2}$$

where $G_i(r) = \sum_{\ell=0}^{r} g_i(\ell)$ is the probability a case diagnosed in period i is reported by period $i+r$.

To estimate α an additional estimating equation is required; we use the common choice (e.g. Lawless 1987)

$$\sum_{i=1}^{T} \frac{\{N_i(T) - \mu_i(T;\boldsymbol{\theta})\}^2}{V\left[\mu_i(T;\boldsymbol{\theta}),\alpha\right]} - T = 0. \tag{2.3}$$

Reasonable choices for the variance function V are $V(\mu,\alpha) = \alpha\mu$ (e.g. McCullagh and Nelder 1989, chap. 11) and $V(\mu,\alpha) = \mu + \alpha\mu^2$ (e.g. Lawless 1987). For the former model α drops out of (2.1) so that $\boldsymbol{\theta}$ is estimable without it; α is then obtained immediately from (2.3) with $\boldsymbol{\theta}$ set equal to its estimate, $\widehat{\boldsymbol{\theta}}$.

The asymptotic covariance matrix for $\widehat{\boldsymbol{\theta}}$ when the $g_i(r)$'s are known is estimated by

$$\widehat{W}_T = \left\{\sum_{i=1}^{T} V\left[\mu_i(T;\theta),\alpha\right]^{-1} \left(\frac{\partial\mu_i(T)}{\partial\boldsymbol{\theta}}\right) \left(\frac{\partial\mu_i(T)}{\partial\boldsymbol{\theta}}\right)'\right\}^{-1}, \tag{2.4}$$

evaluated at $\widehat{\boldsymbol{\theta}}$, $\hat{\alpha}$.

Remark 1. A common approach for the estimation of $\boldsymbol{\theta}$ (e.g. Karon et al. 1988, Rosenberg and Gail 1991) is to adjust the observed counts $N_i(T)$ for reporting delays to obtain

$$\widetilde{N}_i = N_i(T)/G_i(T-i),$$

and then to treat the $\widetilde{N}_i$'s as the responses in a Poisson model or in a procedure similar to that described above. In that case it is assumed that $E(\widetilde{N}_i) = \mu_i(\boldsymbol{\theta})$ and the estimating equations for $\boldsymbol{\theta}$ are the same as (2.1) with $\mu_i(\boldsymbol{\theta})$ replacing $\mu_i(T;\boldsymbol{\theta})$. However, $\mathrm{Var}(\widetilde{N}_i)$ depends on $G_i(T-i)$ so that from this point of view one should still be using (2.1) as is. Treating the $\widetilde{N}_i$'s as the responses tends to underestimate the variance of estimates.

Remark 2. It is well known that functions $\lambda(t;\theta)$ with widely differing shapes over the most recent 3 or 4 years can give similar fits to observed AIDS data, in large part because the probability of getting AIDS within a few years of HIV infection is estimated to be small.

3 Estimation of Reporting Delay Probabilities

Estimates of reporting delay probabilities $G_i(T-i)$ are needed in the preceding section and for model checking and prediction. As noted by many authors, reporting delays r for cases diagnosed in period i and reported by period T are necessarily right-truncated (i.e. $r \leq T - i$) and consequently it is not possible to estimate $G_i(T-i)$ nonparametrically on the basis of the cases diagnosed in period i alone. The way around this is to specify some relationship among probabilities for cases diagnosed in different periods.

Define for each i

$$g_i^*(r) = \frac{g_i(r)}{G_i(r)} \qquad r = 0, 1, 2, \ldots \tag{3.1}$$

and note that for $r < \tau$

$$\frac{G_i(r)}{G_i(\tau)} = \prod_{\ell=r+1}^{\tau} [1 - g_i^*(\ell)]. \tag{3.2}$$

As noted by Kalbfleisch and Lawless (1989, 1991) and others, without further assumptions only the $g_i^*(r)$'s for $r \leq T - i$, and not the $g_i(r)$'s, are estimable nonparametrically from counts n_{ij} with $i \leq j \leq T$. If we assume that reporting delay probabilities do not depend on when the case was diagnosed (so that $g_i^*(r) = g(r)$ for $i \leq r \leq T$) and that $G_i(T) = 1$, then estimation of the $g_i(r)$'s is straightforward (e.g. Kalbfleisch and Lawless 1991). However, for U.S. and other data there is evidence of changes in reporting delay probabilities over time (e.g. Harris 1990, Kalbfleisch and Lawless 1991). One approach (e.g. Harris 1990) is to divide calendar time into intervals and to assume stationary reporting delays within each. We adopt another method, discussed by Lawless (1991), which attempts to estimate reporting delay probabilities using the most recently reported cases. The method assumes that

$$g_i^*(r) = g^*(r) \qquad i + r \geq T - m, \tag{3.3}$$

i.e. that the $g_i^*(r)$'s are stationary for cases diagnosed in the past m periods and into the future. Lawless (1991) obtains the estimates

$$\hat{g}^*(r) = \frac{n_{.r}}{N_{.r}} \qquad r = 1, \ldots, T \tag{3.4}$$

where

$$\begin{aligned} n_{.r} &= \sum_{i=\max(0,T-m-r)}^{T-r} n_{i,i+r} \\ N_{.r} &= \sum_{i=\max(0,T-m-r)}^{T-r} N_i(i+r). \end{aligned}$$

The asymptotic covariance matrix for $\hat{g}^* = (\hat{g}^*(1), \ldots, \hat{g}^*(T))'$ is estimated by

$$\widehat{W}_G = \operatorname{diag}\left(\frac{\hat{g}^*(r)\,[1 - \hat{g}^*(r)]}{N_{.r}}\right). \tag{3.5}$$

Using (3.4) and (3.2) with $\tau = T$, and assuming that $G(T) = 1$, we have estimates

$$\widehat{G}_i(T-i) = \prod_{r=T-i+1}^{T} [1 - \hat{g}^*(r)], \tag{3.6}$$

which can be used in the estimation procedure for $\lambda(t;\boldsymbol{\theta})$ in section 2. The choice of m in the procedure above is discussed in section 5.

We next determine the joint asymptotic covariance matrix for $\widehat{\boldsymbol{\theta}}$ and $\hat{\boldsymbol{g}}^*$ and use it to obtain standard errors for the fitted values and predictions.

4 Estimation and Prediction of Aids Cases

We begin by obtaining the joint asymptotic covariance matrix for $\widehat{\boldsymbol{\theta}}$, $\hat{\boldsymbol{g}}^*$ and $\hat{\alpha}$, where $\hat{\boldsymbol{g}}^*$ is given by (3.4) and where $\widehat{\boldsymbol{\theta}}$, $\hat{\alpha}$ are found by solving the estimating equations (2.1) and (2.3) with $\boldsymbol{g}^*$ estimated by $\hat{\boldsymbol{g}}^*$. For convenience we will write $\mu_i(T)$ for $\mu_i(T;\boldsymbol{\theta}) = \mu_i(\boldsymbol{\theta})G_i(T-i)$ (see (2.2)) and $V_i = V\left[\mu_i(T;\theta), \alpha\right]$

for the variance of $N_i(T)$. Then, from (2.1), (2.3) and (3.4), the estimators $\widehat{\boldsymbol{\theta}}$, $\hat{\boldsymbol{g}}^*$, $\hat{\alpha}$ are the solution to the estimating equations

$$\boldsymbol{u}_1(\boldsymbol{\theta}, \boldsymbol{g}^*, \alpha) = \sum_{i=1}^{T} \left\{ \frac{N_i(T) - \mu_i(T)}{V_i} \right\} \frac{\partial \mu_i(T)}{\partial \boldsymbol{\theta}} = \mathbf{0} \quad (4.1)$$

$$\boldsymbol{u}_2(\boldsymbol{g}^*) = \frac{n_{\cdot r}}{g^*(r)} - \frac{N_{\cdot r} - n_{\cdot r}}{1 - g^*(r)} = 0 \qquad r = 1, \ldots, T \quad (4.2)$$

$$u_3(\boldsymbol{\theta}, \boldsymbol{g}^*, \alpha) = \sum_{i=1}^{T} \frac{\{N_i(T) - \mu_i(T)\}^2}{V_i} - T = 0 \, . \quad (4.3)$$

The asymptotic covariance matrix for $(\widehat{\boldsymbol{\theta}}, \hat{\boldsymbol{g}}^*, \hat{\alpha})$ can be obtained by standard large sample theory for estimating equations (e.g. Inagaki 1973, White 1982). Let $C(\boldsymbol{\theta}, \boldsymbol{g}^*)$ be the $p \times T$ matrix with (u, r) element

$$C_{ur}(\boldsymbol{\theta}, \boldsymbol{g}^*, \alpha) = \sum_{i=T-r+1}^{T} \frac{1}{V_i} \left[\frac{\partial \mu_i(T)}{\partial \theta_u} \right] \left[\frac{\mu_i(T)}{1 - g^*(r)} \right] \quad (4.4)$$

and let $\hat{C} = C(\widehat{\boldsymbol{\theta}}, \hat{\boldsymbol{g}}^*, \hat{\alpha})$. It is shown in the Appendix that the asymptotic covariance matrix of $(\widehat{\boldsymbol{\theta}}, \hat{\boldsymbol{g}}^*)$ is estimated by the matrix $\widehat{W}$ with blocks

$$\begin{aligned} \widehat{\text{asvar}}(\widehat{\boldsymbol{\theta}}) &= \widehat{W}_T + \widehat{W}_T \hat{C} \widehat{W}_G \hat{C}' \widehat{W}_T \\ \widehat{\text{asvar}}(\hat{\boldsymbol{g}}^*) &= \widehat{W}_G \\ \widehat{\text{ascov}}(\widehat{\boldsymbol{\theta}}, \hat{\boldsymbol{g}}^*) &= \widehat{W}_T \hat{C} \widehat{W}_G \end{aligned} \quad (4.5)$$

where $\widehat{W}_T$ and $\widehat{W}_G$ are given by (2.4) and (3.5), respectively.

We remark that if T is large we may want to assume that $G_i(\tau) = 1$ for some $\tau < T$, in which case g^* has dimension $\tau \times 1$. For large T or τ, $\hat{C}$, $\widehat{W}_G$ and $\widehat{W}$ are of large dimension but their entries are easily computed.

We now consider standard errors for fitted values and prediction of AIDS cases. In either case we estimate the expected numbers of cases diagnosed in a time period $[a, b]$ and reported by time $T_0 \geq b$. This equals

$$\mu[a, b; T_0] = \sum_{i=a}^{b} \sum_{j=i}^{T_0} \mu_{ij}$$

$$= \sum_{i=a}^{b} \mu_i(\boldsymbol{\theta}) G_i(T_0 - i).$$

We assume that the required μ_{ij}'s are estimable from $\boldsymbol{\theta}$ and $\boldsymbol{g}*$; in the case of AIDS predictions this sometimes necessitates predicting cases due only to already occurred HIV infections.

Let $\boldsymbol{\phi} = (\boldsymbol{\theta}, \boldsymbol{g}^*)$ and let $\widehat{W}$ be the estimated asymptotic covariance matrix for $\hat{\boldsymbol{\phi}}$ given by (4.5). The estimated asymptotic variance of $\hat{\mu}[a, b; T]$ is $\widehat{W}_M = \hat{\boldsymbol{d}}' \widehat{W} \hat{\boldsymbol{d}}$, where $\boldsymbol{d} = \partial \mu / \partial \boldsymbol{\phi}$ is the $(p + T) \times 1$ vector with entries

$$\frac{\partial \mu[a, b; T_0]}{\partial \theta_u} = \sum_{i=a}^{b} \frac{\partial \mu_i}{\partial \theta_u} G_i(T_0 - i)$$

$$\frac{\partial \mu[a, b; T_0]}{\partial g^*(r)} = \frac{-1}{1 - g^*(r)} \sum_{i=a}^{b} \mu_i G_i(T_0 - i) I(i \geq T_0 - r + 1).$$

where $I(S)$ is the indication function, which equals 1 if S is true and 0 if not.

If $[a, b]$ is a future time period $(a > T)$ then we are interested in prediction of the number of AIDS cases to be diagnosed in $[a, b]$ and reported by time $T_0 \geq b$; we denote this by

$$N[a, b; T_0] = \sum_{i=a}^{b} N_i(T_0). \tag{4.6}$$

We use $\hat{\mu}[a, b; T_0]$ as a point estimate of $N[a, b; T_0]$ and base prediction limits on $N[a, b; T_0] - \hat{\mu}[a, b; T_0]$, which has estimated asymptotic variance

$$\hat{V}_p = \widehat{W}_M + \sum_{i=a}^{b} V \left[\mu_i(T_0, \widehat{\boldsymbol{\theta}}), \hat{\alpha} \right],$$

under the assumptions about the $N_i(T)$'s made in section 2. Variance estimates are also readily developed for cases where $b \leq T$ but $T_0 > T$, i.e. when we are estimating diagnosed but not yet reported AIDS cases.

Table 1. USA Observed and Expected AIDS Counts (rounded), Reported by December 1989.

QUARTERLY PERIOD	OBSERVED COUNT	EXPECTED COUNTS 1a	1b	2a	2b
1977:1–1981:4	372	383	443	411	415
1982:1–2	398	362	329	409	405
1982:3–4	678	673	615	714	702
1983:1–2	1282	1115	1056	1159	1136
1983:3–4	1651	1744	1694	1786	1752
1984:1–2	2562	2605	2564	2632	2590
1984:3–4	3364	3695	3658	3683	3645
1985:1	2195	2338	2321	2309	2296
1985:2	2626	2698	2685	2653	2648
1985:3	3044	3071	3069	3015	3020
1985:4	3173	3463	3477	3399	3417
1986:1	3812	3865	3899	3799	3832
1986:2	4275	4277	4333	4213	4261
1986:3	4734	4696	4774	4636	4699
1986:4	4956	5111	5209	5059	5137
1987:1	5945	5522	5636	5478	5569
1987:2	6417	5923	6046	5890	5987
1987:3	6756	6302	6425	6279	6378
1987:4	6869	6651	6764	6640	6732
1988:1	7398	6964	7056	6966	7042
1988:2	7516	7235	7295	7251	7301
1988:3	7570	7437	7452	7467	7479
1988:4	7277	7546	7505	7590	7555
1989:1	7515	7525	7420	7583	7490
1989:2	7344	7311	7138	7381	7228
1989:3	6160	6506	6281	6578	6379
1989:4	1882	2766	2638	2802	2687
$\sum \frac{(OBS-EXP)^2}{EXP}$		586.1	486.4	606.4	458.9

5 Example

We consider as an example the case of AIDS incidence data for the U.S.A.. Table 1 gives (see column 2) the numbers of AIDS cases diagnosed by quarter and reported by the end of 1989. The counts for the first 20 quarters (1977-81) are grouped and, to save space, the 1982-84 counts are for half-years. Note that these data differ from Table 1 in Rosenberg and Gail (1991) or Table IV in Becker et al. (1991), who show pseudo data obtained by adjusting the AIDS case counts for reporting delays. We have considered several models for the HIV infection intensity $\lambda(t)$ and report here on two:

1. Piecewise constant, with

$$\lambda(t) = \lambda_j \qquad t \in I_j \quad (j = 1, \ldots, 5)$$

where $I_1, \ldots, I_5$ are the five calendar time intervals 1977:1–1980:4, 1981:1–1982:4, 1983:1–1984:4, 1985:1–1987:2, 1987:3–1989:4. It is assumed that $\lambda(t) = 0$ prior to 1977. Rosenberg and Gail (1991) and others consider similar models.

2. Exponential-quadratic, with

$$\lambda(t) = \beta_0 \exp\left\{\beta_1(t - t_0) + \beta_2(t - t_0)^2\right\} \qquad t \geq t_0$$

and $\lambda(t) = 0$ for $t < t_0$. We used $t_0 = 1$, corresponding to 1977:1. Taylor (1989) considers a similar model and, although it is almost certainly inappropriate in the long term, it may provide a reasonable model up to the end of 1989.

There is a good deal of uncertainty about the right hand tail of the reporting delay distribution. Estimates obtained by us here (see line 2 of Table 2) and by Harris (1990) indicate a long tail, with about 13% of reporting delays estimated to exceed 4 years. However, estimates for reporting delays longer than 4 years depend on AIDS cases diagnosed before 1986, and it might be argued that improvements in reporting will lead to only a few recent cases with such long reporting delays.

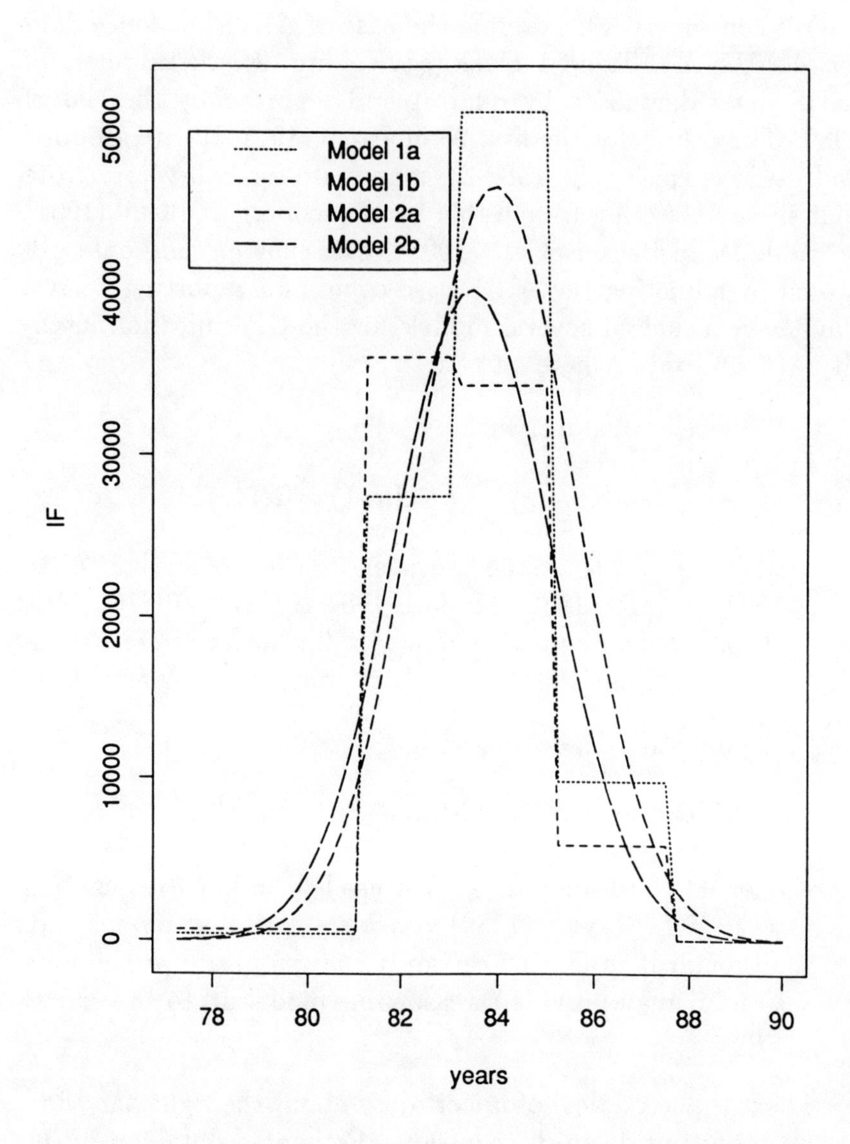

Figure 1. The Estimated HIV Incidence Function

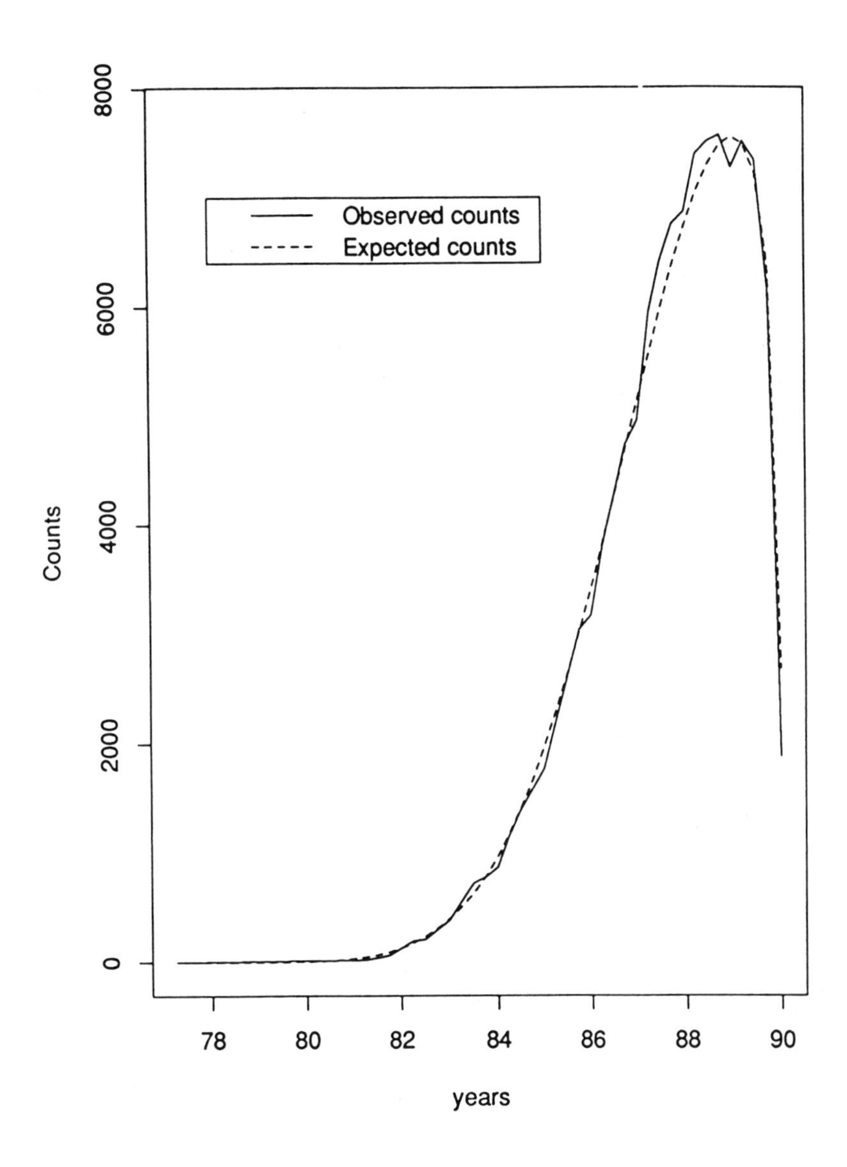

Figure 2. The Expected and Observed AIDS Counts for Model 2b

Indeed, most authors (e.g. Becker et al. 1991, Rosenberg and Gail 1991) truncate the reporting delay distribution at about 4 years. To see the effect on predictions of the assumed upper limit on reporting delays, we report results based on both a "short" reporting delay distribution with all delays assumed to be ≤ 4 years (i.e. $G_i(\tau) = 1$ for $\tau \geq 48$ months) and a "long" reporting delay distribution with delays up to 8 years allowed. In other words, for the former case we in effect predict only future AIDS cases with reporting delays of 4 years or less. Although there is some evidence that reporting delays have lengthened somewhat over the past few years (e.g. Harris 1990), the model fits did not change substantially when we allowed for nonstationarity. Consequently, we show results here with the $g^*(r)$'s assumed constant; this is equivalent to using $m = T$ in (3.3).

We considered several alternatives for the progression probabilities $f_t(s)$ (see (1.3)), including some that allowed for secular changes over time. Assumptions about the $f_t(s)$'s have a great impact on estimates of $\lambda(t)$ and projections (see Bacchetti et al. 1991 for a rather critical discussion) but for simplicity here we report results only for stationary distributions with similar medians. These were discretizations of two models:

a. A Weibull distribution with cumulative distribution function (cdf) $F(s) = 1 - \exp\{-.00211s^{2.516}\}$, as considered by Becker et al. (1991), Rosenberg and Gail (1991) and others.

b. A log logistic distribution with cdf $F(s) = (.1s)^{3.08} / \{1 + (.1s)^{3.08}\}$.

Both models a. and b. have 25th and 50th percentiles equal to 7 and 10 years, respectively, in agreement with estimates from several cohort studies (e.g. see Brookmeyer and Goedert 1989). The log logistic distribution has a longer tail than the Weibull; they are about equally well supported by current data.

To fit the models (i.e. to estimate the $g^*(r)$'s and the parameters in $\lambda(t)$) we took the time periods to be quarter-years, with 1977:1 being $t = 1$ and $T = 52$ representing 1989:4. We used discrete versions of models 1, 2 for $\lambda(t)$ and a, b for $f(s)$.

Estimating the $g^*(r)$'s as in (3.4) we found, in agreement with Harris (1990), that the reporting delay distribution has a long tail, with in excess of 15 percent of cases having a delay of at least 3 years.

Table 2. Estimated Probabilities $\hat{G}(r)$ that the Reporting Delay is $\leq r$ months

r:	6	12	18	24	36	48	60	72	84	96
$\hat{G}(r)$	.55	.69	.75	.79	.84	.87	.90	.92	.96	1.00
$\hat{G}(r)^*$	.63	.79	.86	.91	.96	1.00				

* Assumes that all reporting delays are $\leq$ 48 months

Table 2 (line 2) shows this estimated reporting delay distribution, with reporting delays assumed to be 8 years or less. We show also (line 3) the estimated "short" reporting delay distribution, obtained by truncating the distribution in line 2 at 4 years. The parameters in $\lambda(t)$ were estimated via the quasi-likelihood equations (2.1), with variance function $V[\mu_i, \alpha] = \alpha\mu_i$. The variance parameter α was estimated via (2.3).

Columns 3 to 6 of Table 1 show expected frequencies for models 1a, 1b, 2a, and 2b and the "long" reporting delay distribution. Graphs of the estimated HIV incidence functions $\hat{\lambda}(t)$ for each model are shown in Figure 1. Figure 2 shows expected and observed quarterly AIDS cases, reported by the end of 1989, for model 2b as an illustration of the results in Table 1. It is seen that over the period from about January 1987 to June 1988 the observed cases consistently exceed the expected counts; aside from this the fit of the models is quite good. None of the many models that we explored, including ones that allowed nonstationary reporting delay probabilities and nonstationary incubation probabilities, was able to remove this feature entirely. This feature is not found to the same degree in models fitted by Becker et al. (1991) and Rosenberg and Gail (1991); however, their fits were based on data only to the first quarter of 1988, and used reporting delay-adjusted counts. It is not our objective here to give a highly detailed analysis of AIDS case trends, but it seems likely that a wider variety of models for the incubation distribution and infection intensities has to be considered to explain recent trends. Brookmeyer (1991) and Gail and Rosenberg (1992) provide excellent recent analyses of the U.S. situation.

Table 3. Estimated Numbers of AIDS Cases

Source		Estimated Number of Thousand Cases by the End of 1989		1992		1993	
Model	1a	160	(2.2)	332	(31.8)	394	(59.8)
(Long	1b	159	(2.3)	307	(58.1)	352	(117.6)
R.D.)	2a	160	(4.7)	337	(16.1)	400	(21.8)
	2b	159	(5.6)	313	(19.6)	360	(26.1)
Model	1a	141	(1.6)	288	(27.5)	340	(51.7)
(Short	1b	140	(1.7)	267	(50.6)	304	(102.5)
R.D.)	2a	141	(3.5)	296	(12.2)	351	(16.7)
	2b	141	(4.1)	275	(15.0)	317	(20.2)
CDC[1]		139–144		280–333		330–405	
BWC[2]				363–416			
RG[3]				388–425			

[1] Centers for Disease Control (1990)
[2] Becker et al. (1991)
[3] Rosenberg and Gail (1991)

Table 3 shows predictions of the number of AIDS cases diagnosed (and ultimately reported) to the end of 1989, 1992 and 1993, based on the models fitted above and using the methods of section 4. Standard errors are given in brackets. Note that whether one assumes that future reporting delays are 4 years or less has a large impact on short term projections. Indeed, for the number of cases up to the end of 1989, the difference in the point estimates given by the "long" and "short" reporting delay assumptions dwarfs the standard errors for each case. Also shown are estimates from other sources. In view of the lengthy reporting delays for many cases, it will be several years before projections like those here can be assessed. Regarding short-term projections, we note that models 1a, 1b, 2a and 2b and the "long" reporting delay distribution estimated the number of cases diagnosed in 1990 and reported by the end of 1990 as 27765, 25684, 28224 and 26321, respectively, with standard errors of approximately 2045, 2800, 2240 and 2738. The actual observed number was 26076. The "short" reporting delay distribution gives very similar results. A key point in these estimates and the ones in Table 3 is the rather large standard errors, reflecting the variation due to both reporting delays and incubation times.

6 Additional Remarks

Our objective has been to present a flexible framework for the prediction of reported AIDS cases and to provide realistic standard errors for predictions. We will comment briefly on other sources of uncertainty than those discussed in sections 4 and 5.

We have assumed that progression probabilities $f_t(s)$ are known, although they are of course estimated. Given an estimate $\hat{f}(s)$, say, from a specific study, it is possible to incorporate sampling variation from this into variance estimates for $\hat{\mu}[a, b; T_0]$ or $N[a, b; T_0]$. In view of the variety of studies providing information about $f(s)$ it seems preferable, however, to simply fit models using a plausible range of incubation distributions. Section 5 (see Table 3) illustrates the effect of using two equally plausible distributions which agree closely up to their medians; the effect of changing the medians of the distributions would be even more substantial. Indeed, Bacchetti et al. (1991) argue that progression probabilities for either the entire U.S. population or specific subgroups are currently so uncertain as to render back-calculation unreliable for estimating numbers of HIV-infected persons. We feel that they are perhaps overly pessimistic, but agree that estimation of the pattern and total number of infections by back-calculation is quite uncertain. We have focused here on short term predictions of AIDS cases, which are somewhat less variable. Even so, standard errors for the estimated number of cases only to 1992 are fairly large, and if uncertainty in the progression probabilities is incorporated the estimates verge on being too variable to be much better than crude extrapolation of adjusted case counts.

Another source of much uncertainty, particularly for predictions more than two or three years ahead, is the form of the HIV infection intensity $\lambda(t)$. We have used parametric models for $\lambda(t)$, some of which impose strong assumptions on its shape. Parametric assumptions can to some extent be checked by obtaining nonparametric estimates of the infection curve. Bacchetti et al. (1991), Becker et al. (1991), Becker and Watson (1992), Brookmeyer and Liao (1992) and others discuss a variety of approaches. On current U.S. data such methods produce estimated curves that are qualitatively similar to those in Figure 1, but confidence limits make it clear that there is very little information about $\lambda(t)$ past about 1986. Weakly parametric models which permit a wide variety of shapes reflect this but confidence limits on $\boldsymbol{\theta}$ and $\lambda(t;\boldsymbol{\theta})$ from strongly parametric models which restrict shape severely do not. However, for the latter the uncertainty in $\lambda(t)$ is made clear by fitting models with a variety of shapes. For example, we fitted models that mimic model 2 up to about 1985 but decrease very slowly thereafter; they also gave good fits to the observed U.S. data. Similar results are found in Taylor (1989).

As Table 3 suggests, strongly parametric models such as 2a and 2b give considerably smaller variance estimates for predictions than do weakly parametric models such as 1a and 1b, or nonparametric methods. The former are of course more susceptible to bias so it is sensible to explore models with a variety of plausible shapes for $\lambda(t)$ when making projections. With this proviso, parametric methods are well suited for short term projections of AIDS cases since they are easy to fit and yield prediction limits in a simple way.

Prediction is of course risky in a context where several of the basic process parameters may be undergoing substantial change. Thus, changes in incubation times that are caused by new treatment therapies for HIV-infected persons, changes in reporting delay probabilities, or changes in the probabilities of AIDS cases being diagnosed or reported may have a substantial effect on future AIDS case reports, but be impossible to model accurately with the amount of information currently available.

Finally, there are many other caveats and aspects of AIDS case reporting and prediction which could be discussed, but that is not our purpose. In any event, the important issues have been addressed in numerous reports and papers. Useful references in this regard include Brookmeyer (1991), Brookmeyer and Gail (1988), Brookmeyer and Liao (1990a), Centres for Disease Control (1990), Day et al. (1989) and the Cox Report on AIDS in the U.K. of which it is a part, Jewell (1990), Karon, Dondero and Curran (1988), and Taylor (1989).

APPENDIX

Consider the estimating equations (4.1) – (4.3) and define the partitioned matrices

$$A(\boldsymbol{\theta}, \boldsymbol{g}^*, \alpha) = -E\begin{pmatrix} \frac{\partial u_1}{\partial \theta} & \frac{\partial u_1}{\partial g^*} & \frac{\partial u_1}{\partial \alpha} \\ \frac{\partial u_2}{\partial \theta} & \frac{\partial u_2}{\partial g^*} & \frac{\partial u_2}{\partial \alpha} \\ \frac{\partial u_3}{\partial \theta} & \frac{\partial u_3}{\partial g^*} & \frac{\partial u_3}{\partial \alpha} \end{pmatrix} = \begin{pmatrix} A_{11} & A_{12} & A_{13} \\ A_{21} & A_{22} & A_{23} \\ A_{31} & A_{32} & A_{33} \end{pmatrix}$$

and

$$B(\boldsymbol{\theta}, \boldsymbol{g}^*, \alpha) = \operatorname{cov}\{(\boldsymbol{u}_1', \boldsymbol{u}_2', u_3)'\} = \begin{pmatrix} B_{11} & B_{12} & B_{13} \\ B_{21} & B_{22} & B_{23} \\ B_{31} & B_{32} & B_{33} \end{pmatrix}.$$

Without real loss of generality we write $\boldsymbol{\theta} = (\theta_1, \boldsymbol{\theta}_2')$, where θ_1 is scalar, and assume that $\lambda(t;\boldsymbol{\theta}) = \theta_1 \lambda_1(t;\boldsymbol{\theta}_2)$. Then large sample theory for estimating equations (e.g. Inagaki 1973, White 1982) show the consistency as $\theta_1 \to \infty$ of $(\widehat{\boldsymbol{\theta}}_2, \hat{\boldsymbol{g}}^*, \hat{\alpha})$, that $\hat{\theta}_1/\theta_1$ converges in probability to one, and that the asymptotic covariance matrix for $(\widehat{\boldsymbol{\theta}}, \hat{\boldsymbol{g}}^*, \hat{\alpha})$ is $A^{-1}B(A^{-1})'$. A little algebra shows that

$$\begin{aligned} A_{11} &= \sum_{i=1}^{T} \frac{1}{V_i} \left[\frac{\partial \mu_i(T)}{\partial \boldsymbol{\theta}}\right] \left[\frac{\partial \mu_i(T)}{\partial \boldsymbol{\theta}'}\right] \\ A_{12} &= \sum_{i=1}^{T} \frac{1}{V_i} \left[\frac{\partial \mu_i(T)}{\partial \boldsymbol{\theta}}\right] \left[\frac{\partial \mu_i(T)}{\partial \boldsymbol{g}^{*\prime}}\right] \\ A_{22} &= \operatorname{diag}\left\{\frac{E(N_{.r})}{g^*(r)\,[1-g^*(r)]}\right\} \\ A_{21} &= A_{13} = A_{23} = 0. \end{aligned}$$

It then follows that A^{-1} has the form

$$A^{-1} = \begin{pmatrix} A_{11}^{-1} & D_{12} & 0 \\ 0 & A_{22}^{-1} & 0 \\ D_{31} & D_{32} & A_{33}^{-1} \end{pmatrix} \tag{A1}$$

where $D_{12} = -A_{11}^{-1}A_{12}A_{22}^{-1}$. In addition, we find that

$$\begin{aligned} B_{11} &= \operatorname{cov}(\boldsymbol{u}_1) = A_{11} \\ B_{22} &= \operatorname{cov}(\boldsymbol{u}_2) = A_{22} \\ B_{12} &= B_{21} = 0. \end{aligned} \tag{A2}$$

(To find that $B_{12} = B_{21} = 0$ we note that, conditional on the $N_i(t)$'s, $E(\boldsymbol{u}_2) = \mathbf{0}$, and that $\boldsymbol{u}_1$ depends on the data only through the $N_i(T)$'s.)

The asymptotic covariance matrix of $(\widehat{\boldsymbol{\theta}}, \hat{\boldsymbol{g}}^*)$ is obtained by dropping the last row and column of $A^{-1}B(A^{-1})'$. Utilizing (A1) and (A2), we find by straightforward matrix multiplication that

$$\begin{aligned} \operatorname{asvar}(\widehat{\boldsymbol{\theta}}) &= A_{11}^{-1} + D_{12}A_{22}D_{12}' \\ \operatorname{asvar}(\hat{\boldsymbol{g}}^*) &= A_{22}^{-1} \\ \operatorname{asvar}(\widehat{\boldsymbol{\theta}}, \hat{\boldsymbol{g}}^*) &= D_{12} = -A_{11}^{-1}A_{12}A_{22}^{-1}. \end{aligned} \tag{A3}$$

When $N_{.r}$ is inserted for $E(N_{.r})$ and $\widehat{\boldsymbol{\theta}}$, $\hat{\boldsymbol{g}}^*$, $\hat{\alpha}$ are inserted for the parameters in (A3), the expression (4.5) results.

We note in addition that the estimates just given depend on the validity of both the mean function $\mu_i(T)$ and variance function $V[\mu_i(T;\boldsymbol{\theta}), \alpha]$ for $N_i(T)$. A covariance matrix estimate that is robust to misspecification of the variance function (but not necessarily to non-independence of the $N_i(T)$'s) is produced by the common device (cf. Liang and Zeger 1986) of estimating B_{11} not by A_{11} but by

$$\hat{B}_{11} = \sum_{i=1}^{T} \frac{\{N_i(T) - \hat{\mu}_i(T)\}^2}{\hat{V}_i} \left[\frac{\partial \widehat{\mu_i(T)}}{\partial \boldsymbol{\theta}}\right] \left[\frac{\partial \widehat{\mu_i(T)}}{\partial \boldsymbol{\theta}'}\right] \tag{A4}$$

and $\operatorname{asvar}(\widehat{\boldsymbol{\theta}})$ by

$$\hat{A}_{11}^{-1}\hat{B}_{11}\left(\hat{A}_{11}^{-1}\right)' + \hat{D}_{12}\hat{A}_{22}\hat{D}_{12}'. \tag{A5}$$

This can in particular be used for protection against overdispersion when estimating equations for $\boldsymbol{\theta}$ are based on the Poisson model, i.e. when $V_i = \mu_i(T)$.

Acknowledgments

This research was supported by a grant from the National Institute on Drug Abuse (Grant No. 1-R01-DA 04722, coordinated by the Societal Institute of the Mathematical Sciences).

Bibliography

Bacchetti, P., Segal, M. and Jewell, N.P. (1991). Uncertainty about the incubation period of AIDS and its impact on back calculation. In *AIDS Epidemiology: Methodological Issues*, N.P. Jewell, K. Dietz, and V. Farewell (eds); Boston: Birkhäuser - Boston.

Becker, N.G., Watson, L.F. and Carlin, J.B. (1991). A method of nonparametric back-projection and its application to AIDS data. *Statistics in Medicine* **10**, 1527-1542.

Becker, N. and Watson, L. (1992). Use of empirical transformations in nonparametric back-projection of AIDS incidence data. In *AIDS Epidemiology: Methodological Issues*, N.P. Jewell, K. Dietz, and V. Farewell (eds); Boston: Birkhäuser Boston.

Brookmeyer, R. (1991). Reconstruction and future trends of the AIDS epidemic in the United States. *Science* **253**, 37-42.

Brookmeyer, R. and Damiano, A. (1989). Statistical methods for short-term projections of AIDS incidence. *Statistics in Medicine* **8**, 23-34.

Brookmeyer, R. and Gail, M.H. (1988). A method for obtaining short-term projections and lower bounds on the size of the AIDS epidemic. *Journal of the American Statistical Association* **83**, 301-308.

Brookmeyer, R. and Goedert, J.J. (1989). Censoring in an epidemic with an application to hemophilia-associated AIDS. *Biometrics* **45**, 325-335.

Brookmeyer, R. and Liao, J. (1990a) Statistical modelling of the AIDS epidemic for forecasting health care needs. *Biometrics* **46**, 1151-1163.

Brookmeyer, R. and Liao, J. (1990b). The analysis of delays in disease reporting: methods and results for the acquired immunodeficiency syndrome. *American Journal of Epidemiology* **132**, 355-365.

Brookmeyer, R. and Liao, J. (1992). Statistical methods for reconstructing infection curves. In *AIDS Epidemiology: Methodological Issues*, N.P. Jewell, K. Dietz, and V. Farewell (eds); Boston: Birkhäuser - Boston.

Centers for Disease Control (1990). HIV Prevalence Estimates and AIDS Case Projections for the United States: Report Based upon a Workshop. *Morbidity and Mortality Weekly Report*, No. RR-16, November 30, 1990.

Day, N.E., Gore, S.N., McGee, M.A. and South, M. (1989). Predictions of AIDS epidemic in the UK: The use of the back-projection method. *Philosophical Transactions of the Royal Society of London, Series B* **325**, 123-134.

Gail, M.H. and Rosenberg, P. (1992). Perspectives on using backcalculation to estimate HIV prevalence and project AIDS incidence. In *AIDS Epidemiology: Methodological Issues*, N.P. Jewell, K. Dietz, and V. Farewell (eds); Boston: Birkhäuser - Boston.

Harris, J.E. (1990). Reporting delays and the incidence of AIDS. *Journal of the American Statistical Association* **85**, 915-924.

Inagaki, N. (1973). Asymptotic relations between the likelihood estimating function and the maximum likelihood estimator. *Annals of the Institute of Statistical Mathematics* **265**, 1-26.

Jewell, N.P. (1990). Some statistical issues in the epidemiology of AIDS. *Statistics in Medicine* **9**, 1387-1416.

Kalbfleisch, J.D. and Lawless, J.F. (1989). Inference based on retrospective ascertainment: an analysis of the data on transfusion-associated AIDS. *Journal of the American Statistical Association* **84**, 360-372.

Kalbfleisch, J.D. and Lawless, J.F. (1991). Regression models for right truncated data, with applications to AIDS incubation times and reporting lags. *Statistica Sinica* **1**, 19-32.

Karon, J.M., Dondero, T.J. and Curran, J.W. (1988). The projected incidence of AIDS and estimated prevalence of HIV infection in the United States. *Journal of Acquired Immune Deficiency Syndromes* **1**, 542-550.

Lawless, J.F. (1987). Negative binomial and mixed Poisson regression. *Canadian Journal of Statistics* **15**, 209-225.

Lawless, J.F. (1991). Adjustments for reporting delays and the prediction of occurred but not yet reported events. Unpublished manuscript.

McCullagh, P. and Nelder, J.A. (1989). *Generalized Linear Models.* London: Chapman and Hall.

Pagano, M., DeGruttola, V., MaWhinney, S. and Tu, X.M. (1992). The HIV epidemic in New York City; projecting AIDS incidence and prevalence. In *AIDS Epidemiology: Methodological Issues*, N.P. Jewell, K. Dietz, and V. Farewell (eds); Boston: Birkhäuser - Boston.

Rosenberg, P. and Gail, M.H. (1991). Back-calculation of flexible linear models of the HIV infection curve. *Applied Statistics* **40**, 269-282.

Solomon, P.J. and Wilson, S.R. (1990). Accommodating change due to treatment in the method of back projection for estimating HIV infection incidence. *Biometrics* **46**, 1165-1170.

Taylor, J.M.G. (1989). Models for the HIV infection and AIDS epidemic in the United States. *Statistics in Medicine* **8**, 45-58.

White, H. (1982). Maximum likelihood estimation of misspecified models. *Econometrics* **50**, 1-25.

Department of Statistics and Actuarial Science
University of Waterloo
Waterloo, Ontario
Canada N2L 3G1

Use of Empirical Transformations in Nonparametric Back-projection of AIDS Incidence Data

Niels G. Becker and Lyndsey F. Watson

Abstract: Among methods used for estimating the HIV-infection incidence curve, smoothed nonparametric back-projection has a number of attractive features. Here an empirical transformation is incorporated into the method for the purpose of reducing bias and its effectiveness for reducing bias is studied.

1. Introduction

The discussion is in discrete time, using a month as the unit of time. Let Y_i denote the number of individuals diagnosed with AIDS in month i and N_i the number infected with HIV in month i. We can express $\mu_t = \mathrm{E}(Y_t)$ in terms of $\lambda_i = \mathrm{E}(N_i) \quad (i = 1, \ldots, t)$ by the convolution equation

$$\mu_t = \sum_{i=1}^{t} \lambda_i f_{t-i}, \tag{1.1}$$

where f_i is the probability that the incubation period has length i months. Equation (1.1) is the basis of the method of back-projection, which consists of using observations on the $Y_i \quad (i = 1, \ldots, T)$ and an assumed form for the $f_i \quad (i = 0, \ldots, T-1)$ to estimate the $\lambda_i \quad (i = 1, \ldots, T)$. That is, back-projection gives an estimate of the mean HIV infection incidence over time. The f_i are estimated in practice, and sensitivity analyses must be performed to allow for uncertainties in current knowledge of the incubation distribution.

There are various forms of the method of back-projection. In the parametric approach all the λ_i are expressed in terms of a parameter θ of low dimension and then θ is estimated; see Brookmeyer & Gail (1988) and Taylor (1989). The 'nonparametric' approach allows each λ_i to be a separate parameter. Estimates of the λ_i in the nonparametric setting are unstable in a sense illustrated below, and this difficulty may be overcome by smoothing the estimates in some way.

For estimation of the λ_i we make model assumptions and think in terms of maximising the likelihood function. We assume the N_i to be independent

Poisson variates and take the lengths of incubation periods for infected individuals to be independent random variables. Then the likelihood function corresponding to monthly AIDS counts $y_1, \ldots, y_T$ is given by

$$\prod_{t=1}^{T} \left(\sum_{i=1}^{t} \lambda_i f_{t-i} \right)^{y_t} \exp \left(- \sum_{i=1}^{t} \lambda_i f_{t-i} \right) . \tag{1.2}$$

When studying properties of estimators it is useful to know the true parameter values. For this reason we work with simulated data, in the first instance. The choice of model used for simulation is motivated by properties of the HIV epidemic. The Weibull distribution with survivor function

$$S(x) = \exp(-0.0022x^{2.55}) \qquad x > 0 , \tag{1.3}$$

is chosen for the incubation distribution f. This distribution is chosen because it has the simple Weibull form and is very close to both the distribution estimated by the two-stage approach of Brookmeyer & Liao (1990) and the empirical estimates of Bacchetti & Moss (1990), over the period of time for which data are available. The distribution (1.3) is also close to the Weibull distribution with survivor function $S(x) = \exp(-0.0021x^{2.516})$ estimated by Brookmeyer & Goedert (1989). We take $T = 150$, which is approximately the number of months for which AIDS incidence data are available. In our simulations we assume a number of different forms for the HIV infection intensities λ_i.

We begin by taking $\lambda_i = 100 \quad (i = 1, \ldots, 150)$ for an illustration of the unstable nature of nonparametric maximum likelihood estimates $\hat{\lambda}_i$. Substituting $\lambda_i = 100$ and incubation distribution (1.3) into (1.1) gives $\mu_t = 100\{1 - \exp(-0.0022t^{2.55})\}$. A realisation of AIDS counts $y_1, \ldots, y_{150}$ was simulated, assuming $Y_1, \ldots, Y_{150}$ to be independent Poisson variates with $\mathrm{E}(Y_t) = \mu_t$. The graph of the maximum likelihood estimates $\hat{\lambda}_i$ corresponding to this realisation is shown in Figure 1a. When looking at any graph of estimated HIV infection intensities one must make allowance for the fact the estimates at the right hand end, corresponding to the recent past, are very imprecise. This point and a suggestion for dealing with this imprecision are discussed in Section 4. Even after allowing for the imprecision at the right hand end of the graph we observe that the maximum likelihood estimates, obtained via the EM-algorithm, are unstable in the sense that $\lambda_1, \ldots, \lambda_T$ tend to fluctuate greatly even though the true parameter values are all equal. Estimates from another realisation would show a similar behaviour, with spikes occurring at different locations. It is this property which prompts us to say the estimates are unstable. It is clear that nonparametric maximum likelihood estimation from any given realisation is likely to produce unsatisfactory estimates.

It is interesting to observe that biases, if any, of nonparametric maximum likelihood estimates $\hat{\lambda}_i$ are small. An average of such estimates taken over a number of realisations is quite satisfactory. This is seen from Figure 2a, where the pointwise means of maximum likelihood estimates from 100 realisations are shown together with the corresponding 5, 50 and 95 percentiles. In practice one has just one realisation of AIDS incidence data and it is clear that the unstable nature of the nonparametric maximum likelihood estimates must be overcome by some form of smoothing.

Restricting attention to a parametric family of models is one way of smoothing. This approach is dependent on choosing a suitable family of models, which is not easy because the λ_i are determined largely by behaviour in the community which has changed over time in an unknown way. Smoothing can be imposed on estimates for nonparametric models by maximising a penalised likelihood function (Bacchetti & Jewell, 1991), by use of splines (Rosenberg & Gail, 1991) or by using the EMS algorithm (Becker *et al.*, 1991). Our discussion is given in terms of the EMS-algorithm, but also has relevance to smoothing by other nonparametric methods.

2. Smoothing by the EMS-algorithm

The EM-algorithm, see Dempster *et al.* (1977), is a way of computing maximum likelihood estimates which is particularly useful in situations where one can think of a more complete data set for which maximum likelihood estimation is relatively straightforward. The EMS-algorithm, see Silverman *et al.* (1990), is the EM-algorithm with a smoothing step added. Details of the EMS approach to back-projection of AIDS incidence data are given by Becker *et al.* (1991), and its extension to accommodate age as a covariate is described by Becker & Marschner (1991). We briefly outline the E, M and S steps in the current context.

Consider first the use of the EM-algorithm for the purpose of maximising the likelihood (1.2) with respect to $\lambda_1, \ldots, \lambda_T$. Imagine the more fortunate situation in which we are able to determine when each of the observed AIDS cases was infected. Corresponding to this more complete data set we have the likelihood function

$$\prod_{t=1}^{T}\prod_{i=1}^{t}\{(\lambda_i f_{t-i})^{y_{it}} \exp(-\lambda_i f_{t-i})\} \quad \propto \quad \prod_{i=1}^{T}\lambda_i^{y_{i\bullet}} \exp(-\lambda_i F_{T-i}),$$

where y_{it} denotes the number of individuals infected in month i and diagnosed in month t, $y_{i\bullet} = \sum_{t=i}^{T} y_{it}$ and $F_t = \sum_{i=0}^{t} f_i$. Maximum likelihood estimation for the more complete data is very straightforward, which suggests use of the EM-algorithm for maximising the likelihood (1.2). Following the recipe given by Dempster *et al.* (1977) we find the E and M steps to be

$$\textbf{E}-\textbf{step}: \quad \text{Compute the} \quad \hat{y}_{it} = y_t \frac{\lambda_i^{\text{old}} f_{t-i}}{\sum_{j=1}^{t} \lambda_j^{\text{old}} f_{t-j}}$$

$$\textbf{M}-\textbf{step}: \quad \text{Compute the} \quad \phi_i = \hat{y}_{i\bullet} / F_{T-i} \, .$$

The ϕ_i give the updated values of the estimates after an iteration of the E and M steps. For the EMS-algorithm we obtain updated values of the estimates only after the additional

$$\textbf{S}-\textbf{step}: \quad \text{Compute the} \quad \lambda_i^{\text{new}} = \sum_{j=0}^{k} w_j \phi_{i+j-k/2} \, .$$

The last step smoothes the updated estimates by a moving weighted average. The weights w_j must sum to 1 and would normally be symmetric over the values $0, 1, \ldots, k$. The binomial weights

$$w_i = \binom{k}{i} \Big/ 2^k \qquad i = 0, 1, \ldots, k \, .$$

are a convenient choice.

Figure 1b shows the estimate of the λ_i curve obtained by applying the EMS-algorithm to the same realisation of AIDS counts which led to the maximum likelihood estimate shown in Figure 1a. The binomial weights with $k = 4$ were used in the smoothing step. From a comparison of both Figure 1a with Figure 1b and Figure 2a with Figure 2b, it is evident that estimation from a single realisation of AIDS incidence data is much improved when smoothed nonparametric estimation is used.

3. Bias in Smoothed Nonparametric Estimation

To assess the extent of bias that might arise in EMS back-projection of AIDS incidence data we base a small simulation study on a plausible HIV infection incidence curve. We adopt the curve λ_i^* $(i = 1, \ldots, 144)$, shown by the solid curve in Figure 3a as the true HIV incidence rate. This curve is in fact the estimate of the HIV infection incidence curve obtained by EMS back-projection of the Victorian AIDS incidence data up to December 1990 as reported to the Health Department, Victoria by the end of May 1991.

The incubation distribution (1.3) and the binomial smoothing kernel with $k = 4$ were used in the EMS-algorithm to arrive at λ_i^* $(i = 1, \ldots, 144)$. Now consider simulations in which the curve λ_i^* $(i = 1, \ldots, 144)$ is used as the true mean HIV incidence curve. To generate the simulated realisations we first use λ_i^* and incubation distribution (1.3) in (1.1) to find the corresponding curve of (estimated) mean AIDS counts μ_i^* $(i = 1, \ldots, 144)$. The EMS-algorithm is then used on each of 100 realisations of AIDS counts $y_1, \ldots, y_{144}$, where each realisation is simulated from the Poisson model with means μ_i^* $(i = 1, \ldots, 144)$. The pointwise means of these 100 estimated λ_i curves is shown by the dotted curve in Figure 3a. Also shown in Figure 3a are the pointwise 5, 50 and 95 percentiles corresponding to the 100 estimated curves. We observe that the EMS estimate displays bias which is most pronounced over time periods where the solid curve of Figure 3a displays the greatest curvature. Similar bias is observed in the context of kernel-smoothed density estimation; see Silverman (1986, p. 39).

It seems useful to outline the link between kernel-smoothed density estimation and the EMS approach to smoothed back-projection. Ramlau-Hansen (1983) shows that kernel-smoothed nonparametric estimation can be applied to the estimation of intensities for counting processes. Becker & Yip (1989) illustrate this by obtaining a kernel-smoothed estimate of an infection intensity curve. Use of the weighted average in the EMS approach can be viewed as a discrete version of such kernel smoothing. Kernel-smoothed density estimation has been studied extensively and methods for reducing bias have been proposed; see Silverman (1986, §3.6). The link between kernel-smoothed density estimation and the EMS approach to smoothed back-projection can be used to suggest a way for reducing bias in the latter estimation. Recent work by Wand *et al.* (1991) and Ruppert & Cline (1991) indicates that kernel-smoothing applied to suitably transformed data has some advantages as a method for bias-reduction in density estimation. Ruppert & Cline (1991) propose an approach based on certain empirical transformations in the context of density estimation. Here we adapt their approach to EMS back-projection.

We first try to motivate the proposed approach by an intuitive argument. Observe that smoothing is achieved in the EMS approach by a moving weighted average applied to a sequence of estimates. Suppose we pass a moving average over values λ_i $\;i \in \{\ldots, -1, 0, 1, \ldots\}$. The moving average simply recaptures the original sequence λ_i when all λ_i are equal. In the present context this will also happen when the λ_i lie on a straight line, because we are using symmetric weights. However, it does not happen when the λ_i curve shows nonlinear trends or fluctuations. Instead, the sequence produced by the moving average will tend to fluctuate less than the original sequence. Curvature in the original sequence tends to flatten out by such smoothing. This observation suggests that EMS smoothing has least bias in situations where the true HIV infection intensity has no curvature. We now use a small simulation study to lend empirical support to this suggestion.

EMS back-projection was applied to each of 100 realisations of AIDS counts simulated from the model with $\lambda_i = 100 \quad (i = 1, \ldots, 150)$ and incubation distribution (1.3). The solid curve in Figure 2b shows the graph of the pointwise means of 100 estimated HIV incidence curves. After making due allowance for the imprecision of estimates at the right hand end of the graph, we indeed find little evidence of bias in the estimation of the constant infection intensity.

4. The Wagging Tail

One expects the precision of estimates of the λ_i to decline dramatically as i gets close to T. This is because our only data are AIDS counts and information about recent infection intensities comes only from recent AIDS counts. There will be very few recently infected individuals among recent AIDS cases because the incubation period tends to be long and, furthermore, any recently infected individuals among recent AIDS cases will be indistinguishable from cases infected earlier. This imprecision of estimates of the λ_i for i close to T is reflected in the width of confidence intervals shown in Figures 2a, 2b and 3a.

Inspection of curves of infection intensities estimated from different simulations of AIDS counts reveals that the right hand tail wags dramatically from realisation to realisation, and that the nature of the tail is greatly influenced by the relative sizes of the 2 or 3 most recent AIDS incidences; see Watson (1990). It is clearly unwise to attach much meaning to estimates of λ_i near T. This imprecision is not a fault in the method of estimation. The AIDS incidence data alone simply contain little information about recent infection rates and no amount of statistical ingenuity will overcome this difficulty.

For important tasks such as estimating the total number infected with HIV and predicting AIDS incidence we recommend that the right hand tail of the HIV infection intensity curve be controlled by fixing its value over the last 2 years, say, at a value thought to be sensible. This value should, if possible, be chosen on the basis of additional data such as test results on blood samples of military recruits; see Centers for Disease Control (1990).

It is useful to combine this suggestion with the use of different levels of smoothing over different periods of time. By increasing the level of smoothing over time one can hope to compensate for the decline in precision of the estimates over time. It is important not to increase the level of smoothing too much, because while more smoothing reduces variation it also increases bias when curvature is present. Figure 3b illustrates the result of an application of EMS back-projection in which the level of smoothing increases over time and the estimate is smoothly blended into a level of infection that is assumed to be 5 infections per month for the last 2 years. The pointwise means, 5 and 95 percentiles shown in Figure 3b were obtained from the same 100 realisations generated for the graphs of Figure 3a. In practice the constant level of infection assumed over the last 2 years might be set at each of a pessimistic, intermediary and optimistic level. This seems a sensible way to produce estimates of the number infected with HIV and making predictions of AIDS incidence.

Below we control the wagging tail of estimates of the HIV infection intensity by specifying a constant value for this intensity over the last 24 months of calendar time. Observe, from Figure 3b, that controlling the right hand tail and increasing the level of smoothing with time do not avoid the bias arising from smoothing. We now consider the reduction of bias.

5. Time Transformations and Bias-reduction

Let us think for the moment in terms of a model formulation in continuous time, as this simplifies a discussion of time transformations. The convolution equation (1.1) becomes

$$\mu(t) = \int_0^t \lambda(x) f(t-x)dx \ ,$$

where the minor change in notation is used as a reminder that we are now working in continuous time.

To take advantage of the observation that bias in EMS back-projection is expected to be least when the infection intensities lie on a straight line, we need a time transformation which makes the infection intensities constant on the new time scale. A nonhomogeneous Poisson process with intensity $\lambda(t)$ is changed into a homogeneous Poisson process with constant rate α, say, by the time transformation

$$u = \alpha^{-1}\Lambda(t) = \alpha^{-1}\int_0^t \lambda(x)dx \ , \tag{5.1}$$

where any convenient value may be chosen for α. An individual infected at calendar time t is now considered to be infected at time $u = \alpha^{-1}\Lambda(t)$ on the new time scale. Our data consist of the calendar times of AIDS diagnoses for cases diagnosed by time T. The times of diagnosis on the new time scale lie in $(0, U)$, where $U = \alpha^{-1}\Lambda(T)$. The suggestion is that EMS back-projection applied to the data on the u-scale will, when transformed back to calendar time, result in less bias than EMS back-projection applied directly to data on the t-scale.

The time transformation (5.1) cannot be used in practice because it depends on the unknown intensity function λ, which we are trying to estimate. In real world applications we need to replace Λ by some known function, as discussed below. In simulation studies, on the other hand, it is possible to make direct use of time transformation (5.1), because the infection intensity λ is specified when simulating data, so that Λ is known. Such simulation studies are useful for assessing the potential that time transformations have for reducing bias in nonparametric back-projection.

Consider the time transformation $u = \alpha^{-1}G(t)$, where G is a known increasing function. We now describe the proposed use of such a transformation in more detail. Let $t_1, \ldots, t_n$ denote the calendar times of diagnosis, on a monthly scale but measured to the nearest day, of the n AIDS cases diagnosed by the end of month T. The procedure proposed by Becker *et al.* (1991) consists of grouping the $t_1, \ldots, t_n$, into T successive months and applying the EMS back-projection to the resulting monthly AIDS counts. Let $\hat{\Lambda}_0$ be an estimate of Λ produced by this procedure. The procedure proposed here consists of first computing the $u_i = \alpha^{-1}G(t_i)$, then grouping the u_i by partitioning $(0, U)$ into k intervals of equal length and applying EMS back-projection to the resulting k AIDS counts. In doing so one must work with the incubation distribution on the u-scale. This back-projection gives estimated infection incidences $\hat{\gamma}_1, \ldots, \hat{\gamma}_k$ for the k components intervals of $(0, U)$. To transform these to calendar time infection incidences we first construct an estimate of the continuous cumulative infection intensity function $\Gamma(u)$, by setting $\hat{\Gamma}(i) = \sum_{j=1}^{i} \hat{\gamma}_j$ and using linear interpolation. The corresponding estimated cumulative infection intensity on the calendar time scale is then given by $\hat{\Lambda}(t) = \hat{\Gamma}(G^{-1}(\alpha u)) \quad 0 \le t \le T$. Finally we obtain the estimated monthly infection incidences by computing $\hat{\lambda}_i = \hat{\Lambda}(i) - \hat{\Lambda}(i-1) \quad i = 1, \ldots, T$.

The ideal choice for G is Λ, but this is unknown in real world applications. It is proposed that we use a preliminary estimate of Λ, such as $\hat{\Lambda}_0$ for G, with the expectation that EMS back-projection applied to data on the resulting transformed time scale will produce improved estimates of the λ_i. Having used the empirical time transformation $u = \alpha^{-1}\hat{\Lambda}_0(t)$ to obtain an improved estimate of the mean infection incidence, and therefore an improved estimate $\hat{\Lambda}_1$ of Λ, one can aim at further improvement by repeating the procedure with the new empirical transformation $u = \alpha^{-1}\hat{\Lambda}_1(t)$. Several iterations of this procedure may be used.

6. Applications

To illustrate that the proposed procedure can be useful we apply it to data simulated with the infection intensity λ shown by the solid curve of Figure 4a. This curve was deliberately constructed to be bimodal by taking a mixture of two Normal distributions (with means 4, 7 and standard deviations 1, 1.5, respectively) and keeping the infection intensity constant at 45 over the most recent 3.7 years. An infection intensity with this shape might arise when AIDS cases arise by aggregation of cases from two epidemics which are out of phase.

AIDS counts in calendar time were simulated from the Poisson model with the bimodal infection intensity shown in Figure 4a. The dashed line in Figure 4a gives the estimated curve obtained by EMS back-projection applied directly to these AIDS incidence data. Although moderate smoothing was used for this estimation, it nevertheless caused the two humps to be smoothed out. Note that we controlled the right hand tail of the estimated infection intensity curve by setting the infection incidence at 45 for the last 24 months. For comparison we applied EMS back-projection to AIDS counts for intervals of equal length in the time scale given by $u = 0.01\Lambda(t)$. In the new time scale we controlled the right hand tail of the estimated infection intensity curve by setting the infection incidence at 100 for the last 12 intervals. Transforming back to calendar time produces the estimated infection intensity shown by the dotted curve of Figure 4a. This is seen to give an exceptionally good estimate of the infection intensity, thereby suggesting that time transformations have much potential for improving estimates of the infection intensity.

In practice one does not know Λ and an empirical time transformation is used instead. We use the estimate obtained by EMS back-projection applied to AIDS counts in calendar time, the dashed curve of Figure 4a, to make an empirical time transformation. The time scale arrived at in this way is expected to have an infection intensity which is more nearly constant. Applying EMS back-projection to AIDS counts for 150 intervals of equal length in the new time scale and transforming back to calendar time produces the estimated infection intensity shown by the dotted curve of Figure 4b. This is seen to produce an improvement over the original estimate shown by the dashed curve. In particular, the bias observed in the period prior to time 82 has been reduced. The dotted curve also gives a reasonable estimate of the first hump in the true infection intensity. There is an indication of the presence of the second hump, but this hump is not estimated with precision. Indeed, the performance of the estimate is not good for the recent past.

We have experimented with various assumed values for the infection intensity over the recent past. The EMS approach with empirical time transformation is able to estimate the second hump reasonably accurately when we set the infection intensity at its correct constant value over the most recent 3.7 years. The ability to estimate the second hump deteriorates as we relax this assumption. This is illustrated in Figure 4b, where the correct constant value is assumed over the most recent two years only. The performance of the estimate for recent times tends to deteriorate further when the incorrect constant value is assumed for the infection intensity over the recent past.

Also shown in Figure 4b is the second iterative obtained by repeating the procedure with the time transformation based on the dotted curve. This produces the estimate shown by the dot-dashed curve, which does not differ greatly from the dotted curve, particularly over the more distant past. There is an even clearer indication of the second hump, but a third hump in the more recent past is also (falsely) suggested.

Empirical time transformation is now used on the AIDS incidence data for Victoria, with the aim of reducing bias over time periods where there is curvature in the graph of the infection intensity. In other words, we seek reassurance that the EMS estimate of the infection intensity shown by the solid curve of Figure 3b, has not smoothed out any meaningful bumps in the infection intensity curve. The solid curve in Figure 5 again gives the estimate of the infection intensity as obtained by the EMS approach applied to data in calendar time. This curve is used to make a time transformation and the EMS-algorithm is applied to the AIDS counts on the new time scale, producing the dashed curve in Figure 5.

The estimate given by the solid curve is essentially a smoother version of the dashed curve, and seems to be a reasonable estimate. However, the dashed curve gives a suggestion of where, if at all, the infection intensity might deviate from the solid curve estimate. The dashed curve displays finer detail on which we can focus with a view to gaining further insights. In particular, the dashed curve indicates a small hump in 1983, the source of which can be investigated. One can establish that the hump stems from the first two AIDS cases which preceded the next group of AIDS cases by almost one year. In this instance, therefore, the small hump is merely a consequence of isolated infections which invariably occur during the early stages of an epidemic. In another instance such a hump may have a meaningful interpretation in terms of the infection intensity acting on the community.

The estimate given by the dashed curve indicates a higher infection intensity at the modal time of the solid curve. This is to be expected, although the amount by which the peakedness increases is somewhat unexpected. A second iteration of the EMS approach with empirical time transformation further extends the peak just after 1984.

7. Discussion

It is convenient to use a global smoothing kernel, by which we mean a kernel that does not change over time. However, the lack of precision of estimates in the recent past, a consequence of back-projection, and curvature in the infection intensity are features that benefit from different amounts of smoothing at different time locations. The use of global smoothing kernels together with a time transformation is a convenient way of introducing appropriate levels of smoothing over time. In this way one can accommodate both the need for increased smoothing due to the lack of precision of estimates in the recent past and the need for increased smoothing at times of changing infection intensity. Here we have concentrated only on the bias reduction, apart from the illustration with varying levels of smoothing in Figure 3b.

We used the global smoothing kernel given by the binomial weights with $k = 4$ when applying EMS back-projection to the data in calendar time. When applying EMS back-projection to data in transformed time we used less smoothing, using weights that fall off geometrically. One is able to pick up humps more easily with just one application of EMS back-projection applied to data on the transformed time scale when a low level of smoothing is used at this stage.

The use of empirical time transformations with EMS back-projection has been found to reduce bias and thereby to provide insights into the shape of the infection intensity curve. One can probably gain similar insights by experimenting with the degree of smoothing used on data in calendar time, including no smoothing which amounts to using the EM-algorithm to obtain the nonparametric maximum likelihood estimates. This approach tends to be more time consuming, because the EM-algorithm is much slower to converge and varying the level of smoothing over different time locations involves quite a bit of trial and error. Also, the maximum likelihood estimates can be quite erratic and are very sensitive to assumptions about recent infection intensities, for example.

In short, EMS back-projection applied with global smoothing kernels on an empirically transformed time scale is a relatively efficient and objective tool for exploring the shape of the HIV infection intensity.

Acknowledgements:

The generosity of the AIDS/STD Unit of the Health Department, Victoria, in providing monthly data for the application of Section 6 is gratefully acknowledged.

This work is supported by a CARG project grant from the Department of Community Services and Health, Australia.

References

Bacchetti, P. and Jewell, N.P. (1991). Nonparametric estimation of the incubation period of AIDS based on a prevalent cohort with unknown infection times. *Biometrics*, **47**, 947-960.

Bacchetti, P. and Moss, A.R. (1989). Incubation period of AIDS in San Francisco. *Nature*, **338**, 251-253.

Becker, N.G. and Marschner, I.C. (1991). A method for estimating the age-specific relative risk of HIV infection from AIDS incidence data. *Submitted for publication.*

Becker, N.G., Watson, L.F. and Carlin, J.B. (1991). A method of non-parametric back-projection and its application to AIDS data. *Statistics in Medicine*, **10**, 1527-1542.

Becker, N.G. and Yip, P. (1989). Analysis of variations in an infection rate. *Australian Journal of Statistics*, **31**, 42-52.

Brookmeyer, R. and Gail, M.H. (1988). A method for obtaining short-term projections and lower bounds on the size of the AIDS epidemic. *Journal of the American Statistical Association*, **83**, 301-308.

Brookmeyer, R. and Goedert, J. (1989). Censoring in an epidemic with an application to hemophiliac-associated AIDS. *Biometrics*, **45**, 325-335.

Brookmeyer, R. and Liao, J. (1990) Statistical modelling of the AIDS epidemic for forecasting health care needs. *Biometrics*, **46**, 1151-1163.

Centers for Disease Control (1990). HIV prevalence estimates and AIDS case projections for the US: report based upon a workshop. *Morbidity and Mortality Weekly Report*, **39**, RR-16.

Dempster, A. P., Laird, N. M. and Rubin, D. B. (1977). Maximum likelihood from incomplete data via the EM algorithm (with discussion), *Journal of the Royal Statistical Society, B*, **39**, 1-38.

Ramlau-Hansen, H. (1983). Smoothing counting process intensities by means of kernel functions. *Annals of Statistics*, **11**, 453-466.

Rosenberg, P.S. and Gail, M.H. (1991). Backcalculation of flexible linear models of the HIV infection curve. *Applied Statist.*, **40**, 269-282.

Ruppert, D. and Cline, D.B.H. (1991). Transformation-kernel density estimation – bias reduction by empirical transformations. *Submitted for publication.*

Silverman, B.W. (1986). *Density Estimation for Statistics and data analysis.* London: Chapman and Hall.

Silverman, B.W., Jones, M.C., Wilson, J.D. and Nychka, D.W. (1990). A smoothed EM approach to indirect estimation problems, with particular reference to stereology and emission tomography. *Journal of the Royal Statistical Society, B*, **52**, 271-324.

Taylor, J.M. (1989). Models for the HIV infection and AIDS epidemic in the United States. *Statistics in Medicine*, **8**, 45-58.

Wand, M.P., Marron, J.S. and Ruppert, D. (1991). Transformations in density estimation (with discussion). *Journal of the American Statistical Association*, **86**, 341-361.

Watson, L.F. (1990). *Prediction of AIDS incidence using the method of back-projection.* MSc Thesis, La Trobe University.

Niels G. Becker and Lyndsey F. Watson

Department of Statistics,

La Trobe University,

Bundoora VIC 3083,

Australia

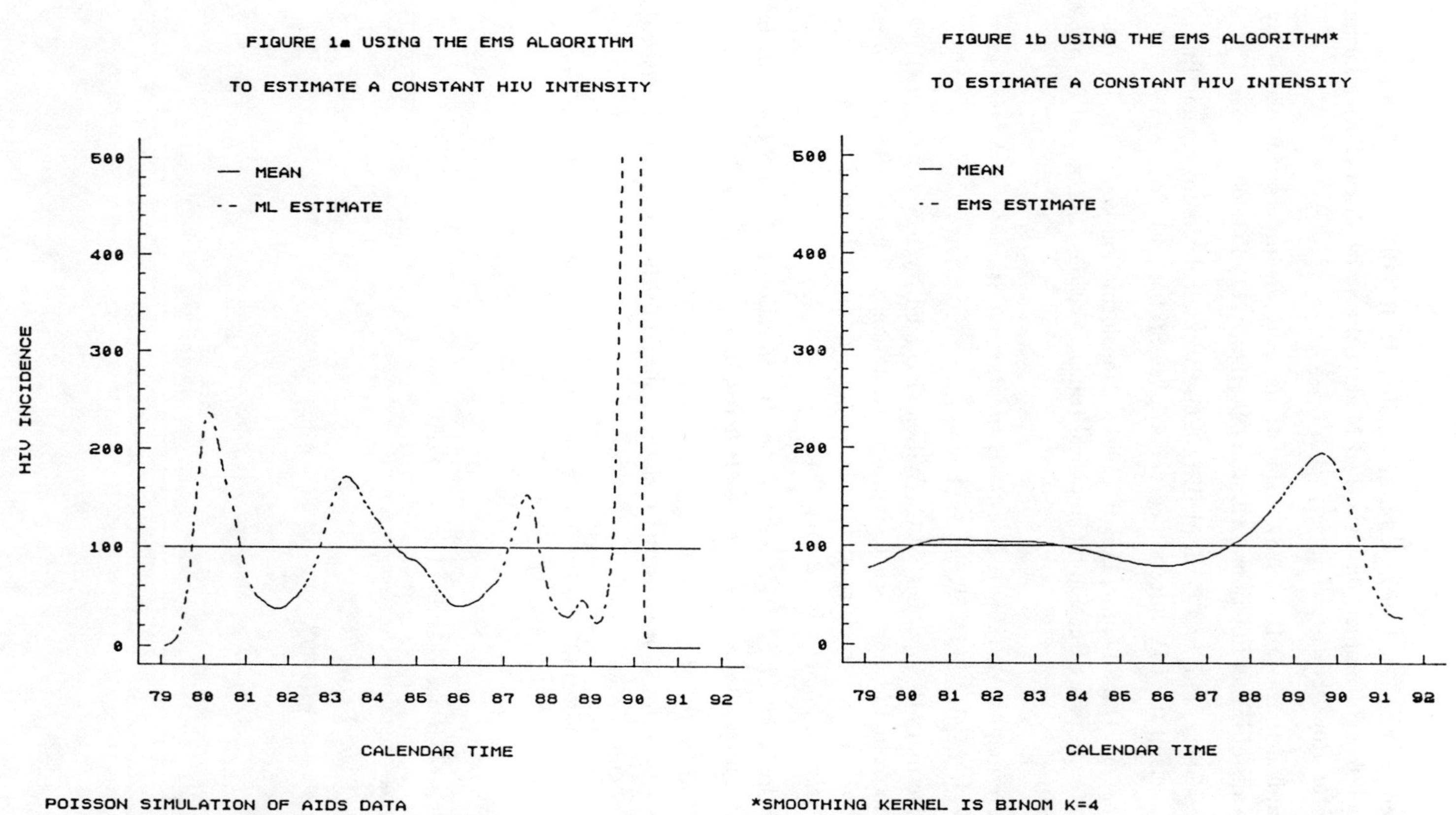
FIGURE 1a USING THE EMS ALGORITHM
TO ESTIMATE A CONSTANT HIV INTENSITY
— MEAN
-- ML ESTIMATE
HIV INCIDENCE
500
400
300
200
100
0
79 80 81 82 83 84 85 86 87 88 89 90 91 92
CALENDAR TIME
POISSON SIMULATION OF AIDS DATA
FIGURE 1b USING THE EMS ALGORITHM*
TO ESTIMATE A CONSTANT HIV INTENSITY
— MEAN
-- EMS ESTIMATE
500
400
300
200
100
0
79 80 81 82 83 84 85 86 87 88 89 90 91 92
CALENDAR TIME
*SMOOTHING KERNEL IS BINOM K=4

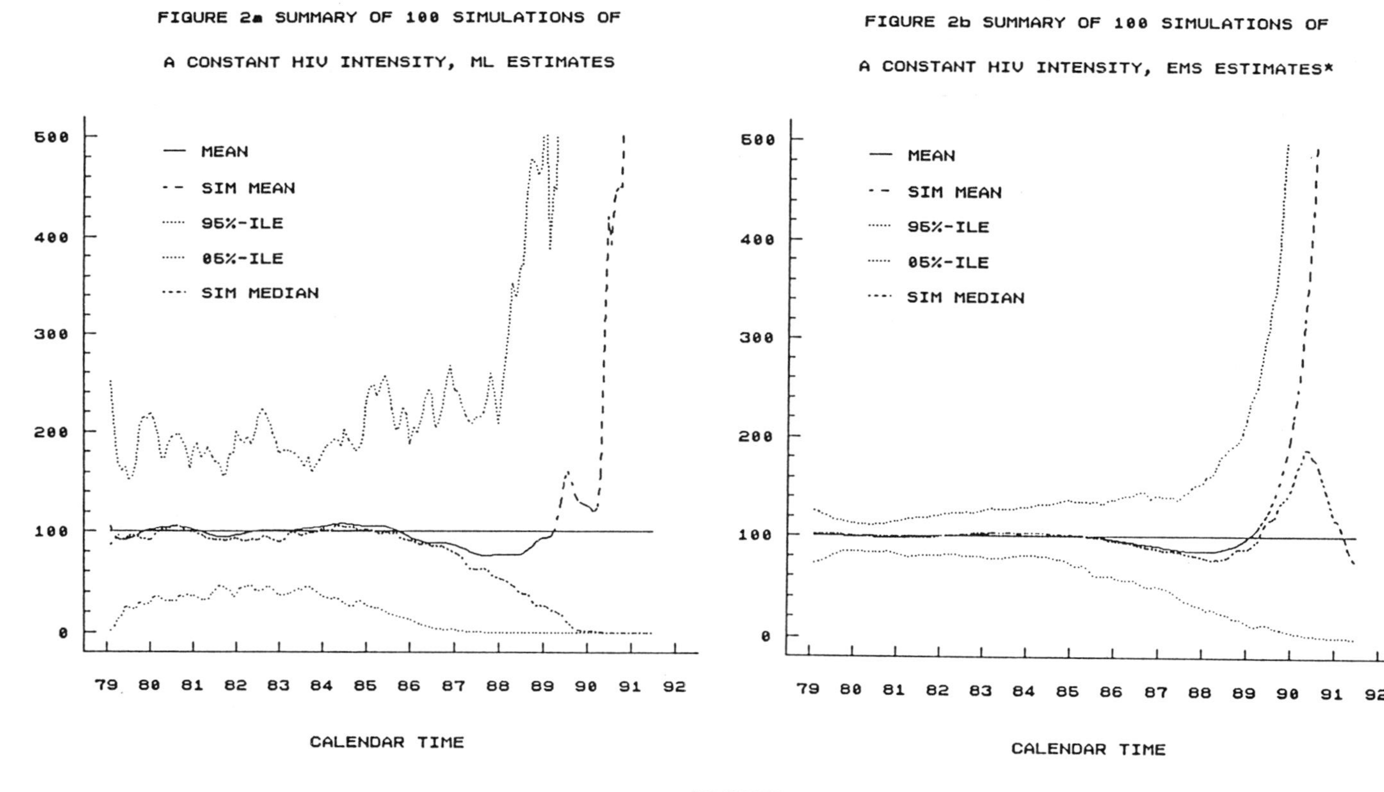
FIGURE 2a SUMMARY OF 100 SIMULATIONS OF
A CONSTANT HIV INTENSITY, ML ESTIMATES
MEAN
SIM MEAN
95%-ILE
05%-ILE
SIM MEDIAN
HIV INCIDENCE
500
400
300
200
100
0
79 80 81 82 83 84 85 86 87 88 89 90 91 92
CALENDAR TIME
FIGURE 2b SUMMARY OF 100 SIMULATIONS OF
A CONSTANT HIV INTENSITY, EMS ESTIMATES*
MEAN
SIM MEAN
95%-ILE
05%-ILE
SIM MEDIAN
500
400
300
200
100
0
79 80 81 82 83 84 85 86 87 88 89 90 91 92
CALENDAR TIME
*SMOOTHING KERNEL IS BINOM K=4

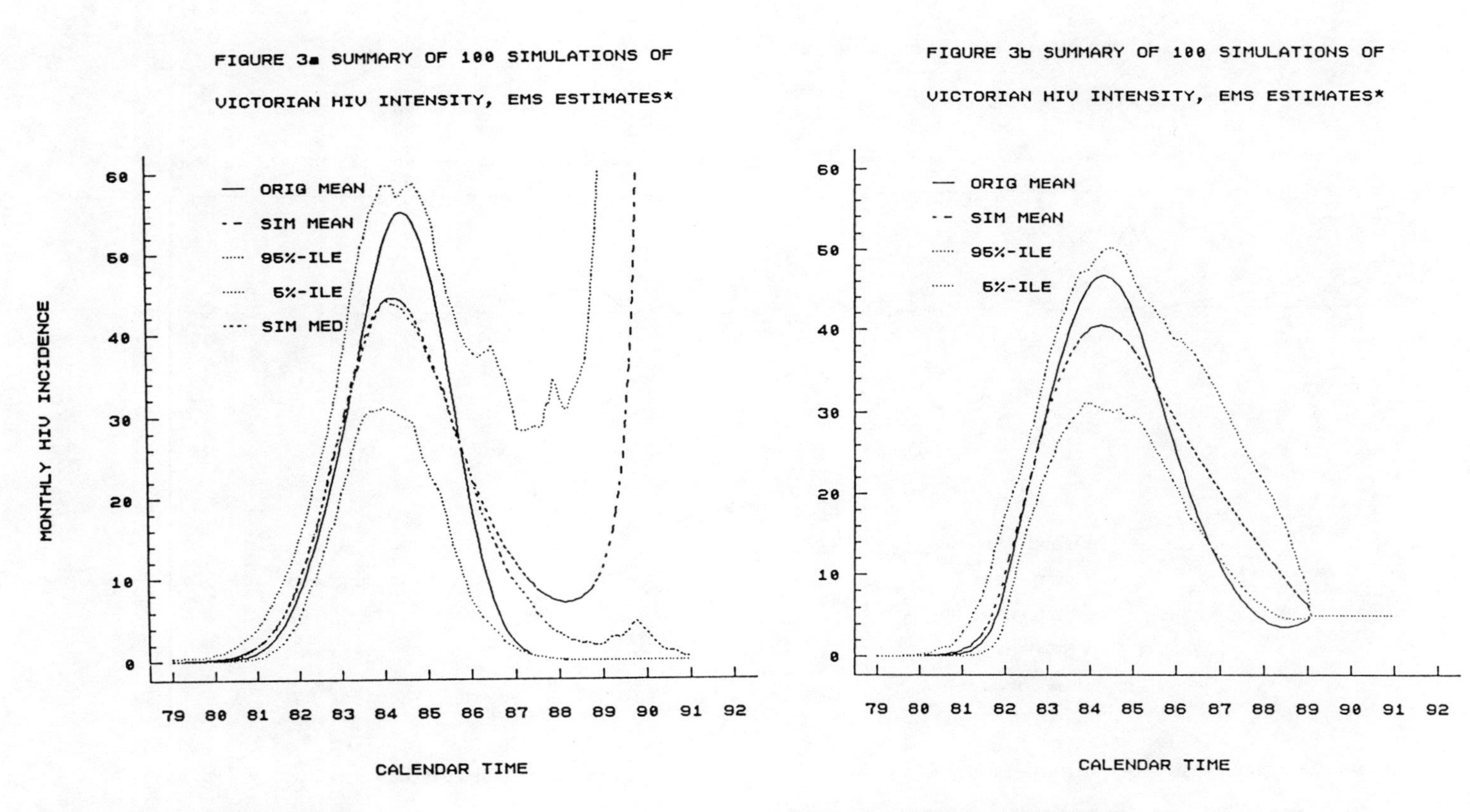

FIGURE 3a SUMMARY OF 100 SIMULATIONS OF VICTORIAN HIV INTENSITY, EMS ESTIMATES*

FIGURE 3b SUMMARY OF 100 SIMULATIONS OF VICTORIAN HIV INTENSITY, EMS ESTIMATES*

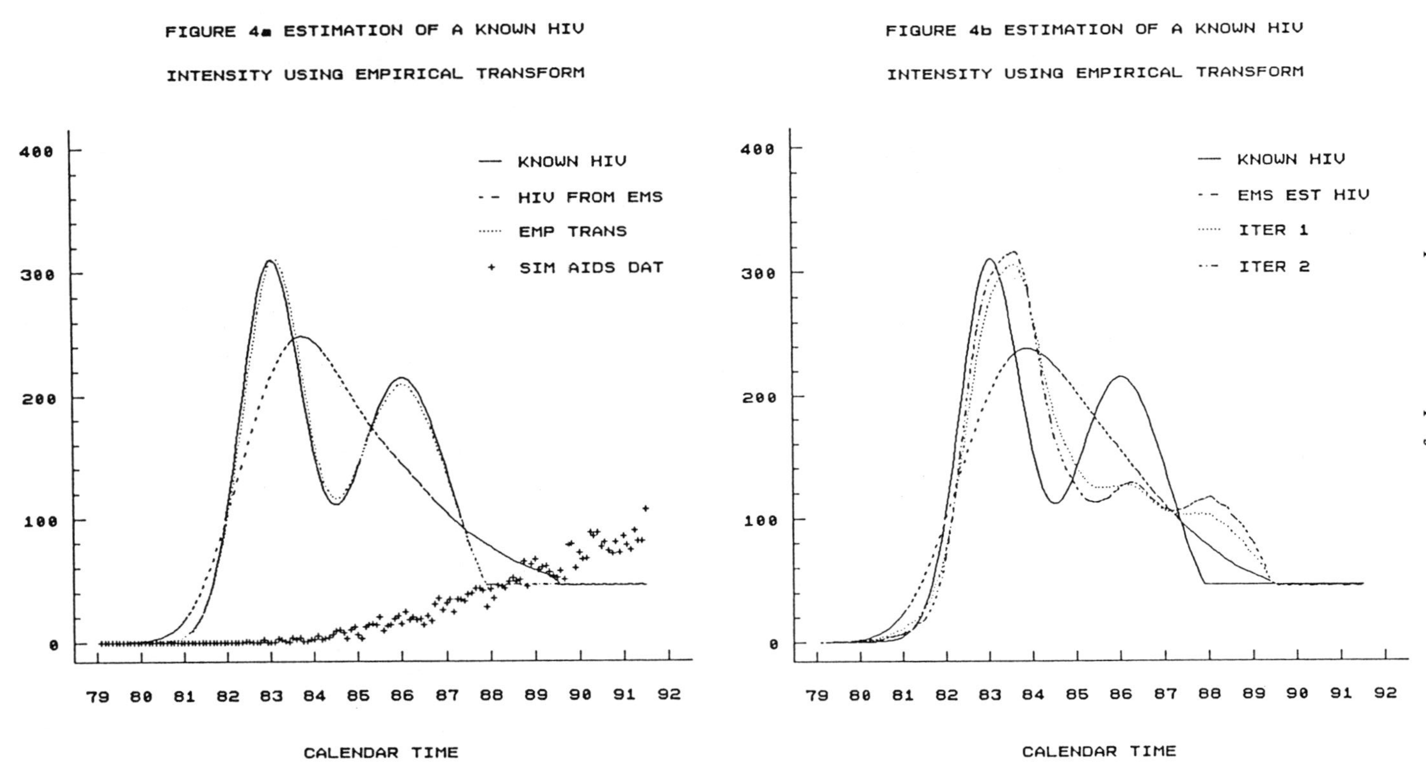
FIGURE 4a ESTIMATION OF A KNOWN HIV
INTENSITY USING EMPIRICAL TRANSFORM
MONTHLY HIV INCIDENCE
400
300
200
100
0
KNOWN HIV
HIV FROM EMS
EMP TRANS
SIM AIDS DAT
79 80 81 82 83 84 85 86 87 88 89 90 91 92
CALENDAR TIME
FIGURE 4b ESTIMATION OF A KNOWN HIV
INTENSITY USING EMPIRICAL TRANSFORM
400
300
200
100
0
KNOWN HIV
EMS EST HIV
ITER 1
ITER 2
79 80 81 82 83 84 85 86 87 88 89 90 91 92
CALENDAR TIME

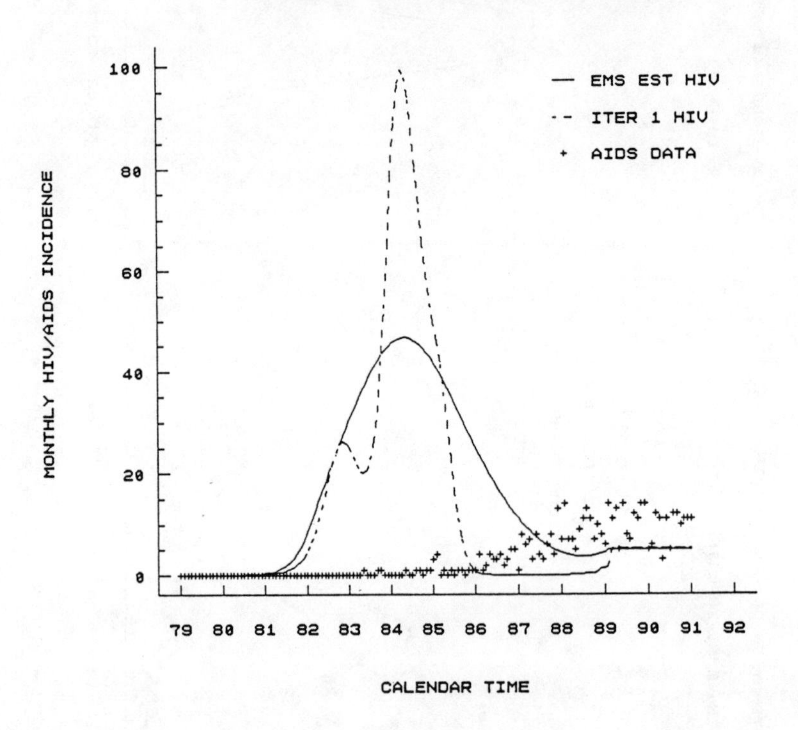
FIGURE 5 ESTIMATION OF THE VICTORIAN HIV
INTENSITY USING EMPIRICAL TRANSFORM
MONTHLY HIV/AIDS INCIDENCE
100
80
60
40
20
0
EMS EST HIV
ITER 1 HIV
AIDS DATA
79
80
81
82
83
84
85
86
87
88
89
90
91
92
CALENDAR TIME

The HIV Epidemic in New York City; Statistical Methods for Projecting AIDS Incidence and Prevalence

Marcello Pagano Victor De Gruttola
Samantha MaWhinney Xin Ming Tu

Abstract

Projections of the incidence and prevalence of diagnosed AIDS cases in New York City through 1995 make use of information from the New York City AIDS Surveillance Registry. The projections are done in three steps: First, adjustment of historic incidence data for observed delays in reporting. Second, estimation of the incidence of HIV infection in New York City during the past several years, based on the adjusted incidence data and external estimates of the latency distribution. Third, projection of future incidence of AIDS based on the estimated incidence of HIV infection. Survival after AIDS diagnosis is estimated from dates of diagnosis and death; these survival estimates are combined with estimated AIDS incidence to project prevalence of AIDS. Because little is known of the incidence of HIV infections since 1986, three alternative scenarios are explored: no new infections since 1986, 5,000 new infections per year, and 10,000 new infections per year. These represent the lower bound and two plausible alternative infection rates.

1 Introduction

Forecasting the incidence and prevalence of the acquired immunodeficiency syndrome (AIDS) caseload for the near future in New York City is important for public health planning. The statistical problems presented by the calculations of these forecasts are the subject of this report.

New York City expends a considerable effort to maintain a surveillance system that provides the information on which our projections are based. Data from this system provide a basis for estimation of the number of AIDS cases which have already been diagnosed but not yet reported, as well as those which will be diagnosed in the near future. Our analysis concerns only AIDS cases which will eventually be reported to the surveillance system. Although some cases will never be reported, other methods need to be developed to overcome this problem. We present statistical methods for projecting AIDS prevalence, using the data available from the surveillance system as well as other sources.

There are three problems in using AIDS surveillance data as the primary source for predicting the future of the epidemic: first, reports of diagnosed AIDS cases are not available immediately to the surveillance system; second, there is usually a long lag between infection with the human immunodeficiency virus (HIV) and diagnosis with AIDS; and, third, survival after diagnosis of AIDS is highly variable.

The first problem is addressed by modeling the reporting delay so that more recent incidence data may be adjusted for this delay. The second problem, that of the long latency, requires more sophisticated modeling approaches. Our goal is to use information from AIDS surveillance to make inference about the prevalence of HIV infection and to make short-term projections. Using the best available estimates of the latency distribution, only about five percent of adults who are infected with the HIV get AIDS within three years of infection. Thus the latest AIDS incidence data reflect information about HIV infection which occurred more than three years ago. This implies that infections which took place in the recent past will not be reflected directly in the available AIDS surveillance data. Of course, we have other information about the nature of the epidemic besides AIDS incidence data, and we must use this understanding in making projections. Since we may never have a population-based, longitudinal, HIV incidence survey, we must extrapolate beyond the present by using history, continuity and arguments external to the data as guides.

The case definition of AIDS was broadened in 1987. This affected the surveillance of the epidemic because some people have been diagnosed as having AIDS who would not have been so classified before 1987. We address this problem below, recognizing that a similar problem will be created by the new definition which should be in place by the beginning of next year.

The actual analyses and predictions were made individually for the groups: (i) men who have sex with men (MSM) excluding intravenous drug users (IVDU), (ii) male IVDU's, (iii) men not known to be in either of the above two categories, (iv) women IVDU, (v) women non-IVDU, and (vi) children less than 13 years of age. This has the advantage of allowing us to model the various sub-epidemics with different parameters when appropriate, however we do not report the sub-analyses individually as the techniques used were common to each of the sub-groups. Rather, we report the analysis for the aggregate of all the groups.

We first correct the data to overcome the reporting lag and the change in definition; we then estimate the HIV incidence; project the AIDS incidence; estimate survival after diagnosis with AIDS; and finally project the AIDS prevalence.

2 Estimating Recent AIDS Incidence Numbers

In order to estimate reporting lag, we treat time as a discrete variable with quarter-year intervals as the unit. Let m_{jk} be the number of AIDS cases diagnosed in quarter j and reported $k-1$ quarters later, for $k = 1, \ldots, 8$. Further, let $m_{j,9}$ be the number of AIDS cases diagnosed in quarter j and reported more than seven quarters later. Let a_j is the number of AIDS cases diagnosed in quarter j, for $j = 1, \ldots, t$. We suppose that beyond a certain time, such as three years for example, the number of unreported, diagnosed cases of AIDS is negligible — see v below. Unfortunately, even with this simplifying assumption, we do not observe all the a_j — the time constraint is such that we do not have enough time to complete the observations. Denote the actual observed a_j by a'_j. Then,

$$\begin{aligned} a'_j &= \sum_{i=1}^{9} m_{ji} \qquad j = 1,\ldots,v, && (1)\\ &= \sum_{i=1}^{8} m_{ji} \qquad j = v+1,\ldots,t-w, && (2)\\ &= \sum_{i=1}^{8+t-w-j} m_{ji} \qquad j = t-w+1,\ldots,t. && (3) \end{aligned}$$

The number v is chosen as that quarter beyond which the $m_{j,9}$ are too close to the end of the observation period to be reliable. Strictly speaking, the a' should indicate their dependence on t, the number of quarters observed, but we have chosen to not clutter up the notation further.

It helps to view the data in a tableau:

$$\begin{array}{lllllll} a'_1 & = m_{11} & \ldots + m_{1\,7-w} & \ldots + m_{17} & + m_{18} & + m_{19} \\ \vdots & & & & & \\ a'_v & = m_{v\,1} & \ldots + m_{v\,7-w} & \ldots + m_{v\,7} & + m_{v\,8} & + m_{v\,9} \\ a'_{v+1} & = m_{v+1\,1} & \ldots + m_{v+1\,7-w} & \ldots + m_{v+1\,7} & + m_{v+1\,8} & \\ \vdots & & & & & \\ a'_{t-w} & = m_{t-w\,1} & \ldots + m_{t-w\,7-w} & \ldots + m_{t-w\,7} & + m_{t-w\,8} & \\ a'_{t-w+1} & = m_{t-w+1\,1} & \ldots + m_{t-w+1\,7-w} & \ldots + m_{t-w+1\,7} & & \\ \vdots & & & & & \\ a'_t & = m_{t\,1} & \ldots + m_{t\,7-w} & & & \end{array}$$

We can use the a'_j to estimate both, the reporting delay distribution, and the a_j.

Model the reporting delay distribution as a multinomial with nine cells, and probabilities p_i, $i = 1,\ldots,9$. To estimate the p_i condition on the a'_i. Thus the log likelihood function can be written:

$$const. + \sum_{i=1}^{9} c_i \ln p_i + s_1 \ln \sum_{i=1}^{9} p_i + s_2 \ln \sum_{i=1}^{8} p_i + \sum_{j=1}^{w} \{r_{t-w+j} \ln \sum_{i=1}^{9-j} p_i\},$$

where

$$
\begin{aligned}
c_i &= \sum_{j=1} m_{ji} \qquad\qquad i = 1, \ldots, 9 \\
s_1 &= \sum_{i=1}^{9} \sum_{j=1}^{v} m_{ji} \\
s_2 &= \sum_{i=1}^{8} \sum_{j=v+1}^{t-w} m_{ji} \\
r_j &= \sum_{i=1} m_{ji} \qquad\qquad j = 1, \ldots, t.
\end{aligned}
$$

The upper limits left out on the summations above indicate that as many terms as possible are included for those summations.

The form of the likelihood is predicated by the fact that the distribution of a subset of cells of a multinomial is again a multinomial.

To allow for the possibility of changes over time in the reporting delay distribution, one can model the p above: define

$$
p_{ji} = Pr(m_{ji} = 1) \qquad i = 1, \ldots, 9,\ j = 1, \ldots
$$

and let them be a function of j. Thus the log likelihood would be

$$
const + \sum_{j=1}^{t} \sum_{i=1} m_{ji}\, ln(p_{ji}).
$$

One possibility, which incorporates the constraints that the p_{ji} are probabilities which sum to one for each j, is the logistic method. Let

$$
\begin{aligned}
p_{ji} &= exp(f(i,j))/\pi_j \qquad i = 1, \ldots, 8 \\
p_{j9} &= 1/\pi_j\,.
\end{aligned}
$$

A possibility for the function f is the linear

$$
f(i,j) = \alpha_i + \beta_i j\,, \tag{4}
$$

which would yield linear plots of $\log(p_{ji}/p_{j1})$ versus j, to aid in model checking, as described in Pagano *et al.* (1991), and shown in Figure 1. Another popular possibility is the proportional hazards model (see Kalbfleisch and Lawless (1991) and references therein) which is also shown in Figure 1. The contrast between the two models is evident.

We chose to use the logistic model with time varying probabilities. Once the appropriate model has been fit, we can estimate the a_j by

$$\begin{aligned}\hat{a}_j &= a'_j & j &= 1,\ldots,v \\ &= a'_j \,/\, (1-\hat{p}_{ji}) & j &= v+1,\ldots,t-w \\ &= a'_j \,/ \sum_{i=1}^{8+t-w-j} \hat{p}_{ji} & j &= t-w+1,\ldots,t\end{aligned}$$

where the $\hat{p}_{ji}$ are the p_{ji} evaluated at the estimated parameters. These $\hat{a}$ are shown in Figure 2 for two models: the first has the β in Equation 4 equal to zero, this corresponds to the methodology used by the Centers for Disease Control, and the second sets the β in Equation 4 equal to their maximum likelihood values. The contrast between the two is evident. We chose to model the lag using the latter since all β estimates tested different from zero. The standard errors of the $\hat{a}_j$ (not shown in the Figure) are available (see Pagano *et al.* 1991).

3 Change in Definition of AIDS

It is impossible to model with a high degree of precision the effect of the change in definition of AIDS that occurred in September of 1987. The reason is that such modeling would require estimation of the distribution of time between development of conditions that qualify as AIDS only under the new definition, AIDS (NDA), and development of AIDS-defining conditions as specified by the old (pre-1987) definition, AIDS (ODA). The change in definition that occurred in 1985 affected mostly children with AIDS, who were very few at that time; therefore, we do not consider the very small impact of this change in definition.

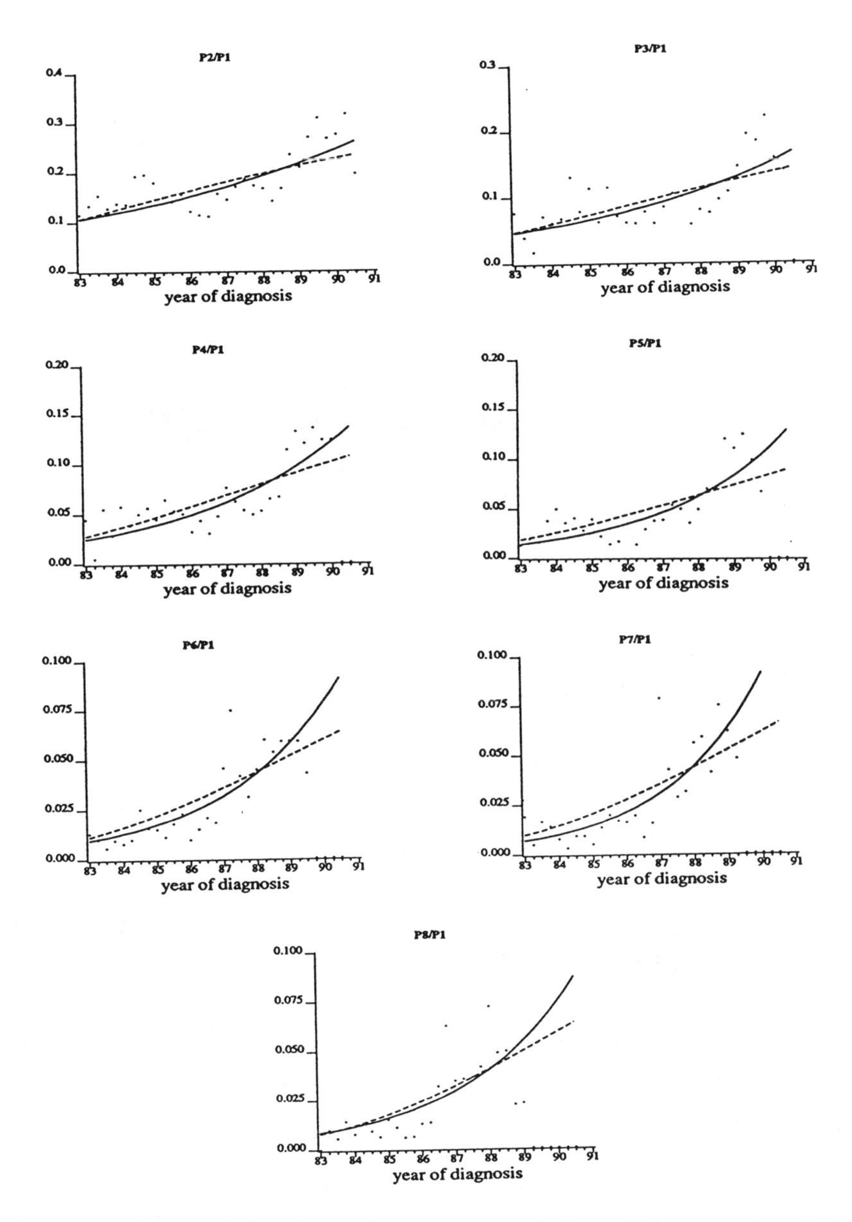

Figure 1: Plots of the data that consist of the cell entries divided by the first cell entry for that year. Superimposed are the fitted multinomial (logistic) model, solid line, and the proportional hazards (Cox) model, dashed line.

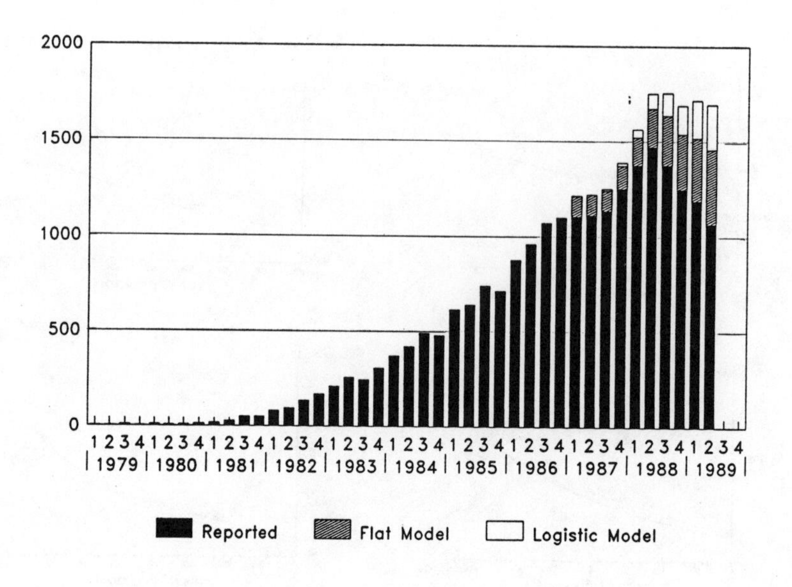

Figure 2: Historical AIDS incidence for New York City through 1989, showing cases actually reported (solid bars), and estimates of cases that will eventually be reported. Two different estimates are used: the "flat model" (hatched bars) and the "logistic model" (open bars.) The flat model assumes that the reporting delays will not vary during the next few years to correspond to the methodology used by the Centers for Disease Control while the logistic model projection is based on past variations in reporting delays.

We have two useful pieces of information that help in assessing the effect of the definitional change. The first is from a review of death certificates from 1986. It revealed that of all people whose death certificates implied that they died of AIDS under either definition, 94 percent of cases would have met ODA criteria, and 6 percent would have met only the NDA criteria. The second is from a review of the New York City AIDS surveillance data base, which revealed that 25 percent of the cases reported in 1989 meet the NDA criterion. Judging from the death certificate results, it appears that about 19 percent of these cases will eventually meet the ODA criterion and the rest will die without ever having met it.

Our correction consists of inflating the number of cases before September 1987 by 6 percent to adjust for the NDA cases that will never be reported. We also assume that 19 percent of the ODA cases actually developed NDA sometime sooner. This analysis assumes that the proportions of NDA and ODA cases has remained fairly constant. We cannot test this hypothesis. It is not known exactly how much sooner the ODA cases developed NDA, so we consider two possibilities: 4 months and 8 months. The reason for these fairly short intervals is that a presumptive diagnosis of PCP (one of the criteria for NDA) usually leads to overt and fairly recognizable disease fairly rapidly, and the wasting and dimentia syndromes are usually very poor prognostic signs.

We modeled the effect of this change by making two corrections. The intent was to move the effect of the definition change back to the beginning of the epidemic. First, all numbers pre-September 1987 were augmented by 6 percent to reflect the estimated number of people who died with the new definition of AIDS before getting the old definition of AIDS. Second, we corrected for the timing of AIDS diagnosis — the time to go from new definition of AIDS to old definition of AIDS — by shifting 19 percent of cases forward two quarters, for all the data through the first two quarters of 1988. To maintain the same total number of cases, the surplus was subtracted from the last two quarters of 1987 and the first two of 1988 according to the ratios 1:3:3:2. These numbers were chosen to reflect the nine months subsequent to the change in definition.

We did not adjust the pediatric numbers since the change of definition should prove to be negligible to infants.

4 HIV Incidence; Estimation and Projections

Let n_j $j = 1, \ldots, T$ be the HIV infection incidence per quarter. Assume that the data we have available are the a_j

$j = 1, \ldots, T$, the AIDS incidence data. The problem is to estimate the infection incidence and to project it into the future. Thus we condition our analysis on the n_j and treat them as parameters to be estimated.

We could proceed with the method outlined in Brookmeyer and Gail(1988), but we did not feel confident about our knowledge of the shape of the distribution of the n_j. Further, we preferred not to assume that the a_j were independent. We choose rather to proceed as follows (see MaWhinney and Pagano, 1991b):

Suppose that x_{jk} are the number of the n_k cases diagnosed in the jth quarter. For a given n_k we can model the vector $(x_{1k}, x_{2k}, \ldots, x_{T+1-k,k})$ as a multinomial random variable with parameter $(p_{1k}, p_{2k}, \ldots, p_{T+1-k,k})$.

In order to evaluate the p_{jk}, we need the latency distribution. Then having obtained the p_{jk}, we have that $\mathcal{E}(x_{jk}) = p_{jk}\, n_k$. So conditional on the values of the n_j, consider the linear model:

$$
\begin{aligned}
a_1 &= x_{11} \\
a_2 &= x_{21} + x_{22} \\
a_3 &= x_{31} + x_{32} + x_{33} \\
&\vdots \\
a_j &= \sum_{k=1}^{j} x_{jk} \\
&\vdots
\end{aligned}
$$

This is not a simple linear model because

$$
var(a_j) = \sum_{k=1}^{j} n_k\, p_{jk}\,(1 - p_{jk}) \tag{5}
$$

$$
covar(a_j, a_{j+m}) = -\sum_{k=1}^{j} n_k\, p_{jk}\, p_{j+m,k} \tag{6}
$$

Define the symmetric matrix Σ whose j^{th} diagonal element is given by Equation 5, and whose $(j, j+m)^{th}$ entry, for positive m is given by Equation 6.

We can obtain the least squares estimates of the n_k:

$$\tilde{n}_k = \frac{a_k - \sum_1^{k-1} \tilde{n}_i\, p_{ki}}{p_{kk}} \tag{7}$$

which can be used to provide an estimate of Σ. One might wish to smooth these estimates to ensure that the estimate of Σ is positive definite.

Equation 7 defines an estimator which is not consistent and is very sensitive to the choice of the p. As an alternative consider the ridge regression estimator defined by:

$$\hat{n} = (W + k\, diag(W))^{-1}\, L^{\top} \Sigma^{-1} a \tag{8}$$

where

$$W = L^{\top}\, \Sigma^{-1}\, L \tag{9}$$

and the lower triangular matrix L has jk element, p_{jk}. The covariance matrix of this estimator is:

$$(W + k\, diag(W))^{-1}\, W\, (W + k\, diag(W))^{-\top} \tag{10}$$

The Generalized Cross-Validation method for choosing the ridge parameter k, was developed by Golub *et al.* (1978). Their method can be expanded to include the case with an arbitrary variance- covariance matrix. The value of k is chosen to be the value which minimizes

$$GCV(k) = \frac{\frac{1}{T} \| (I - A(k)) U^{\top} \mathbf{a} \|^2}{\left[\frac{1}{T} Trace(I - A(k))\right]^2} \tag{11}$$

where

$$A(k) = U^{\top} L\, (W + k\, diag(W))^{-1}\, L^{\top} U \tag{12}$$

and

$$UU^{\top} = \Sigma, \tag{13}$$

is the Cholesky decomposition of Σ.

Note that for each new observation, a, we have a new parameter, n. As a result, we cannot obtain consistent estimators of the parameters unless we reduce the number of parameters so that if their number increases, it does so at a slow enough rate. On the other hand, consistent estimators of the n are not that critical at this point, as our interest in the n are mainly as a means to obtaining projections of the future a's. Consistent estimators of these are important.

The values for the latency distribution (the p's) were obtained from the results of Lifson *et al.* (1989) for all the adult groups. For the pediatric group we used the methods of Auger *et al.* (1988) combined with MaWhinney and Pagano (1991a). The results of the regressions with ridge weight 0.5, are displayed in Figure 3.

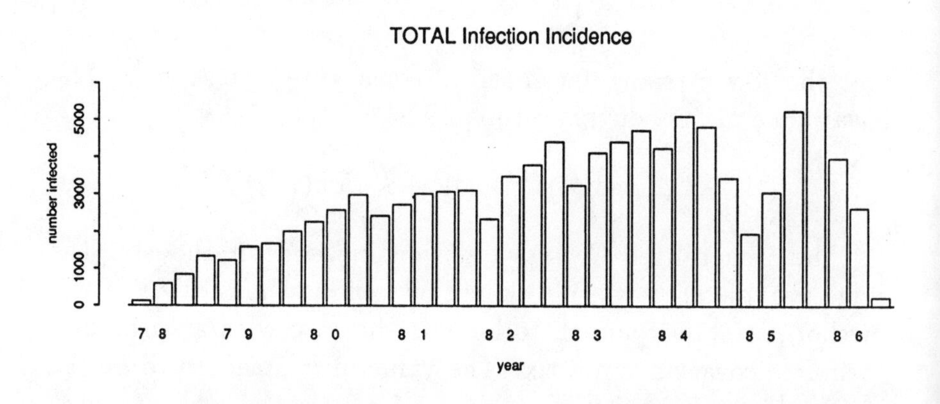

Figure 3: Modeled timing of HIV infection in persons subsequently reported with AIDS. Result of ridge regression with weight 0.5

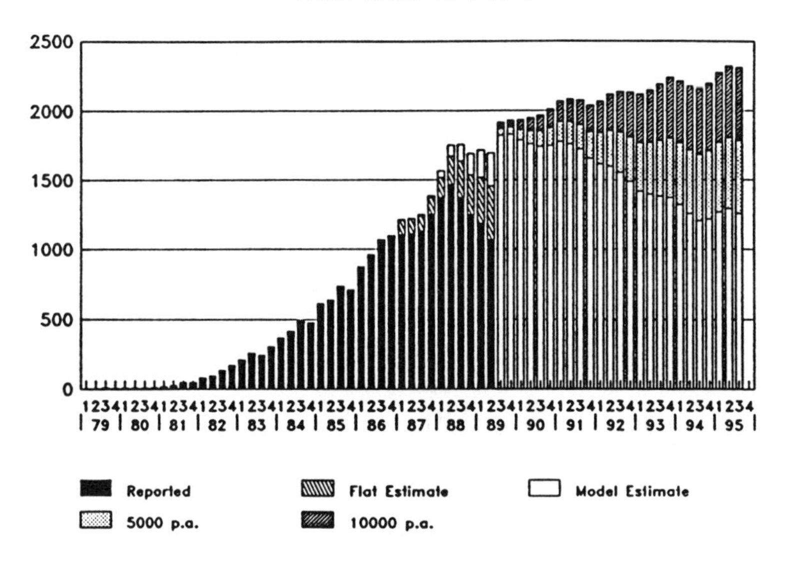

Figure 4: AIDS incidence projections under three HIV infection incidence scenarios, (i) no new infections, (ii) 5,000 new infections *per annum* (p.a.), and (iii) 10,000 new infections *per annum* (p.a.). These accompany the observed and estimated incidence numbers to date; the latter according to the logistic model for reporting.

4.1 Projections

Suppose we have observed the a_j for $j = 1, \ldots, k$ and we wish to predict them for $j = k+1, \ldots, l$. Since,

$$a_j = \sum_{i=1}^{j} x_{ji} \, ,$$

the least squares estimator of a_j is,

$$a_j = \sum_{i=1}^{j} p_{ji}\,\hat{n}_i \qquad j = k+1, \ldots, l.$$

We must distinguish between the $\hat{n}_i$ depending on the value of i. When i is k or less, then $\hat{n}_i$ is available from Equation 7. These methods yield an estimate of 103,000 HIV infected individuals through 1986. Beyond the sample region there are many factors governing the infection rate. One needs to model the incidence of HIV infection in the last two and one-half years, and into the future. Since no one knows what these numbers really are, we have explored three scenarios: one, where there are no further infections — a very conservative lower bound, included to provide a comparison with the earlier backcalculation results — two, an annual infection rate of 5,000 cases, and three, an annual infection rate of 10,000 cases. Scenario two, 5,000 new cases of infection per year, is, in our opinion, very conservative. Scenario three, 10,000 new cases a year, is less than what we estimate the infection rate was in 1986. But 1986 (12,868) was less than 1985 (13,676), which in turn was less than 1984 (18,845). This downward trend may have continued, thus the choice of 5,000 and 10,000. The projections resulting for the three scenarios are displayed in Figure 4.

5 Survival from time of AIDS diagnosis

We estimate survival after AIDS using the New York City AIDS surveillance data base. These data best represent the mix of individuals infected in the City and their health experiences. Results from clinical trials, although very informative, suffer from some selection bias; namely, they represent samples of individuals who are likely to go on clinical trials and have quality medical care readily available. We thus prefered to focus on individuals in the surveillance system.

The approach applies methods similar to those used to determine the reporting lag; above in Section 2 (see Tu *et al.*,

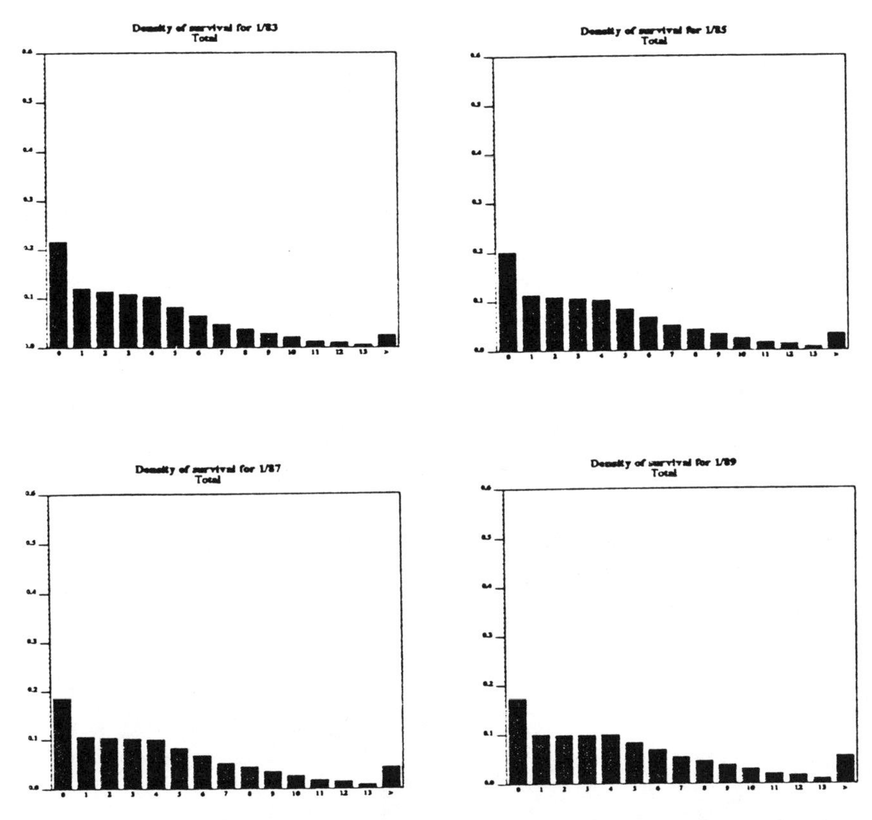

Figure 5: Survival curves for four time points to show the improvement in survival.

1991). The models allow for changes in the survival distribution over time. One shortcoming of this dataset is that the reporting delay distribution of death recording is unavailable. For some reason a common problem amongst AIDS surveillance systems is that they do not record when the date of death was entered into the system; even though they do record when they entered the date of diagnosis. As a result this recording distribution has to be estimated in other ways. We have from Tu *et al.* (1991) an estimate of this reporting delay distribution for the Centers for Disease Control public data set, and we use that estimate. Since New York City represents approximately one-sixth of the epidemic in the United States, this estimate is probably a good approximation. These methods resulted in survival distributions which show a steady improvement in survival since the beginning of the epidemic. An example of this is shown in Figure 5.

6 AIDS Prevalence

Our prevalence projections calculate the convolution of the estimates of AIDS incidence developed above with the estimates of survival calculated in the last section. Of course we do not know what survival will be in the future, so we assume that the survival estimates that apply to 1989 will apply from 1990 to 1995. Since survival is likely to increase, these prevalence projections may be too low. The current and future incidence of HIV infection is also unknown. For that reason, we project prevalence based on three different assumptions about HIV incidence after 1986: 0 per year, 5000 per year and 10,000 per year. The projections of prevalence are displayed in Figure 6.

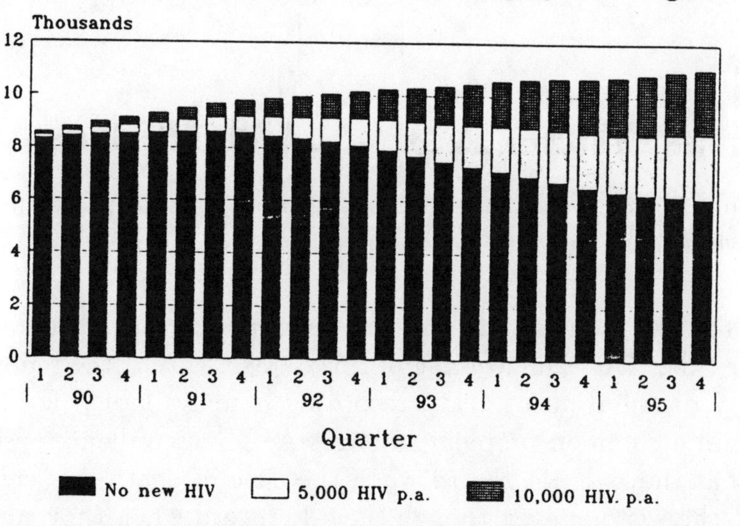

Figure 6: AIDS prevalence projections for six years under three HIV infection scenarios: no new infections, 5,000 new infections *per annum* (p.a.), and, 10,000 new infections *per annum* (p.a.).

Acknowledgements

Research supported in part by grants RO1-AI28076, R29-AI28905 and T32-AI07358 from the NIAID, National Institutes of Health, and a contract from the New York City Department of Health.

Bibliography

Auger I., Thomas P., De Gruttola V., Morse D., Moore D., Williams R., Truman B. and Lawrence C. (1988) "Incubation Period for Pediatric AIDS Patients," *Nature*, **333**: 515-517.

Bacchetti P. and Moss A. (1989) "Incubation Period of AIDS in San Francisco," *Nature*, **338**: 251-253.

Brookmeyer R. and Gail M.H. (1988), "A Method for Obtaining Short-Term Projections and Lower Bounds on the Size of the AIDS Epidemic," *Journal of the American Statistical Association*, **83**, 301-308.

Brookmeyer R. and Goedert J. (1989) "Censoring in an Epidemic with an Application to Hemophilia-Associated AIDS," *Biometrics*, **45**, 325-335.

Kalbfleisch J.D. and Lawless J.F. (1991) "Regression models for right truncated data with application to AIDS incubation times and reporting lags," *Statistica Sinica,* **1**,19-32.

Lifson A., Hessol N., Rutherford G., et al. (1989) "The Natural History of HIV Infection in a Cohort of Homosexual and Bisexual Men: Clinical Manifestations, 1979-1989," Abstract T.A.O.32, Abstracts of the Vth International Conference on AIDS.

MaWhinney S. and Pagano M. (1991a) "Time to AIDS for Children Born to HIV Positive Mothers," Technical Report, Harvard School of Public Health.

MaWhinney S. and Pagano M. (1991b) "Backcalculation Using Regression Decomposition," Technical Report Harvard School of Public Health.

Pagano M., Tu X.M., De Gruttola V. and MaWhinney S. (1991) "Analysis of Censored and Truncated Data: Estimating Reporting Delay Distributions and AIDS Incidence from Surveillance Data," Technical Report, Harvard School of Public Health.

Tu X.M., Meng X. and Pagano M. (1991) "The AIDS Epidemic: Estimating Survival after AIDS Diagnosis from Surveillance Data," Technical Report, Harvard School of Public Health.

Department of Biostatistics,
Harvard School of Public Health,
677 Huntington Avenue,
Boston MA 02115
U.S.A.

Section 2
HIV
Transmission Models

TRIANGLES IN HETEROSEXUAL HIV TRANSMISSION

K. Dietz and D. Tudor

Abstract

A model for HIV transmission is presented which treats concurrent partnerships in the heterosexual population. The basic reproduction number R_0 is calculated as a function of behavorial parameters for the duration of partnerships and for contact rates with primary and secondary partners. The threshold condition for an epidemic, $R_0>1$, is used to derive minimum bounds for the number of partners of an infected index case during the infectious period. If one takes into account the total number of contacts during the infectious period, the values for R_0 are similar for a given number of partners irrespective of whether the partnerships are consecutive or concurrent. To what extent R_0 can be estimated on the basis of behavioral data in a susceptible population is discussed.

1. Introduction

We would like to compare heterosexual HIV transmission with and without concurrent partnerships. The model by Dietz and Hadeler (1988) considers serial monogamy. Waldstätter (1989) allows contacts outside partnerships, but every contact involves a new partner. In the following we describe the formation of pairs and of triangles comprising either two women and one man or two men and one woman. For given contact rates and infection probabilities we calculate the number R_0 of new cases generated by one case in a susceptible population, the number N of partners acquired during the infectious period and the corresponding number C of sexual contacts. In order to compare different transmission patterns we investigate how R_0 depends on N for given C. The calculation of these quantities is based on the methods introduced by Diekmann et al. (1991). The present paper is restricted to constant infectivity.

2. Model assumptions

The demographic model without infection is described by the following equations (see also Fig. 1):

$$\dot{y}_1 = v_1 + s_1\left[(\sigma_0 + \mu_0)p + (\sigma_{2+} + 2\mu_0)q_2\right] - \left[\rho_0 \min(y_1, y_2) + \rho_2 \min(y_1, p) + \mu_0 y_1\right],$$
$$\dot{y}_2 = v_2 + s_2\left[(\sigma_0 + \mu_0)p + (\sigma_{1+} + 2\mu_0)q_1\right] - \left[\rho_0 \min(y_1, y_2) + \rho_1 \min(y_2, p) + \mu_0 y_2\right],$$
$$\dot{p} = \rho_0 \min(y_1, y_2) + (\sigma_{1+} + 2\mu_0)q_1 + (\sigma_{2+} + 2\mu_0)q_2$$
$$-\left[(\sigma_0 + 2\mu_0)p + \rho_1 \min(y_2, p) + \rho_2 \min(y_1, p)\right],$$
$$\dot{q}_1 = \rho_1 \min(y_2, p) - (\sigma_{1+} + 3\mu_0)q_1,$$
$$\dot{q}_2 = \rho_2 \min(y_1, p) - (\sigma_{2+} + 3\mu_0)q_2,$$

where

y_i = number of singles of sex i, $i = 1,2$, where 1 indicates male and 2 female,
p = number of heterosexual pairs,
q_j = number of triangles of type j=1,2, where 1 indicates a two-woman triangle and 2 a two-man triangle,
v_i = recruitment rate of sexually active singles of sex i,
μ_0 = death rate of uninfected individuals,
ρ_0 = pair formation rate,
ρ_j = triangle formation rate of type j,
σ_0 = separation rate of pairs,
σ_{ij} = separation rate of relationships with partner of type k from a triangle of type j, k=1,2, where 1 indicates a primary partner and 2 a secondary partner,
σ_{j+} = $\sigma_{j1}+\sigma_{j2}$
s_i = probability of staying sexually active after becoming single again.

For the pair and triangle formation rate we have chosen the minimum function. Newly recruited singles join the population as singles. They can either form pairs or become a secondary partner of a member of a pair thus forming triangles. Pairs can break up either by the separation of the partners or by the death of one of the partners. They can also become triangles if one of the partners acquires a second

y_2 (–) y_1 [–]

p (–) [–]

[–] (–) [–] q_2 q_1 (–) [–] (–)

Fig. 1 States of the transmission model involving triangles in the absence of infection. Round and square brackets denote females and males, respectively. The minus sign refers to the susceptible state.

partner. A triangle can break up if one of the three partners dies or if either the primary or the secondary relationship is terminated creating a pair and a single. Every individual who becomes single again decides with a certain probability whether to look for a new partner or to stay single.

In order to determine the rates of forming pairs and triangles on a per capita basis we introduce the following notation:

$$\begin{aligned}
&\rho_{01} = \rho_0; \quad \rho_{02} = \rho_0 y_1 / y_2, && \text{if } y_1 \le y_2,\\
&\rho_{01} = \rho_0 y_2 / y_1; \quad \rho_{02} = \rho_0, && \text{if } y \le y_1,\\
&\rho_{11} = \rho_1 y_2 / p; \quad \rho_{12} = \rho_1, && \text{if } y_2 \le p,\\
&\rho_{11} = \rho_1; \quad \rho_{12} = \rho_1 p / y_2, && \text{if } p \le y_2,\\
&\rho_{21} = \rho_2; \quad \rho_{22} = \rho_2 y_1 / p, && \text{if } y_1 \le p,\\
&\rho_{21} = \rho_2 p / y_1; \quad \rho_{22} = \rho_2, && \text{if } p \le y_1.
\end{aligned}$$

Then the following balancing conditions are satisfied:

$$\begin{aligned}
\rho_{01} y_1 &= \rho_{02} y_2,\\
\rho_{12} y_2 &= \rho_{11} p,\\
\rho_{21} y_1 &= \rho_{22} p.
\end{aligned}$$

They ensure that any set of parameters describes consistent rates for males and females.

The calculation of R_0, N, and C requires that we follow an infected individual through all possible states until he or she dies or decides to become sexually inactive. There are 13 states for each sex (see Fig. 2):

1 & 14 = single,
2 & 15 = paired with a susceptible partner,
3 & 16 = paired with an infective partner,
4 & 17 = primary partner of a susceptible partner who has a susceptible secondary partner,
5 & 18 = primary partner of an infective partner who has a susceptible secondary partner,
6 & 19 = primary partner of an infective partner who has an infective secondary partner,
7 & 20 = paired with a susceptible primary partner and with a susceptible secondary partner,
8 & 21 = paired with a susceptible primary partner and with an infective secondary partner,

		14	(+)*	[+]*	1			
	15	(+)*	[−]	(−)	[+]*	2		
	16	(+)*	[+]	(+)	[+]*	3		
(+)*	[−]	(−)	17	4	[−]	(−)	[+]*
(+)*	[+]	(−)	18	5	[−]	(+)	[+]*
(+)*	[+]	(+)	19	6	[+]	(+)	[+]*
[−]	(+)*	[−]	20	7	(−)	[+]*	(−)
[+]	(+)*	[−]	21	8	(−)	[+]*	(+)
[−]	(+)*	[+]	22	9	(+)	[+]*	(−)
[+]	(+)*	[+]	23	10	(+)	[+]*	(+)
(−)	[−]	(+)*	24	11	[+]*	(−)	[−]
(−)	[+]	(+)*	25	12	[+]*	(+)	[−]
(+)	[+]	(+)*	26	13	[+]*	(+)	[+]

Fig. 2 States of the transmission model involving triangles referring to either a male or a female infected index case. Symbols as in Fig. 1. The plus sign refers to the infected state. The index case is indicated by an asterix.

9 & 22 = paired with an infective primary partner and with a susceptible secondary partner,
10 & 23 = paired with an infective primary partner and with an infective secondary partner,
11 & 24 = secondary partner of a susceptible who has a susceptible primary partner,
12 & 25 = secondary partner of an infective who has a susceptible primary partner,
13 & 26 = secondary partner of an infective who has an infective primary partner.

In addition to the demographic parameters we have to introduce parameters relating to the transmission of the infection:

μ_1 = death rate of an infected individual,
h_i = infection probability per contact if the infective partner is of sex i,
β_0 = contact rate within a pair,
β_{jk} = contact rate within a triangle of type j with a partner of type k.

The transition rates between the states are given in Table 1. The negative inverse of the transition matrix provides the sojourn (waiting) times D_{kl} in state l for individuals entering the population in state k.

The basic reproduction number is calculated as the dominant eigenvalue of the following matrix

$$M = \begin{pmatrix} 0 & M_1 \\ M_2 & 0 \end{pmatrix},$$

where M_i, i = 1,2 are 7 x 7 matrices corresponding to the seven possible states in which new cases can be generated. For males these are the states in $I_1 = \{3;5;6;8;9;12;13\}$ and for females in $I_2 = \{16;18;19;21;22;25;26\}$. The elements of one row of M_1, are defined as follows:

$$h_1(\rho_{01}D_{j,1} + \beta_0 D_{j,2});\; h_1\beta_{11}D_{j,7};\; h_1(\rho_{11}D_{j,3} + \beta_{12}D_{j,9});\; h_1(\rho_{21}D_{j,1} + \beta_{22}D_{j,11});\; h_1\beta_{21}D_{j,4};$$
$$h_1(\rho_{11}D_{j,2} + \beta_{12}D_{j,7});\; h_1\beta_{11}D_{j,8},$$

where j is one of the seven initial states for male index cases. M_2 for

Table 1 Transition rates between the states of the transmission model involving triangles. Only the rates for a male index case are given.

$$g_{1,1} = -(\rho_{01} + \rho_{21} + \mu_1);\ g_{1,2} = (1-h_1)\rho_{01};\ g_{1,3} = h_1\rho_{01};\ g_{1,11} = (1-h_1)\rho_{21};\ g_{1,12} = h_1\rho_{21};$$

$$g_{2,1} = s_1(\sigma_0 + \mu_0);\ g_{2,2} = -(\rho_{11} + \rho_{22} + \sigma_0 + h_1\beta_0 + \mu_0 + \mu_1);$$

$$g_{2,3} = h_1\beta_0;\ g_{2,4} = \rho_{22};\ g_{2,7} = (1-h_1)\rho_{11};\ g_{2,8} = h_1\rho_{11};$$

$$g_{3,1} = s_1(\sigma_0 + \mu_1);\ g_{3,3} = -(\rho_{11} + \rho_{22} + \sigma_0 + 2\mu_1);\ g_{3,5} = (1-h_2)\rho_{22};$$

$$g_{3,6} = h_2\rho_{22};\ g_{3,9} = (1-h_1)\rho_{11};\ g_{3,10} = h_1\rho_{11};$$

$$g_{4,1} = s_1(\sigma_{21} + \mu_0);\ g_{4,2} = \sigma_{22} + \mu_0;\ g_{4,4} = -(\sigma_{2+} + h_1\beta_{21} + 2\mu_0 + \mu_1);\ g_{4,5} = h_1\beta_{21};$$

$$g_{5,1} = s_1(\sigma_{21} + \mu_1),\ g_{5,3} = \sigma_{22} + \mu_0;\ g_{5,5} = -(\sigma_{2+} + h_2\beta_{22} + \mu_0 + 2\mu_1);\ g_{5,6} = h_2\beta_{22};$$

$$g_{6,1} = s_1(\sigma_{21} + \mu_1);\ g_{6,3} = \sigma_{22} + \mu_1;\ g_{6,6} = -(\sigma_{21} + \sigma_{22} + 3\mu_1);\ g_{7,2} = \sigma_{11} + \sigma_{12} + 2\mu_0;$$

$$g_{7,7} = -(\sigma_{11} + \sigma_{12} + h_1\beta_{11} + h_1\beta_{12} + 2\mu_0 + \mu_1);\ g_{7,8} = h_1\beta_{12};\ g_{7,9} = h_1\beta_{11};$$

$$g_{8,2} = \sigma_{12} + \mu_1;\ g_{8,3} = \sigma_{11} + \mu_0;\ g_{8,8} = -(\sigma_{11} + \sigma_{12} + h_1\beta_{11} + \mu_0 + 2\mu_1);\ g_{8,10} = h_1\beta_{11};$$

$$g_{9,2} = \sigma_{11} + \mu_1;\ g_{9,3} = \sigma_{12} + \mu_0;\ g_{9,9} = -(\sigma_{11} + \sigma_{12} + h_1\beta_{12} + \mu_0 + 2\mu_1);\ g_{9,10} = h_1\beta_{12};$$

$$g_{10,3} = \sigma_{11} + \sigma_{12} + 2\mu_1;\ g_{10,10} = -(\sigma_{11} + \sigma_{12} + 3\mu_1);$$

$$g_{11,1} = s_1(\sigma_{22} + \mu_0);\ g_{11,2} = \sigma_{21} + \mu_0;\ g_{11,11} = -(\sigma_{21} + \sigma_{22} + h_1\beta_{22} + 2\mu_0 + \mu_1);$$

$$g_{11,12} = h_1\beta_{22};\ g_{12,1} = s_1(\sigma_{22} + \mu_1);\ g_{12,3} = \sigma_{21} + \mu_0;$$

$$g_{12,12} = -(\sigma_{21} + \sigma_{22} + h_2\beta_{21} + \mu_0 + 2\mu_1);\ g_{12,13} = h_2\beta_{21};$$

$$g_{13,1} = s_1(\sigma_{22} + \mu_1);\ g_{13,3} = \sigma_{21} + \mu_1;\ g_{13,13} = -(\sigma_{21} + \sigma_{22} + 3\mu_1).$$

females is defined similarly. In order to calculate the number of new partners during the infectious period of the index case, the left eigenvalue of the matrix M corresponding to the dominant eigenvalue R_0 is used to determine the initial distribution u_i of states of the index case. Then the number of partners, N, is given by

$$N = \sum_{j \in I_1 \cup I_2} u_j\left[(\rho_{01} + \rho_{21})D_{j,1} + \rho_{11}\left(D_{j,2} + D_{j,3}\right)\right].$$

Similarly the number C of contacts during the infectious period is

$$C = N + \sum_{j \in I_1 \cup I_2} u_j\Big[\beta_0\left(D_{j,2} + D_{j,3}\right) + \beta_{21}\left(D_{j,4} + D_{j,5} + D_{j,6}\right)$$
$$+ (\beta_{11} + \beta_{12})\left(D_{j,7} + D_{j,8} + D_{j,9} + D_{j,10}\right) + \beta_{22}\left(D_{j,11} + D_{j,12} + D_{j,13}\right)\Big].$$

For fixed C we want to calculate R_0 as a function of N. We keep all parameters or ratios between parameters fixed except two and vary those two such that C is kept fixed while N varies. Of particular interest is the critical value of N for which $R_0 = 1$, i.e. the minimum number of partners which is necessary to cause an epidemic.

This number of partners is acquired by an index case during the infectious period. It depends on the parameters describing the behaviour of an infected case which does not necessarily agree with the parameters describing the pair formation process of a susceptible individual. One obvious difference is the duration of partnerships which is decreased due to the increased death rate of infected partners. We therefore calculate the number of partners during life time that a susceptible individual would acquire for the same parameters ρ, σ, and s but with death rates of susceptible individuals. Fig. 3 shows the corresponding states for singles, pairs and triangles:

1& 6 single,
2& 7 paired,
3& 8 primary partner,
4& 9 paired with a primary and a secondary partner,
5&10 secondary partner.

The corresponding transition rates are given by the following matrix:

$$\mathrm{G}_0 = \begin{pmatrix} \mathrm{G}_{01} & 0 \\ 0 & \mathrm{G}_{02} \end{pmatrix},$$

where G_{01}=

$$\begin{pmatrix} -(\rho_{01}+\rho_{21}+\mu_0) & \rho_{01} & & & \rho_{21} \\ s_1(\sigma_0+\mu_0) & -(\rho_{11}+\rho_{22}+\sigma_0+2\mu_0) & \rho_{22} & \rho_{11} & \\ s_1(\sigma_{21}+\mu_0) & \sigma_{22}+\mu_0 & -(\sigma_{2+}+3\mu_0) & & \\ & \sigma_{1+}+2\mu_0 & & -(\sigma_{1+}+3\mu_0) & \\ s_1(\sigma_{22}+\mu_0) & \sigma_{21}+\mu_0 & & & -(\sigma_{2+}+3\mu_0) \end{pmatrix},$$

and G_{02} =

$$\begin{pmatrix} -(\rho_{02}+\rho_{12}+\mu_0) & \rho_{02} & & & \rho_{12} \\ s_2(\sigma_0+\mu_0) & -(\rho_{11}+\rho_{22}+\sigma_0+2\mu_0) & \rho_{11} & \rho_{22} & \\ s_2(\sigma_{11}+\mu_0) & \sigma_{12}+\mu_0 & -(\sigma_{1+}+3\mu_0) & & \\ & \sigma_{2+}+2\mu_0 & & -(\sigma_{2+}+3\mu_0) & \\ s_2(\sigma_{12}+\mu_0) & \sigma_{11}+\mu_0 & & & -(\sigma_{1+}+3\mu_0) \end{pmatrix}.$$

The sojourn times are again determined by the negative inverse of this matrix. We assume that newly recruited individuals start as singles. The number of partners for males and females are given by:

$$N_1^- = (\rho_{01}+\rho_{21})D_{1,1} + \rho_{11}D_{1,2},$$

and

$$N_2^- = (\rho_{02}+\rho_{12})D_{6,6} + \rho_{22}D_{6,7}.$$

The number of sexual contacts during lifetime is then

$$C_1^- = N_1^- + \beta_0 D_{1,2} + \beta_{21}D_{1,3} + (\beta_{11}+\beta_{12})D_{1,4} + \beta_{22}D_{1,5},$$

and

$$C_2^- = N_2^- + \beta_0 D_{6,7} + \beta_{11}D_{6,8} + (\beta_{21}+\beta_{22})D_{6,9} + \beta_{12}D_{6,10}.$$

(–)* 6 1 [–]*

(–)* [–] 7 2 (–) [–]*

(–)* [–] (–) 8 3 [–] (–) [–]*
[–] (–)* [–] 9 4 (–) [–]* (–)
(–) [–] (–)* 10 5 [–]* (–) [–]

Fig. 3 States of the transmission model involving triangles for the calculation of the number of partners during a life time. Individuals enter the population in states 1 and 6, respectively. The individuals who are followed up are indicated by an asterix.

One has to realize that surveys of sexual behaviour usually assess the situation among susceptibles. The same parameters describing pair and triangle formation can then lead to different values for N and C for infected individuals.

3. Numerical Results

For all numerical calculations, the following parameter values are held constant: μ_0=0.02 per year, μ_1=0.1 per year, s_1=0.975, s_2=0.95, v_1=2000 per year, v_2=2200 per year.

Three particular relationship formation schemes are considered, each of which can be obtained as a special case of the present model. The "triangles" model allows formation and dissolution of pairs and triples. For this model we set $\rho_0=\rho_1=\rho_2$; $\sigma_{jk}=2\sigma_0$; where ρ_0 and σ_0 are to be chosen as described later. This means that the rate of acquiring a secondary partner is equal to the rate of acquiring a primary partner and that the rate of dissolution of a triangle is twice the separation rate of a pair.
The "pairs only" model considers only the formation and separation of pairs. For this model we set the triangle formation rates equal to zero and the triangle separation rates are taken to be large.
The "Waldstätter" model does allow contacts outside the primary pair, but each of these contacts represents a single (instantaneous) incident, each time with a new partner.

For each of the models described above, only the values of ρ_0 and σ_0 must be supplied. For arbitrary given values of ρ_0 and σ_0, the remaining parameters in the model can be defined while also guaranteeing that the consistency conditions are fulfilled. Then the matrices G,M may be calculated as well as the dominant eigenvalue of M yielding a value for R_0, the basic reproduction number. Using the formula above for C the total number of contacts after infection may then be calculated. Thus, all parameters are defined, C is held constant at the desired level, and the relation between R_0 and N (the expected number of partners during the infectious period) may be plotted by choosing a range of ρ_0 values, calculating the σ_0 values by the secant method to obtain the desired C, then plotting the calculated N versus R_0.

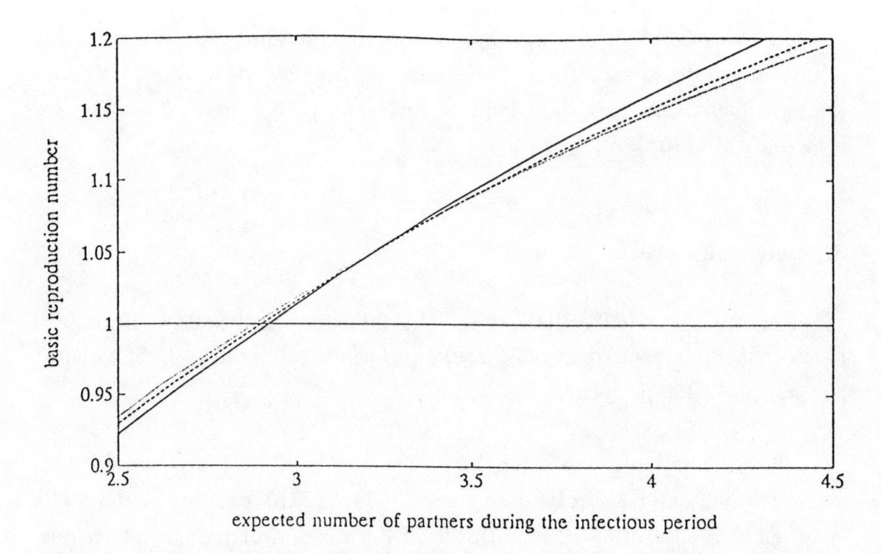

Fig. 4 The basic reproduction number as a function of the mean number of partners during the infectious period for a total of 600 contacts during this time (·····only consecutive partnerships; ------ concurrent partnerships possible; ——— only isolated contacts, each time with a new partner, possible during a primary partnership)

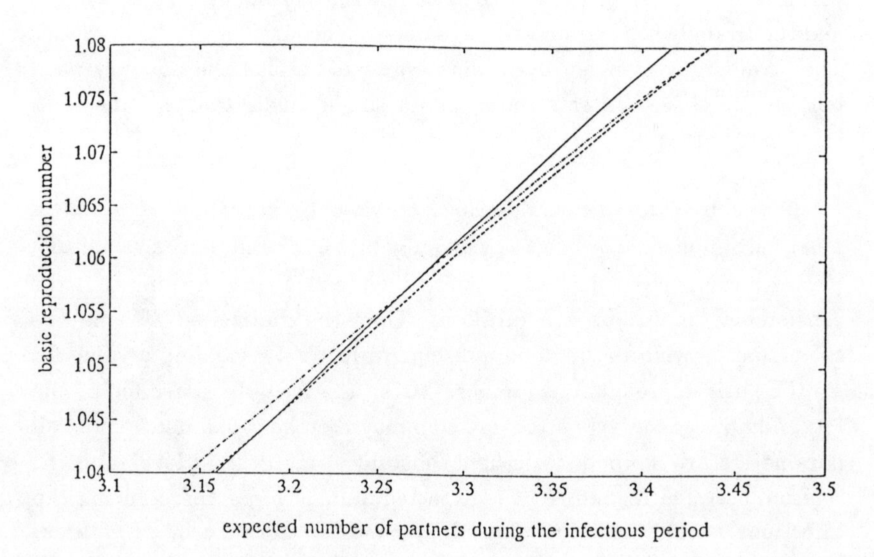

Fig.5 Enlarged section of Fig. 4 around the intersection of the three curves.

The procedure described above was used to produce several graphs such as the one shown in Fig.4. Several sets of values for the probabilities of infection h_1 and h_2 were run as well as for b_0 and C. All the results were consistent in that the relationships between the curves remained the same. For the example in Fig.4 h_1=0.006, h_2=0.002, β_0=100 per year, and C=600. It appears that the three curves intersect in a common point but this is not the case. Figure 5 shows a magnification of the region where the hypothesized intersection would be and it is clear that there is no point common to all three curves. The curve for the model with triangles stays between the other two curves for most values of N. Since the number of contacts during the infectious period is the same for all models and for all values of N, one would expect that for a given value of N, the value of R_0 would be the same, since the average number of contacts divided by the average number of partners is also the same. This should also lead to the same infection probability per partner. This conjecture is also expressed by Weyer (1991). Since his heuristic derivation of the infection probability per partner is given by

$$1-(1-h)^c$$

where c is the average number of contacts per partner, he implicitly assumes that the variance of the number of contacts per partner is zero. In general, the infection probability per partner depends on the distribution of the number, K of contacts per partner. Let f denote the probability generating function of this distribution. Then the infection probability per partner is given by

$$1\text{-}f(1\text{-}h).$$

If we expand this function in powers of h, we get

$$hc-\frac{h^2}{2}\left(\text{var}(K)+c^2-c\right)+o\left(h^2\right).$$

If the infection probability per contact is small (h is estimated between 10^{-3} and 10^{-2}), one sees that the variance of K has a small negative influence on the infection probability per partner, that is to say, increasing the variance of the number of contacts per partner decreases the infection probability, but only slightly. Therefore it is not surprising that the three curves in Fig. 4 are very close together. The differences which can be noticed are partly due to the fact that the number of contacts per *new* partner may also be different for the three models, mainly because the duration of partnerships varies and therefore also the number of contacts with the source of infection of the index case. Since the source of infection is already infected, all contacts with the source are therefore "wasted" from the point of view of counting secondary cases and should be subtracted from the total number of contacts in order to calculate the average number of contacts per new partner. These calculations will be reported elsewhere.

4. Concluding remarks

The present model was motivated by the results of surveys of sexual behaviour in England and the U.S. which estimate the cumulative incidence of concurrent partnerships at about 50% for males and 30% for females (Sally Blower, personal communication). Thus, the phenomenon is widespread enough that it could not be ignored. The present analysis shows that the calculation of the basic reproduction number is hardly affected by concurrent partnerships provided, of course, that one has reliable estimates of the underlying parameters, especially of the number of partners and the total number of contacts during the infectious period.

This assumption is, however, very much in doubt since the usual surveys of sexual behaviour collect data mainly from susceptible individuals or from individuals whose state of infection is unknown. If one uses these data to estimate behavioral parameters such as the duration of partnerships, or lengths of time between partnerships, or number of contacts during partnerships, then it is not clear to what extent these estimates are relevant to infected individuals. During a prolonged partnership, the index case may experience the loss of a partner due to the infection which may in the worst case lead to an increase in the number of new partners per unit of time or, in the best case, to a complete withdrawal from having unprotected sexual contacts. Even if no partner is lost due to the infection, there may be a reduction in the rate of sexual contacts due to appearance of HIV disease symptoms. Therefore, it is not clear at all to what extent data from sexual behaviour surveys among susceptibles are relevant to the calculation of R_0. Most likely they would lead to an overestimate, but an underestimate is not totally to be excluded. Thus, recent attempts to assess R_0 for the heterosexual population on the basis of surveys of sexual behaviour must be interpreted cautiously, especially if the resulting estimates are close to one. Numerical results using the formulas given above for calculating the number of partners in a susceptible population will be given elsewhere.

Acknowledgements

The first author was supported in part by NATO grant (D.890350) and the second author by the Deutsche Forschungsgemeinschaft (Di 308/5-1).

References

Diekmann, O., Dietz, K., Heesterbeek, J.A.P. (1991). The basic reproduction ratio for sexually transmitted diseases. Part I: Theoretical considerations. *Mathematical Biosciences* **107**, 325-339.

Dietz, K., Hadeler, K.P. (1988). Epidemiological models for sexually transmitted diseases. *Journal of Mathematical Biology*, **26**, 1-25.

Waldstätter, R. (1989). Pair formation in sexually-transmitted diseases. In *Mathematical and Statistical Approaches to AIDS Epidemiology,* (ed. C. Castillo-Chavez), *pp.*260-274. Springer, Berlin (*Lecture Notes in Biomathematics,* **83**).

Weyer, J. (1990). Über das Ansteckungspotential HIV-infizierter Personen. *AIDS-Forschung*, **5**, 31-40.

Klaus Dietz
Department of Medical Biometry
Eberhard-Karls-University
Westbahnhofstr. 55
W7400 Tübingen
Germany

David Tudor
Synthelabo Recherche
31, avenue Paul Vaillant-Couturier
92225 Bagneux CEDEX
France

Structured Population Models for HIV Infection Pair Formation and Non-constant Infectivity

K.P.Hadeler

Abstract: The spread of a sexually transmitted disease with long incubation period such as HIV is modeled in a population which is structured by age, sex, and duration of infection. Since empirical evidence shows that in the HIV situation infectivity varies considerably from the moment of infection to the onset of AIDS, the effects of non-constant infectivity are studied in detail. A characteristic eigenvalue problem is derived which determines stability or instability of the uninfected state of the population. For the case of constant population size the basic reproduction number is calculated. The dependence of this number on the infectivity is studied by analytical and numerical methods. The results indicate that non-constant infectivity leads to a lower basic reproduction number when compared to a constant infectivity obtained by appropriate averaging.

The classical model, in continuous time, for the evolution of an age-structured population is the Lotka-Sharpe or McKendrick model. This model assumes the form of a renewal equation (Sharpe and Lotka 1911, Lotka 1922) or of a hyperbolic partial differential equation with boundary condition (McKendrick 1926), for the function $x(t,a)$ which is the age distribution of the population at time t (see the monograph by Webb 1985 for a modern treatment). The variable a is the chronological age. The continuous time model is extremely useful for the qualitative study of the behavior of populations. For the treatment of actual data one uses discrete versions (the typical time step is one year) which are known as Leslie or Lexis models (see Keyfitz 1985).

The differential equation (subscripts denote partial derivatives)

$$x_t + x_a + \mu(a)x = 0 \tag{1a}$$

describes aging and age-dependent death, whereas the boundary condition

$$x(t,0) = \int_0^\infty b(a)x(t,a)da \tag{1b}$$

describes the recruitment of newborn individuals. Since the work of Feller (1941) it is known that, under mild conditions on the mortality function $\mu(a)$ and the fertility function $b(a)$, for a large class of initial data $x(0,a)$ the solution $x(t,a)$ is asymptotic to an exponential function $\bar{x}(a)\exp(\lambda t)$, where $\bar{x}(a)$ is the stationary age distribution, and λ is the exponent of growth of the total population.

Generally it is understood that the model (1) should be seen as a model for the female population only, as a model for the replication of mothers to daughters. If the equations are seen as a model for the total population then it is difficult to interpret the fertility $b(a)$. It has been observed rather early (Kuczynski 1932) that contradictions arise if the model is applied to the female part and the male part of a population separately. Hence there is some need for an appropriate model for a two-sex population. The formulation of such a model, known as the two-sex problem, has met great difficulties. It has even been questioned that this problem is reasonable at all (Parlett 1972). It appears that it is important and interesting although there may be not only one possible model.

Models for two-sex populations have been formulated. In these models aging, birth, and death are assumed as linear processes (it is assumed that crowding effects do not exist, thus birth and death of individuals are seen as events independent of other individuals) whereas pair formation is a nonlinear interaction. The main difficulty in model design is the appropriate definition of a pair formation law.

Based on the work of Keyfitz and others (see Keyfitz 1985) the most complete description of a model for a two-sex population has been given by Hoppensteadt (1975) (see also Hadeler 1989a, Arbogast and Milner 1989). In this model there are three state variables. The function $x(t,a)$ is the distribution of female singles of chronological age a, the function $y(t,b)$ is the distribution of single males of chronological age b, and $p(t,a,b,c)$ is the distribution of pairs where the female partner has age a, the male partner has age b, and the pair has existed for a time interval of length c. The model has the form of three hyperbolic differential equations together with boundary conditions. Due to the linearity of the birth and death law the differential equations themselves are linear, also the boundary conditions describing birth are linear, the only nonlinearity is the pair formation law which enters the boundary condition for the function p at $c = 0$. The equations read

$$\begin{aligned}
&x_t+x_a + \mu_x(a)x + \int_0^\infty p(t,a,b,0)db \\
&\qquad - \int_0^\infty \int_c^\infty \mu_y(b)p(t,a,b,c)dbdc - \int_0^\infty \int_c^\infty \sigma(a,b,c)p(t,a,b,c)dbdc = 0, \\
&y_t+y_b + \mu_y(b)y + \int_0^\infty p(t,a,b,0)da \qquad\qquad (2a)\\
&\qquad - \int_0^\infty \int_c^\infty \mu_x(a)p(t,a,b,c)dadc - \int_0^\infty \int_c^\infty \sigma(a,b,c)p(t,a,b,c)dadc = 0, \\
&p_t+p_a + p_b + p_c + \mu_x(a)p + \mu_y(b)p + \sigma(a,b,c)p = 0,
\end{aligned}$$

together with boundary conditions for the recruitment of singles

$$\begin{aligned}
x(t,0) &= \int_0^\infty \int_c^\infty \int_c^\infty b_x(a,b,c)p(t,a,b,c)dadbdc, \\
y(t,0) &= \int_0^\infty \int_c^\infty \int_c^\infty b_y(a,b,c)p(t,a,b,c)dadbdc,
\end{aligned} \qquad (2b)$$

and the formation of pairs

$$
\begin{aligned}
p(t,a,c,c) &= 0,\\
p(t,c,b,c) &= 0,\\
p(t,a,b,0) &= \phi(x,y)(t,a,b).
\end{aligned}
\tag{2c}
$$

Notice that the newly formed pairs $p(t,a,b,0)$ enter equations (2a) linearly. All equations are linear with the exception of the third boundary condition in (2c).

The coefficient functions, mortalities $\mu_x(a)$, $\mu_y(b)$, fertilities $b_x(a)$, $b_y(b)$, separation rate $\sigma(a,b,c)$, are nonnegative. Their qualitative behavior reflects the modelling assumptions for the population considered. The pair formation function ϕ is a function which defines the number of newly formed pairs (per unit of time) of female partners of age a and male partners of age b for given distributions of singles $x(t,a)$, $y(t,b)$. Thus ϕ maps a pair of densities $x(a)$ and $y(b)$ into a function $p(a,b,0) = \phi(x,y)(a,b)$ of two variables a, b (of course, in the time evolution all these quantities depend also on the chronological time t). There are some general views about what properties a pair formation function should have. $p(a,b,0)$ is nonnegative, $p(a,b,0)$ vanishes if either $x(a)$ or $y(b)$ vanishes, $\phi(x,y)$ should be homogeneous of degree 1. A rather well established candidate for a pair formation function is the generalized harmonic mean

$$
\phi(x,y)(a,b) = \frac{m(a,b)x(a)y(b)}{\int_0^\infty g(a)x(a)da + \int_0^\infty h(b)y(b)db}. \tag{3}
$$

Here the weight functions g and h are positive, the function $m(a,b)$ is nonnegative.

The function (3) can be seen as a mixing model for different classes. Of course one can introduce, in addition to age and sex, other characters to structure the population, in particular with respect to social behavior (see, e.g., Jacquez et al. 1988, 1989, Busenberg and Castillo-Chavez 1989, Castillo-Chavez and Blythe 1989, Sattenspiel and Simon 1988, Ng and Anderson 1989). Here we shall consider only age and sex as structure variables.

The mathematical analysis of the model (2) meets great difficulties. Waldstätter (1990) has proved that the initial value problem is well posed and that, under suitable conditions, the solutions exist for all $t \geq 0$. If all coefficients are constant then, by integration of the equations, one can make a transition to an ordinary differential equations model for the total number X of single females, the total number Y of single males, and the total number of pairs P. This model has been formulated already by Kendall (1949) (actually a somewhat simpler version, without separation of pairs). The qualitative behavior of the o.d.e. model has been completely analyzed in Hadeler, Waldstätter, Wörz-Busekros (1988). Waldstätter (1990) has also analysed a related problem studied by Yellin and Samuelson (1974). There are always two trivial exponential solutions describing a purely female and a purely male population, respectively. In addition there is at most one two-sex exponential solution. If the latter exists then it is globally stable and the two pure states are unstable. Furthermore it can be shown that the two-sex solution exists whenever the parameters are sufficiently symmetric with respect to the two sexes. Of course the exponents of the two pure states are always negative. As the exponent of the exponential solution in the model (1), the exponent of the two-sex solution can be of either sign.

Computer simulations show that, for realistic sets of parameters, the solutions of the general equations (2) approximate exponential solutions of the form

$$x(t,a) = \bar{x}(a)e^{\lambda t}, \quad y(t,b) = \bar{y}(b)e^{\lambda t}, \quad p(t,a,b,c) = \bar{p}(a,b,c)e^{\lambda t}. \tag{4}$$

These "persistent" solutions describe populations with a stable distribution of age and sex classes for which the total population grows exponentially. It can also be conjectured that for sufficiently symmetric choices of the parameters there should be always at least one stable two-sex exponential solution. These claims have not been proved so far. One complication of the general case as compared to the ordinary differential equations case is the loss of monotonicity: An increase of the population (by immigration, say) may lead to a decrease of newly formed pairs in certain age classes, in particular if the immigrants and the residents have different age distributions. In Hadeler (1990) a special case has been considered: The population is split into adults (age $> \tau$) and children (age $< \tau$). Parameters are constant within each of these two classes. Children do not form pairs. Then the parameter τ plays the role of a maturation period. Under these conditions the model (2) can be reduced to a system of three coupled delay equations

$$\begin{aligned}
\dot{x}(t) &= b_x e^{-\mu_x \tau} p(t-\tau) + (\mu_y + \sigma)p(t) - \mu_x x(t) - \varphi(x(t), y(t)),\\
\dot{y}(t) &= b_y e^{-\mu_y \tau} p(t-\tau) + (\mu_x + \sigma)p(t) - \mu_y y(t) - \varphi(x(t), y(t)),\\
\dot{p}(t) &= -(\mu_x + \mu_y + \sigma)p(t) + \varphi(x(t), y(t)).
\end{aligned} \tag{5}$$

For the model (5) one can indeed show that there is at most one exponential two-sex solution which is at least locally stable whenever it exists.

Kendall's o.d.e. model is obtained from (5) for $\tau = 0$,

$$\begin{aligned}
\dot{x} &= b_x p + (\mu_y + \sigma)p - \mu_x x - \varphi(x,y),\\
\dot{y} &= b_y p + (\mu_x + \sigma)p - \mu_y y - \varphi(x,y),\\
\dot{p} &= -(\mu_x + \mu_y + \sigma)p + \varphi(x,y).
\end{aligned} \tag{6}$$

In the following we shall be mainly interested in the symmetric case where all parameters are independent of the sexes. Then $\varphi(x,x) = \rho x$ with some parameter $\rho > 0$. If we consider a symmetric situation where the female and the male compartment have the same size then the equations become linear, and it is sufficient to consider the variables x and y,

$$\begin{aligned} \dot{x} &= (b+\mu+\sigma)p - (\mu+\rho)x, \\ \dot{p} &= -(2\mu+\sigma)p + \rho x. \end{aligned} \tag{7}$$

This system has an exponential solution $(\bar{x}, \bar{p})\exp(\hat{\lambda}t)$ where

$$\hat{\lambda} = -\mu + \frac{1}{2}\sqrt{(\mu+\sigma+\rho)^2 + 4\rho b} - \frac{\mu+\sigma+\rho}{2}. \tag{8}$$

The coefficients $\bar{x}$, $\bar{p}$ are easily obtained from the corresponding linear system.

Of particular importance is the case of constant population size which is characterized by $\hat{\lambda} = 0$ or, equivalently, by

$$\rho(b+\mu+\sigma) - (\mu+\rho)(2\mu+\sigma) = 0.$$

Notice that in the pair formation model the case of constant population size does not occur for $b - \mu = 0$ (as in linear population models), since only individuals in pairs produce offspring. Of course one could consider a model with constant recruitment (as in Dietz 1988 or Dietz and Hadeler 1988).

Although there are models which consider jointly demography and disease transmission (see, e.g., Busenberg and Hadeler 1990), most models for the transmission of infectious diseases do not distinguish between sexes, even if the disease is sexually transmitted. K.Dietz (1987) has pointed out that two susceptible individuals who form a pair (without any sexual contact outside the pair bond) are practically immune, although not immune in the medical sense. Thus, neglecting the fact that a large portion of the population is engaged, at least temporally, in stable pairs, will generally lead to an overestimation of the transmission rate in a heterosexual population. In Dietz and Hadeler (1988) this view has been further explored in a model for a two-sex population (without age structure and with constant recruitment) in which the two sexes and infected/uninfected individuals have been distinguished. The basic assumptions were that at a given moment, each individual is either single or a member of a pair, and that the disease can only be transmitted within a pair consisting of an infected and an uninfected partner. Within the framework of this model a threshold condition has been derived for the stability of the uninfected state of the population. The critical parameters in the model are, of course, the transmission probabilities, but the rate of pair formation and separation as well. In the HIV infection the length of the incubation period has the same order of magnitude as the generation time of the population. Also there seems to be a demographic impact if the disease establishes itself in the heterosexual population. Therefore it makes sense to consider the spread of the disease within the framework of a demographic model. In Hadeler and Ngoma (1990) the model of Dietz and Hadeler (1988) has been extended by dropping the assumption of constant recruitment. In Hadeler (1989b) a general model for the spread in an age structured population has been presented.

There are empirical data supporting the view that the infectivity of an HIV carrier is not constant. The infectivity seems to be high shortly after the individual has been infected, then rather low over an extended period, and ultimately high again. Thus one should introduce variable infectivity into the model as well. Assuming constant infectivity will possibly again lead to an overestimation of the rate of transmission.

Thus, in addition to chronological age, for infected individuals the time since infection has to be recorded. We introduce the following independent variables: a the age of a female, b the age of a male, c the duration of a pair, α duration of the infection in a female, β duration of the infection in a male. These variables satisfy the inequalities $a \geq c$, $b \geq c$, $a \geq \alpha$, $b \geq \beta$.

The state variables are: $x(a)$ noninfected single females, $y(b)$ noninfected single males, $u(a,\alpha)$ infected single females, $v(b,\beta)$ infected single males, $P(a,b,c)$ pairs with both partners noninfected, $Q(a,b,c,\beta)$ pairs, only male partner infected, $R(a,b,c,\alpha)$ pairs, only female partner infected, $S(a,b,c,\alpha,\beta)$ pairs of two infected partners.

The following are the parameter functions:

$\mu_x(a)$, $\mu_y(b)$ mortality of noninfected females and males of age a and b, respectively,
$\mu_u(a,\alpha)$, $\mu_v(b,\beta)$ mortality of infected females and males depending on age and duration of infection,
$\sigma_P(a,b,c)$, $\sigma_Q(a,b,c,\beta)$, $\sigma_R(a,b,c,\alpha)$, $\sigma_S(a,b,c,\alpha,\beta)$ separation rates of the different types of pairs depending on demographic and infection state,
$b_P(a,b,c)$, $b_Q(a,b,c,\beta)$, $b_R(a,b,c,\alpha)$, $b_S(a,b,c,\alpha,\beta)$ birth rates of the different types of pairs,
ν_x, ν_y sex-ratio coefficients,
$\kappa_x(a,\alpha)$, $\kappa_y(b,\beta)$ the infection rate within a pair.

Finally ϕ is the pair formation function. As indicated earlier it is not at all clear what this function should be. Following the general idea of harmonic means one can choose

$$\begin{aligned}
\phi_P(x,y,u,v)(a,b) &= m_P(a,b)x(a)y(b)/N,\\
\phi_Q(x,y,u,v)(a,b,\beta) &= m_Q(a,b,\beta)x(a)v(b,\beta)/N,\\
\phi_R(x,y,u,v)(a,b,\alpha) &= m_R(a,b,\alpha)u(a,\alpha)y(b)/N,\\
\phi_S(x,y,u,v)(a,b,\alpha,\beta) &= m_S(a,b,\alpha,\beta)u(a,\alpha)v(b,\beta)/N,
\end{aligned}$$

where (in the following we omit multiple integral signs)

$$\begin{aligned}
N = \int_0^\infty & g(a)x(a)da + \int_0^\infty h(b)y(b)db\\
&+ \int_0^\infty g_1(a,\alpha)u(a,\alpha)dad\alpha + \int_0^\infty h_1(b,\beta)v(b,\beta)dbd\beta.
\end{aligned}$$

The first four partial differential equations describe the evolution of the four types of singles,

$$
\begin{aligned}
&x_t + x_a + \mu_x x + \int_0^\infty P(a,b,0)db + \int_0^\infty Q(a,b,0,\beta)dbd\beta \\
&- \int_0^\infty (\mu_y + \sigma_P)Pdbdc - \int_0^\infty (\mu_v + \sigma_Q)Qdbdcd\beta = 0, \\
&y_t + y_b + \mu_y y + \int_0^\infty P(a,b,0)da + \int_0^\infty R(a,b,0,\alpha)dad\alpha \\
&- \int_0^\infty (\mu_x + \sigma_P)Pdadc - \int_0^\infty (\mu_u + \sigma_R)Rdadcd\alpha = 0, \\
&u_t + u_a + u_\alpha + \mu_u u + \int_0^\infty R(a,b,0,\alpha)db + \int_0^\infty S(a,b,0,\alpha,\beta)dbd\beta \\
&- \int_0^\infty (\mu_y + \sigma_R)Rdbdc - \int_0^\infty (\mu_v + \sigma_S)Sdbdcd\beta = 0, \\
&v_t + v_b + v_\beta + \mu_v v + \int_0^\infty Q(a,b,0,\beta)da + \int_0^\infty S(a,b,0,\alpha,\beta)dad\alpha \\
&- \int_0^\infty (\mu_x + \sigma_Q)Qdadc - \int_0^\infty (\mu_u + \sigma_S)Sdadcd\alpha = 0,
\end{aligned}
\tag{9a}
$$

Similarly, the next four equations describe the evolution of pairs,

$$
\begin{aligned}
&P_t + P_a + P_b + P_c + [\mu_x + \mu_y + \sigma_P]P = 0, \\
&Q_t + Q_a + Q_b + Q_c + Q_\beta + [\mu_x + \mu_v + \sigma_Q]Q + \kappa_x Q = 0, \\
&R_t + R_a + R_b + R_c + R_\alpha + [\mu_u + \mu_y + \sigma_R]R + \kappa_y R = 0, \\
&S_t + S_a + S_b + S_c + S_\alpha + S_\beta + [\mu_u + \mu_v + \sigma_S]S = 0.
\end{aligned}
\tag{9b}
$$

The recruitment of newborns is governed by the boundary conditions

$$
\begin{aligned}
&x(t,0) = \nu_x \int_0^\infty (b_P P + b_Q Q d\beta + b_R R d\alpha + b_S S d\alpha d\beta)dadbdc, \\
&y(t,0) = \nu_y \int_0^\infty (b_P P + b_Q Q d\beta + b_R R d\alpha + b_S S d\alpha d\beta)dadbdc, \\
&u(t,a,0) = 0, \\
&v(t,b,0) = 0,
\end{aligned}
\tag{9c}
$$

where the possibility of vertical transmission has been excluded. Finally, the boundary conditions for pairs are given by

$$
\begin{aligned}
&P(t,a,b,0) = \phi_P(x,y,u,v)(t,a,b), \\
&Q(t,a,b,0,\beta) = \phi_Q(x,y,u,v)(t,a,b,\beta), \\
&Q(t,a,b,c,0) = 0, \\
&R(t,a,b,0,\alpha) = \phi_R(x,y,u,v)(t,a,b,\alpha), \\
&R(t,a,b,c,0) = 0, \\
&S(t,a,b,c,\alpha,0) = \kappa_y R(t,a,b,c,\alpha), \\
&S(t,a,b,c,0,\beta) = \kappa_x Q(t,a,b,c,\beta), \\
&S(t,a,b,0,\alpha,\beta) = \phi_S(x,y,u,v)(t,a,b,\alpha,\beta).
\end{aligned}
\tag{9d}
$$

Notice that the boundary conditions for these variables, at $c = 0$, contain the only nonlinearities within this system. Thus the contact between a susceptible and an infected individual is modeled by the nonlinear boundary condition for the variable Q or R, respectively, whereas the event of infection is desribed by the transition from Q or R to S in the equations (9a).

We expect that this general model will have the properties of the o.d.e. models investigated by Dietz (1987), Dietz and Hadeler (1988), Hadeler and Ngoma (1990) as well as the properties of the age structure model (2) which both appear as special cases. Thus we expect, for realistic choices of the parameters, the existence of an exponential solution describing the asymptotic behavior of an uninfected population

$$x(t,a)=\bar{x}(a)e^{\lambda t},\quad y(t,b)=\bar{y}(b)e^{\lambda t},\quad P(t,a,b,c)=\bar{p}(a,b,c)e^{\lambda t},$$

$$u\equiv 0,\ v\equiv 0,\ Q\equiv 0,\ R\equiv 0,\ S\equiv 0.$$

Then we expect a threshold phenomenon for critical parameters such as pair formation rate or infection rate of the following kind: when the parameter exceeds the threshold then the uninfected exponential solution loses stability and an infected exponential solution appears.

Computer simulation shows that this is what actually happens.

Several authors have studied the effects of variable transmission rates, e.g., Thieme and Castillo-Chavez (1989). K.Dietz has proposed to this author to study the effects of variable infectivity in a model with pair formation. In order to get an idea about the possible effects of variable infectivity we consider a case where all demographic parameters are constant. Then we can neglect the effects of age structure and the duration of the infection is the essential independent variable. Specializing the model (9) we introduce now the variables $X(t)$, $Y(t)$, $u(t,\alpha)$, $v(t,\beta)$, $P(t)$, $Q(t,\beta)$, $R(t,\alpha)$, $S(t,\alpha,\beta)$. Notice that some of these variables are scalars, others are one- or two-dimensional distributions. Using a harmonic mean law with identical weights (sexual partners do not discriminate between uninfected and infected) we obtain the following set of equations,

$$\begin{aligned}
&\dot{X}+\mu X+2\frac{\rho}{N}X\Big(Y+\int_0^\infty v\,d\beta\Big)=bT+(\mu+\sigma)P+(\bar{\mu}+\sigma)\int_0^\infty Q\,d\beta,\\
&\dot{Y}+\mu Y+2\frac{\rho}{N}\Big(X+\int_0^\infty u\,d\alpha\Big)Y=bT+(\mu+\sigma)P+(\bar{\mu}+\sigma)\int_0^\infty R\,d\alpha,\\
&u_t+u_\alpha+\bar{\mu}u+2\frac{\rho}{N}u\Big(Y+\int_0^\infty v\,d\beta\Big)=(\mu+\sigma)R+(\bar{\mu}+\sigma)\int_0^\infty S\,d\beta,\\
&v_t+v_\beta+\bar{\mu}v+2\frac{\rho}{N}\Big(X+\int_0^\infty u\,d\alpha\Big)v=(\mu+\sigma)Q+(\bar{\mu}+\sigma)\int_0^\infty S\,d\alpha,\\
&\dot{P}+(2\mu+\sigma)P=2\frac{\rho}{N}XY,\\
&Q_t+Q_\beta+(\mu+\bar{\mu}+\sigma)Q=2\frac{\rho}{N}Xv-\kappa(\beta)Q,\\
&R_t+R_\alpha+(\bar{\mu}+\mu+\sigma)R=2\frac{\rho}{N}uY-\kappa(\alpha)R,\\
&S_t+S_\alpha+S_\beta+(2\bar{\mu}+\sigma)S=2\frac{\rho}{N}u(t,\alpha)v(t,\beta),
\end{aligned}\tag{10a}$$

$$N = X + Y + \int_0^\infty u d\alpha + \int_0^\infty v d\beta,$$
$$T = P + \int_0^\infty Q d\beta + \int_0^\infty R d\alpha + \int_0^\infty \int_0^\infty S d\alpha d\beta, \tag{10b}$$
$$u(t,0) = 0, \quad v(t,0) = 0, \quad Q(t,0) = 0, \quad R(t,0) = 0, \tag{10c}$$
$$S(t,\alpha,0) = \kappa(\alpha) R(t,\alpha), \quad S(t,0,\beta) = \kappa(\beta) Q(t,\beta). \tag{10d}$$

Here the parameters b, μ, ρ, σ are the same as in (7), $\bar{\mu} \geq \mu$ is the mortality of infected, and the function κ is the infection rate depending on the time since infection.

This is a homogeneous system. In general the total population is not constant. The problem with constant population size (of the uninfected population) can be obtained as the special case for $\hat{\lambda} = 0$. For a general theory of homogeneous equations, in the finite dimensional case, see Hadeler (1992). Within the present paper we shall not deal with the analytical problems that are posed by the fact that equations (10) define an infinite-dimensional system.

Of course there is an uninfected exponential solution with exponent $\hat{\lambda}$ given by (8) and $(X, Y, u, v, P, Q, R, S) = (X, X, 0, 0, P, 0, 0, 0)$ where $X = \bar{x}$, $P = \bar{p}$. We linearize the system at this trivial solution. Then $\hat{\lambda}$ is also an eigenvalue of the linearization. The uninfected exponential solution is stable if the other eigenvalues λ of the linearization satisfy the condition $Re(\lambda - \hat{\lambda}) < 0$. Hence the uninfected solution loses stability when one of the eigenvalues different from $\hat{\lambda}$ passes through $\hat{\lambda}$. In this case we expect the bifurcation of a stable infected exponential solution. In general, i.e., if $\bar{\mu} > \mu$, the exponent of this solution will be smaller than $\hat{\lambda}$.

In the case of constant population size we have $\hat{\lambda} = 0$. Hence the uninfected stationary solution loses stability if one of the eigenvalues (other than the trivial eigenvalue 0) passes through 0.

We denote the deviations from equilibrium by the variables x, y, u, v, p, q, r, s. In view of the symmetry of the problem it is sufficient to keep the variables x, u, p, q, s. We omit the calculations and arrive at the system

$$\begin{aligned}
&\dot{x} + \mu x + \rho x = bT + (\mu + \sigma)p + (\bar{\mu} + \sigma)\int_0^\infty q d\alpha, \\
&u_t + u_\alpha + \bar{\mu} u + \rho u = (\mu + \sigma) q + (\bar{\mu} + \sigma) \int_0^\infty s d\beta, \\
&\dot{p} + (2\mu + \sigma)p = \rho(x - \int_0^\infty u d\alpha), \\
&q_t + q_\alpha + (\mu + \bar{\mu} + \sigma) q = \rho u - \kappa(\alpha) q(\alpha), \\
&s_t + s_\alpha + s_\beta + (2\bar{\mu} + \sigma) s = 0,
\end{aligned} \tag{11a}$$

$$T = p + 2\int_0^\infty q d\alpha + \int_0^\infty \int_0^\infty s d\alpha d\beta, \tag{11b}$$

$$u(t,0) = 0, \quad q(t,0) = 0, \quad s(t,\alpha,0) = \kappa(\alpha) q(\alpha), \quad s(t,0,\beta) = \kappa(\beta) q(\beta). \tag{11c}$$

We notice that the equation for s becomes independent of the other variables reflecting the fact that near the onset of infection the contacts between infected individuals do not play a role.

We consider the eigenvalue problem of the partial differential system (11), i.e., we look for exponential solutions of (11). We find that this problem can be decomposed (as usual in bifurcation problems in epidemiology). We can first determine the variables u, q, s, and then x, p. The problem for the three infected variables which will give the desired bifurcation condition reads

$$\begin{aligned} &u_\alpha + (\rho + \bar{\mu} + \lambda)u = (\mu + \sigma)q + (\bar{\mu} + \sigma)\textstyle\int_0^\infty s d\beta, \\ &q_\alpha + (\mu + \bar{\mu} + \sigma + \lambda)q = \rho u - \kappa(\alpha)q, \\ &s_\alpha + s_\beta + (2\bar{\mu} + \sigma + \lambda)s = 0, \end{aligned} \tag{12a}$$

$$u(0) = 0, \quad q(0) = 0, \quad s(\alpha, 0) = \kappa(\alpha)q(\alpha), \quad s(0, \beta) = \kappa(\beta)q(\beta). \tag{12b}$$

This is a homogeneous stationary problem for three variables. We have to find nontrivial solutions. We first solve the equation for s, a linear hyperbolic equation in the positive orthant with boundary data (in terms of q on the axes). The solution is

$$s(\alpha, \beta) = \begin{cases} \kappa(\alpha - \beta)q(\alpha - \beta)\exp(-\tilde{\sigma}\beta), & \alpha > \beta, \\ \kappa(\beta - \alpha)q(\beta - \alpha)\exp(-\tilde{\sigma}\alpha), & \alpha < \beta, \end{cases} \tag{13}$$

where

$$\tilde{\sigma} = 2\bar{\mu} + \sigma + \lambda. \tag{14}$$

We define the function

$$\eta(\alpha) = \textstyle\int_0^\infty s(\alpha, \beta)d\beta. \tag{15}$$

After elementary calculations we find

$$\eta(\alpha) = \int_0^\alpha e^{-\tilde{\sigma}(\alpha - \tau)}\kappa(\tau)q(\tau)d\tau + \int_0^\infty \kappa(\tau)q(\tau)d\tau \cdot e^{-\tilde{\sigma}\alpha}, \tag{16}$$

from where

$$\dot{\eta} + \tilde{\sigma}\eta = \kappa(\alpha)q, \tag{17}$$

and

$$\eta(0) = \textstyle\int_0^\infty \kappa(\alpha)q(\alpha)d\alpha. \tag{18}$$

Now we can replace the last equation of (12a) by equation (17). Then the eigenvalue problem (12) of a partial differential equation has been reduced to that of an ordinary differential equation for the functions u, q, and η,

$$\begin{aligned} &u_\alpha + (\bar{\mu} + \rho + \lambda)u = (\mu + \sigma)q + (\bar{\mu} + \sigma)\eta, \\ &q_\alpha + (\bar{\mu} + \mu + \sigma + \lambda)q = \rho u - \kappa(\alpha)q, \\ &\eta_\alpha + (2\bar{\mu} + \sigma + \lambda)\eta = \kappa(\alpha)q, \end{aligned} \tag{19a}$$

$$u(0) = 0, \quad q(0) = 0, \quad \eta(0) = \int_0^\infty \kappa(\alpha) q(\alpha) d\alpha. \tag{19b}$$

This is a system of three linear equations with one side condition.

The structure of this problem is the following. The differential equations (19a) have a unique solution for every initial data. Choose the initial data $u(0,\lambda) = 0$, $q(0,\lambda) = 0$, $\eta(0,\lambda) = 1$. Compute the solution $u(\alpha,\lambda)$, $q(\alpha,\lambda)$, $\eta(\alpha,\lambda)$ and the quantity $\mathcal{R}(\lambda) = \int_0^\infty \kappa(\alpha) q(\alpha,\lambda) d\alpha$. Determine λ such that $\mathcal{R}(\lambda) = 1$. Then λ is an eigenvalue.

Since (19) reduces the stability problem of the uninfected solution of (10) to a finite-dimensional problem, (19) can be seen as a kind of "characteristic problem", similar to a characteristic equation. We shall see in a moment that in a special case a reduction to a "true" characteristic equation is possible.

Thus we can formulate the first result.

Result 1: *Suppose that in the general model* (9) *the coefficients are symmetric with respect to the sexes, and constant, with the exception of the transmission rate. Then the model assumes the form* (10). *The stability of the noninfected solution is governed by the characteristic problem* (19)*: Determine the leading eigenvalue λ_0 of the problem* (19). *If $\lambda_0 < \hat{\lambda}$ then the uninfected solution is stable. If $\lambda_0 > \hat{\lambda}$ then the uninfected solution is unstable.*

The case of constant population size is characterized by $\hat{\lambda} = 0$, i.e., the birth rate b (which does not enter the system (19)) is adapted to the other parameters in such a way that net population growth is zero. In this case the critical value for λ_0 is zero.

Result 2: *In the case of constant population size the uninfected state is stable if the leading eigenvalue λ_0 of the system* (19) *is negative. The uninfected state is unstable if the leading eigenvalue is positive.*

This result leads immediately to a formula for the basic reproduction number. The basic reproduction number $\mathcal{R}_0$ is the number of infected which is produced by one infected individual during its lifetime in a totally susceptible population.

Result 3: *The basic reproduction number $\mathcal{R}_0$ (for constant population size) can be obtained in the following way. Solve the initial value problem*

$$\begin{aligned} u_\alpha + (\bar{\mu} + \rho) u &= (\mu + \sigma) q + (\bar{\mu} + \sigma)\eta, \\ q_\alpha + (\bar{\mu} + \mu + \sigma) q &= \rho u - \kappa(\alpha) q, \\ \eta_\alpha + (2\bar{\mu} + \sigma)\eta &= \kappa(\alpha) q, \\ u(0) = 0, \quad q(0) &= 0, \quad \eta(0) = 1, \end{aligned} \tag{20}$$

and compute

$$\mathcal{R}_0 = \int_0^\infty \kappa(\alpha) q(\alpha) d\alpha, \tag{21}$$

or, equivalently,

$$\mathcal{R}_0 = (2\bar{\mu} + \sigma)\int_0^\infty \eta(\alpha)d\alpha - 1. \tag{22}$$

The uninfected state is stable for $\mathcal{R}_0 < 1$ *and unstable for* $\mathcal{R}_0 > 1$.

In the special case where the coefficient $\kappa(\alpha)$ is constant we can integrate (19a) and, using (19b), we obtain a system of linear equations for the variables

$$\bar{u} = \int_0^\infty u d\alpha, \quad \bar{q} = \int_0^\infty q d\alpha, \quad \bar{\eta} = \int_0^\infty \eta d\alpha,$$

namely

$$\begin{aligned} (\bar{\mu} + \rho + \lambda)\bar{u} &= (\mu + \sigma)\bar{q} + (\bar{\mu} + \sigma)\bar{\eta}, \\ (\mu + \bar{\mu} + \sigma + \kappa + \lambda)\bar{q} &= \rho\bar{u}, \\ (2\bar{\mu} + \sigma + \lambda)\bar{\eta} &= 2\kappa\bar{q}. \end{aligned} \tag{23}$$

Equations (23) represent the eigenvalue problem of the matrix

$$C = \begin{pmatrix} -(\bar{\mu} + \rho) & \mu + \sigma & \bar{\mu} + \sigma \\ \rho & -(\bar{\mu} + \mu + \sigma + \kappa) & 0 \\ 0 & 2\kappa & -(2\bar{\mu} + \sigma) \end{pmatrix}. \tag{24}$$

This problem has been derived in Hadeler and Ngoma (1990), formula (4.31). The matrix C has nonnegative off-diagonal elements. Hence the Perron-Frobenius theory applies. There is a positive eigenvector which corresponds to the eigenvalue with maximal real part. Thus in the case of constant κ the spectral problem (19) reduces to an eigenvalue problem of a matrix. Notice that the matrix of the differential equation (19a) and the matrix C differ by a factor "2" in the second element of the third row.

Now we return to the case of a variable coefficient $\kappa(\alpha)$. Adding the equations (19a) one finds that

$$u(\alpha) + q(\alpha) + \eta(\alpha) = e^{-(\bar{\mu}+\lambda)\alpha}\big(u(0) + q(0) + \eta(0)\big).$$

Thus one can reduce the problem to

$$\begin{aligned} \tilde{u}_\alpha + \rho\tilde{u} &= (\mu + \sigma)\tilde{q} + (\bar{\mu} + \sigma)\tilde{\eta}, \\ \tilde{q}_\alpha + (\mu + \sigma)\tilde{q} &= \rho\tilde{u} - \kappa(\alpha)\tilde{q}, \\ \tilde{\eta}_\alpha + (\bar{\mu} + \sigma)\tilde{\eta} &= \kappa(\alpha)\tilde{q}, \end{aligned} \tag{25a}$$

$$\tilde{u}(0) = 0, \quad \tilde{q}(0) = 0, \quad \tilde{\eta}(0) = \int_0^\infty \kappa(\alpha)e^{-(\bar{\mu}+\lambda)\alpha}\tilde{q}(\alpha)d\alpha. \tag{25b}$$

This problem is essentially two-dimensional. It is not obvious that the general case of (25) can be further reduced.

Now consider the special case where $\bar{\mu} = \mu$. We introduce a new variable

$$w = q + \eta \tag{26}$$

and find that the variables u and w satisfy a linear system with constant coefficients

$$\begin{pmatrix} u \\ w \end{pmatrix}_\alpha = \begin{pmatrix} -(\mu+\rho+\lambda) & \mu+\sigma \\ \rho & -\tilde{\sigma} \end{pmatrix} \begin{pmatrix} u \\ w \end{pmatrix}. \tag{27}$$

The eigenvalues of the matrix are $-(\mu+\lambda)$ and $-(\tilde{\sigma}+\rho)$. Thus the general solution is

$$\begin{pmatrix} u \\ w \end{pmatrix} = c_1 \begin{pmatrix} \mu+\sigma \\ \rho \end{pmatrix} e^{-(\mu+\lambda)\alpha} + c_2 \begin{pmatrix} -1 \\ 1 \end{pmatrix} e^{-(\tilde{\sigma}+\rho)\alpha}.$$

We are interested in the solution which satisfies the initial conditions $u(0) = 0$, $w(0) = 1$ which is

$$\begin{aligned} u(\alpha) &= \frac{\mu+\sigma}{\mu+\sigma+\rho}\left(e^{-(\mu+\lambda)\alpha} - e^{-(\tilde{\sigma}+\rho)\alpha}\right), \\ w(\alpha) &= \frac{1}{\mu+\sigma+\rho}\left(\rho e^{-(\mu+\lambda)\alpha} + (\mu+\sigma)e^{-(\tilde{\sigma}+\rho)\alpha}\right). \end{aligned} \tag{28}$$

We use the explicit representation of u to find an explicit formula for q from the second equation in (19a),

$$q(\alpha) = \frac{\rho(\mu+\sigma)}{\mu+\sigma+\rho}\int_0^\alpha e^{-\int_\tau^\alpha(\tilde{\sigma}+\kappa(\nu))d\nu}\left(e^{-(\mu+\lambda)\tau} - e^{-(\tilde{\sigma}+\rho)\tau}\right)d\tau\cdot\eta(0). \tag{29}$$

This expression can be introduced into the last condition of (19b),

$$1 = \frac{\rho(\sigma+\mu)}{\sigma+\mu+\rho}\int_0^\infty \kappa(\alpha)\int_0^\alpha e^{-\int_\tau^\alpha(\tilde{\sigma}+\kappa(\nu))d\nu}\left(e^{-(\mu+\lambda)\tau} - e^{-(\tilde{\sigma}+\rho)\tau}\right)d\tau d\alpha.$$

By simple manipulations we arrive at the characteristic equation

$$\begin{aligned} \frac{\rho(\mu+\sigma)}{\mu+\sigma+\rho}\int_0^\infty \kappa(\alpha)e^{-\lambda\alpha}\int_0^\alpha & e^{-(2\mu+\sigma)(\alpha-\tau)-\int_\tau^\alpha \kappa(\nu)d\nu} \\ & \times\left(e^{-\mu\tau} - e^{-(2\mu+\sigma+\rho)\tau}\right)d\tau d\alpha = 1. \end{aligned} \tag{30}$$

Equation (30) can be applied in several ways.

First of all it is a characteristic equation which governs the stability of the uninfected exponential solution. This solution is linearly stable if the roots λ satisfy the inequality $Re(\lambda - \hat{\lambda}) < 0$. Hence the critical situation occurs when the characteristic equation has the root $\lambda = \hat{\lambda}$, i.e., when

$$\begin{aligned} \frac{\rho(\mu+\sigma)}{\mu+\sigma+\rho}\int_0^\infty \kappa(\alpha)e^{-\hat{\lambda}\alpha}\int_0^\alpha & e^{-(2\mu+\sigma)(\alpha-\tau)-\int_\tau^\alpha \kappa(\nu)d\nu} \\ & \times\left(e^{-\mu\tau} - e^{-(2\mu+\sigma+\rho)\tau}\right)d\tau d\alpha = 1. \end{aligned} \tag{31}$$

Equation (31) is the threshold condition on the parameters.

Since many other studies consider the case of constant population size, we look at that case in more detail. For constant population size we have $\hat{\lambda} = 0$. Then the condition (31) reads

$$\frac{\rho(\mu+\sigma)}{\mu+\sigma+\rho}\int_0^\infty \kappa(\alpha)\int_0^\alpha e^{-(2\mu+\sigma)(\alpha-\tau)-\int_\tau^\alpha \kappa(\nu)d\nu} \times \left(e^{-\mu\tau} - e^{-(2\mu+\sigma+\rho)\tau}\right) d\tau d\alpha = 1. \tag{32}$$

The left hand side of equation (32) is the basic reproduction number $\mathcal{R}_0$.

One cannot immediately see that the expression (32) is monotone in κ, as it should be. By partial integration one can transform the equation and obtain

Result 4: *In the case $\bar{\mu} = \mu$ the basic reproduction number is given by*

$$\mathcal{R}_0 = \frac{\rho(\mu+\sigma)}{\mu+\sigma+\rho}\left[\frac{\mu+\sigma+\rho}{\mu(2\mu+\sigma+\rho)} - (2\mu+\sigma) \times \int_0^\infty\int_0^\alpha e^{-(2\mu+\sigma)(\alpha-\tau)-\int_\tau^\alpha \kappa(\nu)d\nu}\left(e^{-\mu\tau} - e^{-(2\mu+\sigma+\rho)\tau}\right) d\tau d\alpha\right]. \tag{33}$$

From this representation one sees the monotonicity immediately.

In the case of constant κ equation (30) is equivalent to the cubic equation

$$\frac{\kappa\rho(\sigma+\mu)}{(2\mu+\sigma+\kappa+\lambda)(\mu+\lambda)(2\mu+\sigma+\rho+\lambda)} = 1. \tag{34}$$

This equation has been discussed in detail by Hadeler and Ngoma (1990).

Of course the assumption $\bar{\mu} = \mu$ is not realistic for the HIV infection. Nevertheless this special case throws some light on how the system might behave in the general case.

We return to the general case. We discuss a slight extension of the model and the results. In Dietz and Hadeler (1988) there is a discussion how a pair should be defined. These authors had defined that a pair starts with one sexual contact (with a probability of transmission if one partner is susceptible and the other infected). If this definition is applied all equations from problem (9) onward have to be slightly modified. We have to interpret the parameter $\kappa(\alpha)$ as the product of a contact rate (assumed constant) and a transmission probability (variable) and we have to account for those newly formed pairs in which infection occurs at the first instant. In order to keep the notation of Dietz and Hadeler (1988) we call the transmission probability $h(\alpha)$ and the contact rate β (not to be confused with the independent variable used earlier). Then the system corresponding to (19) reads

$$\begin{aligned} u_\alpha + (\bar{\mu} + \rho + \lambda)u &= (\sigma + \mu)q + (\sigma + \bar{\mu})\eta, \\ q_\alpha + (\mu + \bar{\mu} + \sigma + \lambda)q &= \rho(1 - h(\alpha))u - \beta h(\alpha)q, \qquad (35a) \\ \eta_\alpha + (2\bar{\mu} + \sigma + \lambda)\eta &= \rho h(\alpha)u + \beta h(\alpha)q, \end{aligned}$$

$$u(0) = 0, \quad q(0) = 0, \quad \eta(0) = \int_0^\infty h(\alpha)\big(\beta h(\alpha)q(\alpha) + \rho u(\alpha)\big)d\alpha. \qquad (35b)$$

We repeat how the basic reproduction number (for constant population size) can be computed from this three-dimensional problem. Solve the initial value problem of (35a) (with $\lambda = 0$) for the initial condition $u(0) = 0$, $q(0) = 0$, $\eta(0) = 1$, and compute

$$\mathcal{R}_0 = \int_0^\infty h(\alpha)\big(\beta q(\alpha) + \rho u(\alpha)\big)d\alpha. \qquad (36)$$

Since (19) or (35) is just a simple linear system it should be easy to discuss the qualitative dependence of the basic reproduction number on the model parameters, in particular to check whether the basic reproduction number depends in a monotone way on the infection rate κ, also in the case of differential mortality $\bar{\mu} > \mu$. So far we have not been able to give an analytic proof.

K.Dietz has asked whether there is a systematic change in the basic reproduction number for nonconstant infectivity, in particular if the basic reproduction number for $\kappa(\alpha)$ can be compared with the basic reproduction number for the constant $\bar{\kappa} = \bar{\mu}\int_0^\infty \kappa(\alpha)\exp(-\bar{\mu}\alpha)d\alpha$. We have studied simple cases with computer simulation where $\kappa(\alpha)$ assumes large values near $\alpha = 0$ and for large α, and small values in an intermediate interval. We have chosen $\mu = 0.1$, $\bar{\mu} = 0.25$, $\rho = 1$, $\sigma = 1.9$, and

$$\kappa(\alpha) = \begin{cases} \kappa_0 & \text{if } \alpha \notin (\alpha_1, \alpha_2), \\ \kappa_0 - \kappa_1 & \text{if } \alpha \in [\alpha_1, \alpha_2], \end{cases}$$

depending on four parameters $\alpha_1, \alpha_2, \kappa_0, \kappa_1$. Fig.1 shows $\mathcal{R}_0$ as a function of α_2, where $\kappa_0 = 1.1$, $\kappa_1 = 1.0$, $\alpha_1 = 3$, and α_2 ranges from 3 to 20 in equidistant steps. Fig.2 shows $\mathcal{R}_0$ as a function of κ_1. Here $\alpha_1 = 3$, $\alpha_2 = 20$, $\kappa_0 = 2$, and κ_1 ranges from 0 to κ_0. In both cases $\mathcal{R}_0$ (continuous line) is a decreasing function of the parameter, and the corresponding value for constant κ (dashed line) is indeed larger. Hence it seems that variable infectivity leads to a lower basic reproduction number.

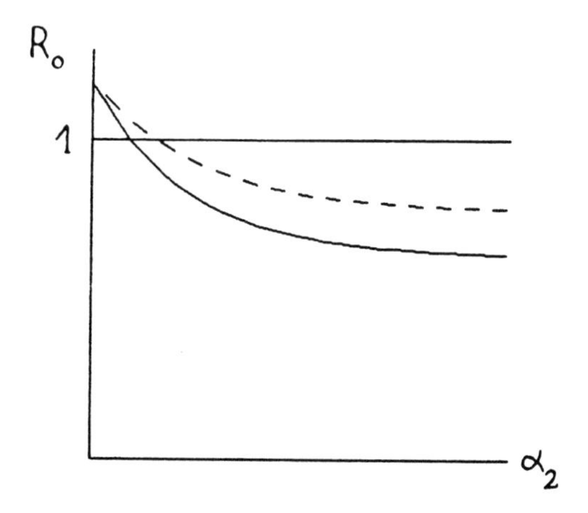

Fig.1: Dependence of $\mathcal{R}_0$ on α_2

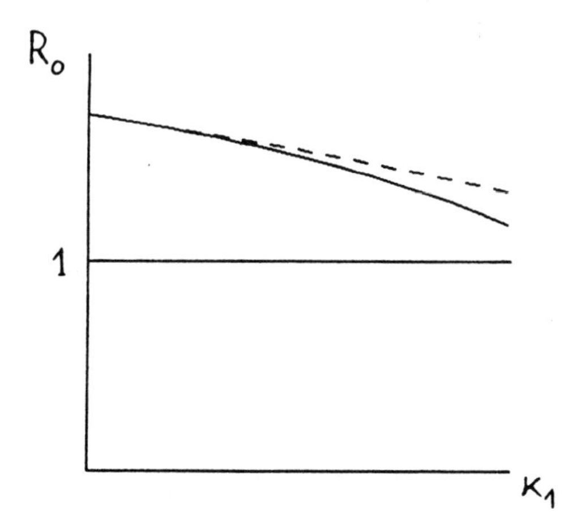

Fig.2: Dependence of $\mathcal{R}_0$ on κ_1

Acknowledgement: The author thanks Johannes Müller for extensive discussions.

References

Arbogast, T., Milner F.A. (1989) A finite-difference method for a two-sex model of population dynamics. SIAM J. Numer. Anal. 26, 1474-1486

Busenberg, S., Castillo-Chavez, C. (1989) Interaction, pair formation and force of infection in sexually transmitted diseases. In: C. Castillo-Chavez (1989), 289-300

Busenberg, S., Hadeler, K.P. (1990) Demography and epidemics. Math. Biosc. 101, 63-74

Castillo-Chavez, C. (Ed.) (1989) Mathematical and Statistical Approaches to AIDS Epidemiology. Lecture Notes in Biomath. 83, Springer Verlag

Castillo-Chavez, C., Blythe, S.P. (1989) Mixing framework for social/sexual behavior. In: Castillo-Chavez (1989), 275-285

Castillo-Chavez, C., Cooke, K., Huang, Levin, S.A. (1989) Results on the dynamics for models for the sexual transmission of the human immunodeficiency virus. Applied Math. Letters 2, 327-331

Dietz, K. (1987) Epidemiological models for sexually transmitted infections. Proc. First World Congress Bernoulli Soc., Tashkent 1986, Vol. II, 539-542, VNU Science Press, Utrecht

Dietz, K. (1988) On the transmission dynamics of HIV. Math.Biosc. 90, 397-414

Dietz, K., Hadeler, K.P. (1988) Epidemiological models for sexually transmitted diseases. J. Math. Biol. 26, 1-25

Feller, W. (1941) On the integral equation of renewal theory. Ann. Math. Stat. 12, 243-267

Hadeler, K.P. (1989a) Pair formation in age structured populations. Proc. Workshop on Selected Topics in Biomathematics (eds. A.Kurzhanskij, K. Sigmund) Laxenburg, Austria 1987, Acta Appl.Math. 14, 91-102

Hadeler, K.P. (1989b) Modeling AIDS in structured populations. Bull. Int. Stat. Inst. 53, Book 1, 83-99

Hadeler, K.P. (1990) Homogeneous delay equations and models for pair formation. Preprint Center for Dynamical Systems, Georgia Institute of Technology, J.Math.Biol, to appear.

Hadeler, K.P. (1992) Periodic solutions of homogeneous equations. J.Diff. Equ. 95, 183-202

Hadeler, K.P., Ngoma, K. (1990) Homogeneous models for sexually transmitted diseases. Rocky Mtn. J. Math. 20, 967-986

Hadeler, K.P., Waldstätter, R., Wörz-Busekros, A. (1988) Models for pair formation in bisexual populations. J. Math. Biol. 26, 635-649

Hoppensteadt, F. (1975) Mathematical Theories of Populations: Demographics, Genetics and Epidemics. Regional Conference Series in Applied Mathematics 20, SIAM, Philadelphia

Jacquez, J.A., Simon, C.P., Koopman, J., Sattenspiel, L., Perry, T. (1988) Modeling and analysing HIV transmission: The effect of contact patterns. Math. Biosc. 92, 119-199

Jacquez, J.A., Simon, C.P., Koopman, J., Structured Mixing: Heterogeneous mixing by the definition of activity groups. In: C. Castillo-Chavez (1989), 301-315

Kendall, D.G. (1949) Stochastic processes and population growth. J. Roy. Statist. Soc. Ser.B., 11, 230-264

Keyfitz, N. (1985) Applied Mathematical Demography, 2nd ed., Springer Verlag

Kuczynski, R.R. (1932) Fertility and Reproduction. p. 36-38, New York, Falcon Press
Lotka, A.J. (1922) The stability of the normal age distribution. Proc. Nat. Acad. Sci. 8, 339-345
McKendrick, A.G. (1926) Applications of mathematics to medical problems. Proc. Edinb. Math. Soc. 44, 98-130 (1926)
Ng, T.W., Anderson, R.M. (1989) A model for the demographic impact of AIDS in devoloping countries: Age-dependent choice of sexual partners. Bull. Int. Stat. Inst. 53, Book 4, 425-448
Parlett, B. (1972) Can there be a marriage function? In: T.N.T.Greville (Ed.) Population Dynamics, Academic Press
Sattenspiel, L., Simon, C.P. (1988) The spread and persistence of infectious diseases in structured populations. Math. Biosc. 90, 341-366
Sharpe, F.R., Lotka, A.J. (1911) A problem in age distribution. Phil.Mag. 21, 435-438
Thieme, H.R., Castillo-Chavez, C. (1989) On the role of variable infectivity in the dynamics of the human immunodeficiency virus epidemic. In: Castillo-Chavez (1989), 157-176
Waldstätter, R. (1989) Pair formation in sexually transmitted diseases. In: C. Castillo-Chavez (1989), 260-274
Waldstätter, R. (1990) Models for Pair formation with Applications to Demography and Epidemiology. Dissertation Universität Tübingen 1990
Webb, G.F. (1985) Theory of Nonlinear Age-dependent Population Dynamics. M. Dekker
Yellin, J., Samuelson, P.A. (1974) A dynamical model for human population. Proc.Nat. Acad.Sci. USA 71, No.7, 2813-2817

Universität Tübingen
Lehrstuhl für Biomathematik
Auf der Morgenstelle 10
D-7400 Tübingen

WEAK LINKAGE BETWEEN HIV EPIDEMICS IN HOMOSEXUAL MEN AND INTRAVENOUS DRUG USERS

Herbert W. Hethcote and James W. Van Ark

Summary

Since homosexual men who are also intravenous drug users interact sexually with homosexual men and share needles with intravenous drug users, they are a potential transfer linkage between the HIV epidemics in homosexual men and intravenous drug users. One theory is that these HIV epidemics are not crucially linked by homosexual intravenous drug users so that neither epidemic is feeding or sustaining the other. A simulation model with HIV transmission and progression to AIDS is formulated for three risk groups. Evidence based on fitting this model to AIDS incidence data in New York City supports the theory that neither HIV epidemic sustains the other. Thus the HIV epidemics in homosexual men and intravenous drug users are only weakly linked and can be modeled as separate epidemics.

1. Introduction

The largest number of AIDS cases in the United States have occurred in homosexual men and intravenous drug users (IVDUs). The transmission mechanisms for HIV in these groups are needle-sharing between IVDUs and homosexual intercourse. Since homosexual men who are also IVDUs have both possible transmission mechanisms and interact with both homosexual men and IVDUs, they could be an important transmission link between these two groups. It is conceivable that a primary HIV epidemic in one of these groups could sustain a secondary HIV epidemic in the other group through the linkage provided by the homosexual IVDUs. The goal of this paper is to evaluate the relative importance of HIV transmissions by homosexual IVDUs and to decide if they form an essential linkage between the HIV epidemics in homosexual men and IVDUs.

A geographic analysis of where HIV epidemics in homosexual men and IVDUs are occurring together and separately suggests that these epidemics are not strongly connected. Major HIV epidemics in homosexual men are occurring throughout the United States, but major epidemics in IVDUs are focused in the Northeast region of the U.S. (NE region). If epidemics in homosexual men generally sustained epidemics in IVDUs, then there would be major epidemics in IVDUs throughout the U.S., and this has not occurred. If HIV epidemics in IVDUs generally sustained HIV epidemics in homosexual men, then the minor epidemics in IVDUs outside the NE region would probably cause only minor HIV epidemics in homosexual men in these areas, and this has not occurred since there are major HIV epidemics in homosexual men in many places outside the NE region. Thus it does not appear likely that HIV epidemics in either homosexual men or IVDUs are supporting HIV epidemics in the other. It is possible that the reason why major HIV epidemics in IVDUs are occurring in the NE region but not elsewhere is that the needle-sharing and other IVDU behaviors are different in the NE region. Thus it seems desirable to investigate possible connections between epidemics in homosexual men and IVDUs more thoroughly in the NE region. The most AIDS cases in the NE region occur in New York City (NYC), so it seems appropriate to use NYC to test the theory that the epidemics are essentially independent and separate.

During the early phase of the HIV epidemic in homosexual men and IVDUs, the HIV transmission process was probably like a random or stochastic process. In this early phase the homosexual IVDUs may have been involved in the seeding of HIV in the populations of homosexual men and IVDUs (Battjes, Dickens and Amsel, 1989). The stochastic nature of the beginning of the HIV epidemic is not of interest here. The main concern is the role of homosexual IVDUs when the epidemics are established and growing. Although many simplifying assumptions are necessary in order to use a deterministic model for an HIV epidemic, this type of model is well-suited as a quantitative descriptor of an epidemiological process. A deterministic HIV epidemiological model has been developed for a population of homosexual men in Hethcote, Van Ark, and Longini (1991) and applied to homosexual men in San Francisco in Hethcote, Van Ark, and Karon (1991). This model is generalized here to the three risk groups: homosexual men, homosexual IVDUs, and IVDUs. Then this model is used to explore the importance of homosexual-IVDUs in connecting the HIV epidemics in homosexual men and IVDUs.

How can one test the theory that the HIV epidemics in homosexual men and IVDUs are not crucially linked by homosexual IVDUs and are essentially separate epidemics? The approach used here is to first fit one risk group models to the AIDS incidence data in NYC for homosexual men and IVDUs separately; then the three risk group model for homosexual men, homosexual IVDUs, and IVDUs is fit to the AIDS incidence data. If the parameter values and the general pattern of HIV incidences obtained in the simultaneous fitting of the three risk groups are similar to those obtained in the separate fits, then the homosexual IVDUs are not a crucial link between the other two groups, and their HIV epidemics can be treated separately.

The model for the progression of HIV-infected persons to AIDS in Section 2 is based on CD4 cell counts. The model of Hethcote, Van Ark, and Longini (1991) for HIV transmission dynamics in a population of homosexual men is described briefly in Section 3 and extended to a model for the three risk groups linked by homosexual and needle-sharing contacts in Section 4.

Information on HIV and AIDS in NYC is given in Section 5, and parameter values are estimated in Section 6. Fits of the one group model to the NYC populations of homosexual men and IVDUs are found in Sections 7 and 8. Section 9 presents the simultaneous fitting to the AIDS incidence data for the three risk groups. A key conclusion in Section 10 is that the HIV epidemics in homosexual men and IVDUs are not strongly connected by the homosexual IVDUs. Thus the HIV epidemics in homosexual men and IVDUs can be modeled separately. This separation of the HIV epidemics in homosexual men and IVDUs is likely to also hold in racial/ethnic subgroups and in other regions.

2. Modeling the Progression of HIV-Infected Persons to AIDS

Since people who are infected with HIV seem to progress through various stages or phases towards AIDS and death due to AIDS (Redfield et al., 1986; Seligman et al., 1987), a natural model for this progression is through a sequence of five clinical phases (Hethcote, 1987; Longini et al., 1989, 1990). The first phase is the pre-antibody period, in which a person is infected, but not antibody seropositive. The second phase includes persons who are infected and antibody seropositive, but are asymptomatic. The third phase (symptomatic) occurs when the person develops an abnormal hematologic indicator and/or prodromal illnesses such as persistent generalized lymphadenopathy or oral candidiasis. The fourth phase is clinical AIDS, and the fifth phase is death due to AIDS. A progression model using stages based on these clinical phases was presented in Hethcote, Van Ark, and Longini (1991) and used in Hethcote, Van Ark, and Karon (1991) for modeling HIV/AIDS in homosexual men in San Francisco.

As information about the effects of HIV on the immune system has accumulated, it has become clear that the progress towards AIDS coincides with a decline in the number of $CD4^+$ T-lymphocytes (T4 cells). Thus T4 cell count intervals can be used as stages and the progression through these stages can be measured. Longini et al. (1991) have used a continuous-time Markov process to model the decline of T4 cells in HIV-infected persons. A staged progression model based on T4 cell counts is probably more precise since it is based on quantitative laboratory measurements instead of clinical symptoms.

The $CD4^+$ T-lymphocytes (T4 cells) are a primary target of HIV in the host, and the decline in T4 cells is an important indicator of progression towards AIDS. Longini et al. (1991) defined six stages of HIV infection

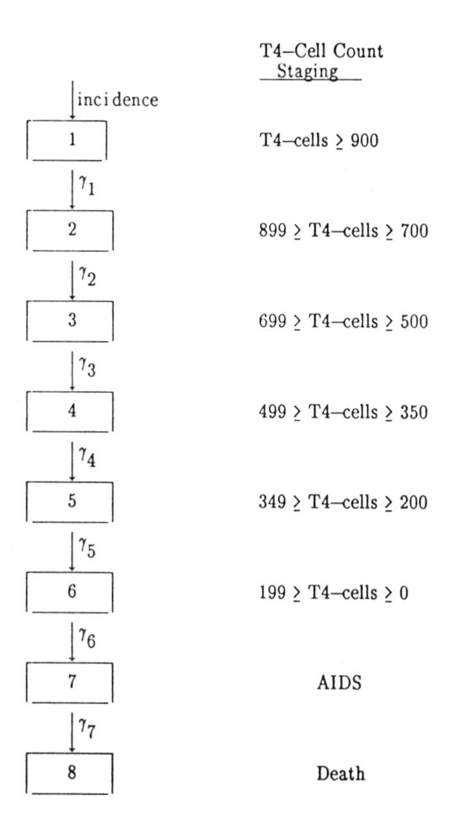

Figure 2.1. The staged model based on T4-cell counts for progression to AIDS and death when there are 7 infectious stages (6 stages before AIDS).

for individuals who have not yet been diagnosed with AIDS (technically, who have developed an opportunistic infection corresponding to the Walter Reed stage six (Redfield et al., 1986)). These six stages correspond to T4 cell count intervals given in Figure 2.1 and Table 2.1. The transition rates between these stages were estimated from data on 1796 HIV-positive individuals in the United States Army using a continuous-time Markov process model. The transition rate constants and mean waiting times are given in Table 2.1.

The estimated mean waiting time from seroconversion to when the T4 cell count is persistently below 500 is 4.1 years, the mean waiting time until it is below 200 is 8.0 years, and the mean waiting time from seroconversion to AIDS diagnosis (technically, diagnosis with Walter Reed stage 6 opportunistic infection) is 9.6 years. The data were also analyzed for three age groups (≤ 25, 26–30, and > 30), and although the progression rates were the same for T4 cell counts ≥ 500, the two older groups progressed faster when T4 cell counts were < 500. Although age is a cofactor, it is not considered in our model.

It seems likely that T4 cell counts will become the most widely used marker for HIV progression. They are currently used as indicators for starting zidovudine, other antiviral treatments and PCP prophylaxis with aerosol pentamidine. The T4 cell counts will probably also be used as surrogate endpoints can significantly shorten the clinical trials needed for testing and approval of drugs and vaccines (Machado, Gail and Ellenberg, 1990).

Table 2.1. Estimated parameters, γ, and mean waiting times, μ, in each stage of infection with no cofactors. Standard errors are in parentheses.

Stage i	T4–cell count interval	Transition rate $\hat{\gamma}_i$ in months^{-1}	Mean waiting time $\hat{\mu}_i$ in years	Cum. waiting time in years
1	> 899	0.0764 (0.0051)	1.1 (0.1)	1.1 (0.1)
2	700 – 899	0.0665 (0.0033)	1.3 (0.1)	2.4 (0.1)
3	500 – 699	0.0499 (0.0021)	1.7 (0.1)	4.1 (0.1)
4	350 – 499	0.0429 (0.0019)	1.9 (0.1)	6.0 (0.1)
5	200 – 349	0.0408 (0.0022)	2.0 (0.1)	8.0 (0.2)
6	1 – 199	0.0529 (0.0035)	1.6 (0.1)	9.6 (0.2)

Payne et al. (1989) reported a median survival time of 12.5 months for 4524 AIDS patients in SF between July 1981 and December 1987. Survival time is the time from diagnosis of AIDS to death. Lemp et al. (1990) reported a median survival time of 12.1 months for patients in the SF Vaccine Trial Cohort; but this was 14.4 months for patients diagnosed in 1986 and 1987 (presumably due to therapy or better care). Thus the median survival time of AIDS patients (without therapy) seems to be approximately one year. In the modeling here a 12.5 month median survival time is used; this corresponds to a mean survival time of 18.0 months, and a transition rate constant equal to 0.0555. This transition rate constant has no effect on AIDS incidence, but it does affect the AIDS prevalence and the AIDS death rate. The incidence of a condition such as HIV infection or developing AIDS is the number of persons contracting the condition per unit time, which is not the same as the prevalence, which is the number of people with the condition at the given time.

3. The HIV Transmission Dynamics Model for Homosexual Men

Individuals are either susceptible to HIV infection or infectious. The infectious period is unknown, but the virus seems to persist in the host indefinitely since it can be isolated from the blood for many years after the infection (Curran et al., 1988). No evidence to the contrary exists; therefore HIV infectivity is assumed to continue for life. The population considered first consists of homosexual men who change male sex partners frequently, i.e., at least once every few years. This group is subdivided into men who have many different male sex partners (very active) and those who have only a few different partners (active). Although some modelers have used more sexual activity levels or risk groups in theoretical studies (Jacquez et al., 1988; Blythe and Anderson, 1988; Castillo-Chavez et al., 1989; Kaplan and Lee, 1990), the two activity levels used here do not introduce lots of parameters which cannot be estimated and are consistent with the existence of a small fraction of homosexual men who are very active sexually.

Consider the flow diagram for homosexual men shown in Figure 3.1. Table 3.1 contains a list of the parameters and variables used in the model. For simplicity, the number of infectious stages shown in Figure 3.1 is four instead of the seven stages shown in Figure 2.1. The population size is Q, the number of very active men is $QV = F \times Q$, and the number of active men is $QA = (1 - F) \times Q$. The numbers of susceptible persons are SV and SA for the very active and active groups, respectively. The five compartments X(I) in Figure 3.1 correspond to four infectious stages (including the AIDS stage) and the death stage among very active people while the compartments Y(I) are analogous for active people. The sum of the left column of compartments in Figure 3.1 is always QV and the sum of the middle column is QA so that the very active and active population sizes are conserved.

Men in the first three Z(I) compartments are those who have moved from the region after they were infected with HIV. When men in these three Z(I) compartments eventually develop AIDS, they are placed in the ZAIDS compartment. The compartment Z(4) consists of those who emigrated from the region after they had AIDS but who would still be counted as local AIDS cases. The compartments X(5), Y(5) and Z(5) contain men who have died of AIDS, and the transfers between these compartments are merely to balance the flows so that the total very active and active populations remain constant. Since men who have died of AIDS are included in the total very active and active population sizes, the fraction of these populations which are still alive and sexually active will decrease as more men in those populations die.

Natural deaths (not related to HIV infection) occur in each compartment with rate constant μ with balancing inflows μQV and μQA into the susceptible compartments. Let δ be the turnover rate constant corresponding to the normal migration of sexually active homosexual men. The

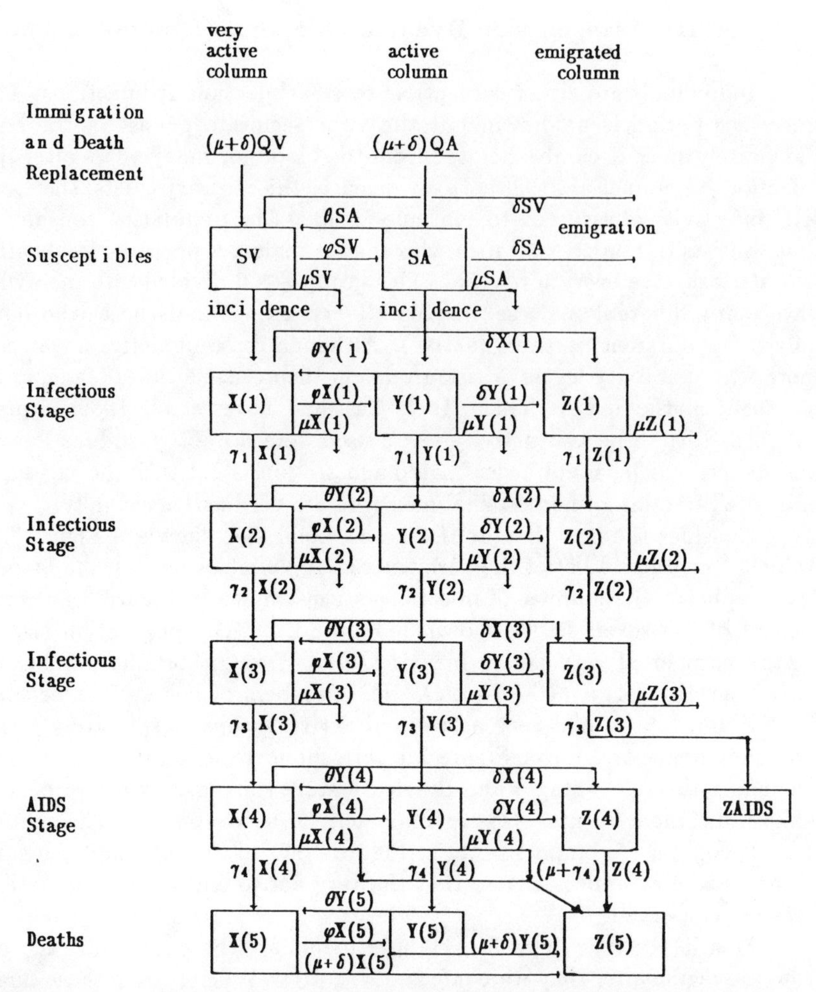

Figure 3.1. Diagram with compartments and transfers in the simulation model.

emigrations from the very active and active groups are balanced by immigration δQV and δQA into the very active and active susceptibles. In addition to geographic migration, the turnover could also be due to initiation or cessation of homosexual activity. The transfer rate constant of Font IBMcorresponds to the natural movement of homosexual men from sexually very active status to active status. There are balancing transfers from the active to the very active compartments with a transfer rate constant of $\theta = \varphi \times QV/QA$.

As in Section 2, the parameters γ_i in Figure 3.1 govern the movement through the stages of HIV infection to AIDS and death due to AIDS. These transfer rate constants correspond to negative exponential waiting times in the compartments with mean waiting times equal to $1/\gamma_i$. Based on similarities to the clinical staging model used in Hethcote, Van Ark, and Longini (1991), stages 2 to 3 in Figure 2.1 are called asymptomatic and stages 4 to 6 are called symptomatic. People in stage 1 may have an acute influenza-like illness in a pre-antibody phase.

Table 3.1. List of parameters and variables.

Population Size and Turnover Rate Constants

- Q = total population size
- F = fraction of population who are sexually very active
- R = ratio of partnership rates for very active and active men
- μ = natural mortality rate constant
- δ = migration rate constant
- ϕ = transfer rate constant from very active to active states

Stages of the Infection

- m = number of infectious stages
- γ_k = rate constant for progression from stage k to stage k+1
- ω_k = relative infectivity of stage k men compared with asymptomatic men
- ρ_k = relative sexual activity of stage k men compared with asymptomatic men

Sexual Activity

- STD = starting date of the epidemic
- QH = probability of transmission to partners by infected asymptomatic men
- PAS = average number of partners per month at start
- STR = starting date for reduction in average number of partners per month
- STP = stopping date for reductions
- RDN = yearly reduction factor
- η = fraction of new partnerships distributed by proportionate mixing

Variables (functions of time)

- SV = number of susceptible very active men
- SA = number of susceptible active men
- X(k) = number of very active men in stage k
- Y(k) = number of active men in stage k
- Z(k) = number of emigrated men in stage k

Individuals in some phases cease sexual activity or adopt protective measures when they learn of their HIV status because of a desire to avoid infecting others; others cease sexual activity because they are ill due to HIV-related symptoms. Let PA be the average number of partners per month for asymptomatic infected men. Let ρ_k be the relative sexual activity of those in stage k compared to asymptomatic infected men, so $\rho_k PA$ is the average number of homosexual partners per month for stage k infected men.

The infectiousness of individuals in the stages leading to AIDS seems to vary. People in the pre-antibody, symptomatic and AIDS stages seem to be more infectious than people in the asymptomatic stages (Longini et al., 1989). If QH is the probability of transmission of HIV infection to a partner by an infected asymptomatic man and ω_k is the relative infectivity of those in stage k, normalized so $\omega_k = 1$ for asymptomatics, then the probability of transmission for infected persons in stage k is $\omega_k QH$. All of the ω_k are equal for men in the symptomatic stages. Since there are many types of sexual interactions in a homosexual partnership, QH is a simplified composite or average of many factors such as the numbers and types (anal, oral, receptive, insertive, unprotected, safer) of contacts per partner. Although very active people may tend to have shorter length partnerships with fewer contacts than active people, the contacts of very active people may have higher risk of transmission. The quantity QH is really the proportion of partners of infected asymptomatic men who are infected, but it is usually called the probability of transmission.

Data on sexual behavior and gonococcal proctitis for homosexual men in large cities suggest that partnership formation rates for homosexual men have changed (CDC; 1990a, 1990b). A simple way to model this phenomenon is to assume that the average number PA of different partners per month is first constant, then decreases as a geometric sequence, and then is constant again. A geometric sequence is the discrete approximation to a negative exponential decrease in partnership rates suggested by the gonococcal proctitus data in SF (Pickering et al., 1986; Hessol et al., 1989; Kohn, personal communication, 1990). In the model, the number of partners per month before reduction starts is PAS, the date at which reduction starts is STR, the date at which reduction stops is STP, and the yearly reduction factor is RDN. The number of different partners per month is $PH = PA/(1 + F(R - 1))$ for the fraction $1 - F$ of the population which is active and $R \times PH$ for the fraction F which is very active. The monthly effective contact rate is the product of the contact rate (the number of different partners per month) and the proportion of partnerships resulting in transmission.

One method of specifying the contact rates between subpopulations in an epidemiological model is with proportionate mixing (Hethcote and Yorke, 1984; Nold, 1980; Dietz and Schenzle, 1985; Hethcote and Van Ark, 1987). In this method each group has a sexual activity level, and the new partners of a person are distributed among the groups in proportion to the activity levels of the groups. Alternatively, a person may be more likely to choose a sexual partner with the same level of sexual activity. This is now called preferred mixing (Jacquez et al.,1988; Blythe and Castillo-Chavez, 1989).

Since data have not been found on mixing patterns in homosexual men, a more general form of mixing is used here. Let η be the fraction of the new partnerships distributed by proportionate mixing among all groups so that the fraction $1-\eta$ of new partnerships occur internally to each group. The incidences of HIV infection in the active and very active groups due to the internal mixing in each group are, respectively,

$$\left[\sum_{i=1}^{m} (1-\eta) \times \rho_i \times PH \times \omega_i \times QH \times Y(i)\right] \times \frac{SA}{QA - Y(m+1)},$$

$$\left[\sum_{i=1}^{m} (1-\eta) \times \rho_i \times R \times PH \times \omega_i \times QH \times X(i)\right] \times \frac{SV}{QV - X(m+1)}.$$

Now consider the fraction η of new partnerships distributed by proportionate mixing among all groups (Hethcote and Van Ark, 1987, eq. 6.6). The activity levels for the active and very active subpopulations are the numbers of partners per month, PH and $R \times PH$, respectively. The average number of partnership formations in the population per month is

$$C = PH \times (QA - Y(m+1)) + R \times PH \times (QV - X(m+1))$$

so that the incidences in the active and very active subpopulations due to proportionate mixing are

$$\sum_{i=1}^{m} \eta \times \rho_i \times PH \times \omega_i \times QH \times [R \times x(i) + Y(i)] \times \frac{PH \times SA}{C},$$

$$\sum_{i=1}^{m} \eta \times \rho_i \times PH \times \omega_i \times QH \times [R \times X(i) + Y(i)] \times \frac{R \times PH \times SV}{C},$$

respectively. The total incidences in the active and very active subpopulations are the sums of the internal incidences and the external proportionate mixing incidences.

The monthly change in the number of people in a compartment in Figure 3.1 is equal to the monthly inflows minus the monthly outflows. Thus the model consists of simultaneous nonlinear difference equations corresponding to the compartments in Figure 3.1. The HIV epidemic starts with one infected person entering the very active stage 1 compartment on the starting date STD and then progresses in one-month time steps.

4. The HIV Transmission Dynamics Model for Three Risk Groups

Sections 2 and 3 have focused on modeling the transmission dynamics of HIV and the progression to AIDS for homosexual men. This model is now expanded to include three major risk groups: homosexual (and bisexual) men, homosexual (and bisexual) men who are intravenous drug users, and intravenous drug users (IVDUs). In this model the homosexual men have homosexual partnerships within their own group and also with homosexual-IVDUs. The IVDUs have needle-sharing partnerships with other IVDUs and also with homosexual-IVDUs. Figure 4.1 summarizes the risk groups and possible routes of transmission of HIV infection.

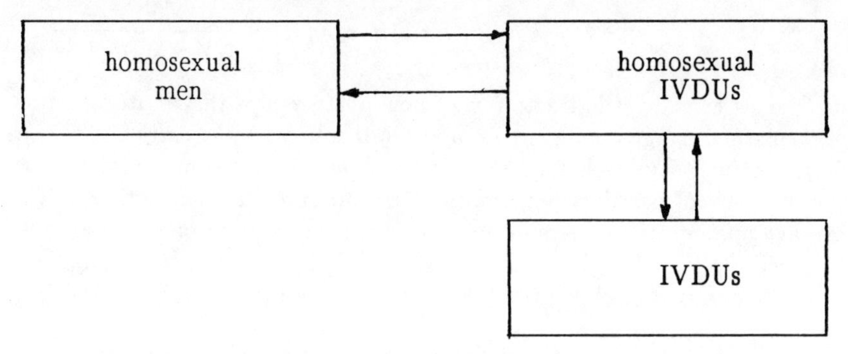

Figure 4.1. Risk groups and infection transmission connections.

Recall that the homosexual men are subdivided into active and very active subpopulations. In the modeling of homosexual men in San Francisco (SF), the 10% of the homosexual men in the very active class were ten times as sexually active as those in the active class (the parameters $F = .10$ and $R = 10$). Here the IVDU population is also subdivided into these two activity level classes based on their number of needle-sharing partners per month. The needle-sharing contacts are modeled in a way analogous to the homosexual contacts in that there is an average number of new needle-sharing partners per month and there are probabilities of transmission per new needle-sharing partner that are dependent on the stage of infection of the partner just as for homosexual partners. As indicated previously the homosexual-IVDUs have both homosexual partners and needle-sharing partners.

The progression of HIV infecteds to AIDS has been developed carefully as a sequence of stages in Section 2 and the same progression is used for all adult risk groups in this general model. The progression variables and parameters in Figure 3.1 and Table 3.1 now exist for all three risk groups: the homosexual men with suffix H, the homosexual-IVDUs with suffix B

for both, and the IVDU population with suffix D for drug user. All populations are subdivided into very active and active subgroups where the activity is either sexual or needle-sharing partnership formation. For example, the quantities for homosexual men are QVH, SVH, $XH(1), \cdots, XH(8)$, QAH, SAH, $YH(1), \cdots, YH(8)$, $ZH(1)$, $ZH(6)$ and $ZAIDSH$. The suffixes H, B, and D are also used for other parameter values. For example, QHH and QHD are the probabilities of transmission of HIV infection by an infective in an asymptomatic stage during a homosexual partnership and a needle-sharing partnership. The quantities PAH and PAD are the average number of new homosexual and needle-sharing partnerships per month.

As in the model for homosexual men, the fraction ETAD of new needle-sharing partnerships are distributed by proportionate mixing and the fraction (1 - ETAD) of new partnerships occur internally to each group. The total incidences in the active and very active subpopulations are the sums of the internal incidences and the external proportionate mixing incidences. The incidences with suffixes H and D on the variables and parameters are used for homosexual partners and needle-sharing partners. The homosexual-IVDUs are considered to have both homosexual partnerships and needle-sharing partnerships. The incidence in the homosexual-IVDUs with suffix B is the sum of both the homosexual and needle-sharing incidences.

It may seem strange to use the same form for the incidence terms for homosexual men and for IVDUs; however, this same form is based on the following similarities. People in both groups do form partnerships that consist of one or more contacts (homosexual or needle-sharing). Bath houses or gay bars might be analogous to shooting galleries as places where multiple partnerships occur. The number of contacts and duration of partnerships vary greatly in both populations so that the very active and active categories are a simplification for both populations. People in both populations can have multiple simultaneous partnerships and the incidence terms account for this somewhat since this behavior could correspond to frequent partner change. Thus the incidence term above is a simplication for both populations, but probably is reasonable for both populations.

The fit criteria of the simulations must be specified for this general model. The first criterion for the simulations is that the parameter values must be consistent with the *a priori* parameter estimates obtained from data. Since estimates of HIV incidence are generally not available, the second criterion is that the yearly AIDS incidences in the risk groups in the simulations must be close to the yearly AIDS incidence data. Many of the parameter values in the model are fixed at their estimated values, but some are allowed to vary to give the best fit. For example, the population sizes of the homosexual men and IVDUs are fixed, but the population size of the homosexual-IVDUs is varied in order to obtain the best fit to the AIDS incidence data in this population. The migration rates and natural mortality rates are fixed at the estimated values. The parameters related to the progression through the stages (λ_i for $i = 1, 2, \cdots, 7$) are all fixed and equal to the values found in Section 2. Other fixed parameter values are the probabilities (or proportions) of transmission QHH and QHD per asymptomatic partner, the parameters ω_k which multiply these QH values to determine the probability of transmission by a stage k infective and the parameters ρ_k which are the fractions still active in stage k.

The predicted AIDS cases in the three risk groups in the NYC model must be close to the delay-adjusted AIDS incidence. The number of AIDS cases per year are not linearly independent so that a hypothesis of the chi-square goodness of fit test is not satisfied. Nevertheless the chi-square value of the sum of the squares of the observed minus the expected divided by the expected values is computed as a measure of the fit. Separate chi-square sums are also computed for each of the three risk groups.

The fitting procedure involves choosing parameter values sequentially with those subject to the most uncertainty chosen last or adjusted to fit the AIDS incidence data. Fixed values are used for many parameters such as population sizes, migration rates, natural mortality rates, number of stages, stage transition rates, probabilities of transmission by asymptomatic infectives, multiplying factors for probability of transmission and fractions still active in the stages, activity level fractions and ratios, and the transfer rate constants between the activity levels.

After the parameters above are fixed, the reduction starting times (year and month) NYSTRH , NMSTRH, NYSTRD, and NMSTRD are chosen and the size NSIZEB of the homosexual-IVDU population is chosen. Rough guesses are made for six parameters:the initial average numbers of partners per month (PASH and PASD), the yearly reduction factors (RDNH and RDND) and the external mixing fractions (ETAH and ETAD). A computer program finds the values of these six parameters which minimize the sum of the chi-square values for the homosexual men, homosexual-IVDUs and IVDUs.

5. Data on HIV and AIDS Incidence in New York City

The incidences of AIDS in New York City (NYC) and San Francisco (SF) given in Table 5.1 have been adjusted for reporting delays and for the 1987 change in the AIDS surveillance definition. The delay-adjusted incidence data as reported by October 1, 1991 were supplied by John Karon and Debra Hansen in the Division of HIV/AIDS, Center for Infectious Diseases, Centers for Disease Control (CDC). Patients are said to satisfy the consistent case definition of AIDS if they have a diagnosis (definitive or presumptive) of a disease in the pre-1987 case definition. Based on a study of homosexual men in SF a procedure was developed for estimating when the nonconsistent cases would later meet the consistent case definition (Hethcote, Van Ark and Karon, 1991). This procedure has been used to obtain the total adjusted consistent cases in Table 5.1 as the sums of the consistent and the modified nonconsistent cases. The data has not been adjusted for underreporting.

Note that the pattern of yearly AIDS incidence for homosexual men in NYC is similar to the patterns for homosexual men in SF for the first five years in the sense that the ratios of incidences in succeeding years are similar. After the first five years, the AIDS incidence in homosexual men in NYC seems to grow faster than in SF. The AIDS incidence in homosexual men in SF is approximately equal to that in NYC about one year earlier so the NYC epidemic undoubtedly started earlier. A Los Angeles Times article (Steinbrook, 1988) suggested that the AIDS incidences in white homosexual men in NYC, SF and Los Angeles were reaching plateaus in about 1988. The simulation modeling in Hethcote, Van Ark, and Karon (1991) suggested that the AIDS incidence in homosexual men in SF reached a plateau in about 1989 and may decline in the future.

Table 5.1. The AIDS incidence by categories in New York City is adjusted for reporting delays and the 1987 AIDS definition change. The adjusted AIDS incidence in homosexual men in San Francisco is included for comparison.

Year	homosexual men	homosexual IVDUs	IVDUs	homosexual men–SF
1979	5	1	0	0
1980	23	3	5	2
1981	95	9	21	22
1982	272	45	115	86
1983	577	73	276	228
1984	1017	82	503	442
1985	1463	142	871	678
1986	2068	167	1314	1010
1987	2321	206	1754	1275
1988	2489	174	2326	1285
1989	2451	180	2542	1338
1990	2378	158	2895	1551

The pattern for about the first five years for AIDS incidence in IVDUs in NYC is similar to that for homosexual men in NYC one year earlier, but after five years the incidence in IVDUs continues to grow instead of leveling off or reaching a peak. Indeed, the AIDS incidence in IVDUs jumps significantly in 1988 and then increases slowly. The AIDS incidence in homosexual-IVDUs in NYC is roughly 7 to 9% of that in homosexual men with larger differences in a few years. Thus the AIDS incidence pattern in homosexual men in NYC who are also IVDUs is similar to that for homosexual men in NYC.

In modeling the HIV prevalence in IVDUs it is significant that some HIV positive IVDUs are dying from HIV-related causes that do not meet the AIDS definition. These causes include pneumonia, endocarditis and tuberculosis. Stoneburner et al. (1988) estimated these HIV-related deaths by comparing observed narcotics-related deaths in 1982 to 1986 with those that would be expected without the AIDS epidemic and those reported as AIDS-related deaths. The number of IVDUs was assumed to be constant from 1979 to 1986 and AIDS-related cases were subtracted so that the average annual narcotics- related deaths for 1979 to 1981 was 488 deaths per year. Thus 2440 narcotics-related deaths would be expected for 1982 to 1986. Hence of the actual 6157 narcotics-related deaths in 1982 to 1986, 2440 were expected and 1197 were AIDS-related deaths, so that the excess deaths were 2520. Stoneburner at al. (1988) provide evidence that these 2520 excess deaths are HIV-related, but they occur in people who do not satisfy the definition of having AIDS.

In February 1989, the NYC Department of Health (NYCDOH, 1989) gave revised estimates of the number of NYC residents in various risk groups who were HIV-positive. Their estimated ranges were 33,015 to 75,998 for men who have sex with men (MSM), 60,000 to 90,000 male IVDUs, 20,000 to 30,000 female IVDUs, 10,000 to 15,000 other men, 1,000 to 20,000 other women and 1600 to 4400 children. Their estimated range for MSM were obtained in three ways. Assuming 15% underreporting, they compared white and other categories of MSM in NYC with MSM in San Francisco. Using back-calculation, they obtained the estimate of 33,015. By direct calculation with 30% to 50% positivity and a risk population estimate of about 150,000, they obtained a range of 42,406 to 75,998 for HIV prevalence in MSM. The IVDU estimates are based on 40% to 60% prevalence in a population of 200,000 IVDUs where one quarter of them are women. They note that there is some evidence for a leveling off of HIV prevalence in IVDUs beginning in 1985 (DesJarlais et al., 1989).

6. Parameter Estimations for New York City

The linkage between the HIV epidemics in homosexual men and IVDUs in NYC is analyzed in later sections. The simulation modeling needs *a priori* estimates and initial estimates for parameter values for the three group model consisting of homosexual men, homosexual IVDUs, and IVDUs. These estimates are used in fitting the model or as initial estimates of parameters that are adjusted in the fitting process.

6.1 Estimates of Population Sizes and Turnover

Estimates of the population size of the homosexual men in NYC have ranged up to 500,000, but the estimate in 1988 was reduced to about 100,000 (Lambert, 1988). A recent estimate of the NYC Department of Health of this population size is about 150,000 (NYC DOH, 1989). In the NYC model the size of the population of sexually active homosexual men is taken to be 100,000. The migration rate with equal immigration and emigration is taken to be 5% per year as it was in the SF model (Hethcote, Van Ark, and Longini, 1991).

Friedland and Klein (1987) note that ninety percent of the IVDUs are heterosexual, implying that 10% are homosexual. If there are about 200,000 IVDUs in NYC, then there would be about 20,000 homosexual-IVDUs in NYC, but this estimate is very crude. In a study of homosexual men (Darrow et al., 1987), 20% said that they had injected drugs and 60% of the drug users said that they had shared hypodermic needles. Since 12% of these homosexuals were needle-sharing IVDUs, roughly 12,000 of the 100,000 would be homosexual-IVDUs who share needles. Due to the uncertainty of the size of the homosexual-IVDU population, this size is taken as a variable in the NYC model which is to be determined to fit the homosexual-IVDU AIDS data.

Many papers (e.g., Friedland and Klein, 1987; Selwyn et al., 1987; Drucker, 1986) have given 200,000 as the approximate size of the IVDU population in NYC; however, it is not clear if these are independent estimates or are all based on one original source. Dolan et al. (1987) found that 59% of 193 in a drug abuse treatment program (1983-1985) reported that they had shared needles. Other studies of IVDUs in treatment programs found that 66% (Mulleady and Green, 1985) and 68% (Black et al., 1986) reported needlesharing. Of course, these percentages may be unrealistically low since they are based on self-reporting of people in treatment programs. Darrow (personal communication, 1988) states that nearly all IVDUs share needles. Schuster (1988) reports that 70% to 90% of IVDUs are needle-sharers. If 20,000 (10% of 200,000 IVDUs) are homosexuals, and 30,000 (17% of the remaining 180,000 IVDUs) do not share needles, then the size of the nonhomosexual needle-sharing IVDU population in NYC would be 150,000. In the rest of this paper IVDU will mean non-homosexual needle-sharing IVDUs, and the size of this population in the NYC model is taken to be 150,000.

It is not clear whether the size of the needle-sharing population has changed with time. Kozel and Adams (1986) reported that the number of heroin users seems to have remained reasonably stable, but the number of people injecting forms of cocaine has increased. Others found that needle-sharing among drug users has decreased. Des Jarlais et al. (1987, 1988, 1989) found that 54% of 59 IVDUs in a treatment program in 1985 reported some risk reduction in needle-sharing; 75% in 1986 and 85% in 1987 reported some AIDS reduction behavior. Of course, self-reported changes of these IVDUs may be biased. In the model the number of needle-sharing IVDUs is fixed at 150,000, but it would be possible to change this size with time if more information becomes available.

Since three-fourths of all IVDUs in the United States are male (Des-Jarlais et al., 1988) it is assumed that this fraction is also true for needle-sharers in NYC. This means that there are about 37,500 female IVDUs and 112,500 male IVDUs in NYC. Friedland and Klein (1987) state that 30% to 50% of the IVDU women have engaged in prostitution.

The migration or turnover rates in homosexual men and in IVDUs in NYC are difficult to estimate. One study found an annual inactivation rate of 13- 25% for IVDUs who died, relocated outside of NYC, or ceased all intravenous drug use (Drucker and Vermund, 1989). Another study (Des Jarlais et al., 1989) of a 1987 subject group found that 11% had begun injecting illicit drugs after 1980 and 4% had begun after 1984; thus the entry rate was about 2% per year. The high exit rate is not consistent with the low entry rate. As a compromise, the migration rate is chosen as 5% per year, which is the same as for homosexual men.

The transfer rates between the very active and active classes is estimated to be 5% per year as in the SF model (Hethcote, Van Ark, and Longini, 1991). The natural mortality rate in all four risk groups is taken to be $\mu = 0.000532$ which is the value used in the SF model for homosexual men. This corresponds to the death rate of men aged 45-54. Although not all people in the risk groups are men or are in this age bracket, this slightly higher death rate is suitable for people in these groups with a somewhat risky lifestyle.

6.2 Estimation of Parameters Related to the Stages

Very little information seems to be available for the progression of IVDUs from HIV infection to AIDS. Thus it is assumed that all adults who become infected progress through the T4-cell count stages to AIDS as described in Section 2. The probabilities ω_k of transmission by a person in stage k and relative sexual or needle-sharing activity ρ_k of a stage k individual are assumed to be the same as those for the baseline parameter for SF homosexual men set in Table 6.1 from Hethcote, Van Ark, and Longini (1991). The fixed parameters in Table 6.1 are based on many data sources and sexual behavior surveys; the optimization parameters are those values which give the best fit to the HIV and AIDS incidence estimates for SF.

Table 6.1. Baseline parameter set

Parameter	Value
Fixed Parameters	
Population size	Q = 56,000
Natural mortality rate constant	$\mu = 0.000532$
Monthly migration percentage	$\delta = 0.05/12$
Monthly activity level change rate constant	$\phi = 0.05/12$
Probability of transmission	QH = 0.05
Mean times in phases	2.2, 52.6, 62.9, and 18.0 mo.
Very active fraction	F = 0.10
Activity level ratio	R = 10
Relative weights ($\omega \times \rho$) of transmission in 4 phases	2, 1, 1.5, and 7.5
Number of stages	m = 7
Optimization Parameters	
Starting date of the epidemic	STD = October 1975
Reduction starting date	STR = August 1981
Reduction stopping date	STP = December 1986
External mixing fraction	$\eta = 0.82$
Average number of partners per month before STR	PAS = 0.75
Yearly reduction factor	RDN = 0.61

6.3. Sexual Behavior Parameter Estimates

The AIDS incidence pattern for homosexual men in NYC in Table 5.1 is similar to that of homosexual men in SF about 1 year later. Thus the *a priori* estimates for homosexual men are the baseline parameter values for SF given in Table 6.1 except that the NYC population size is 100,000 and the epidemic starting date is one year earlier.

6.4. Needle-Sharing Behavior Parameter Estimates

Needle-sharing seems to occur primarily within a particular group. In a study of IVDUs in NYC, Selwyn et al. (1987) found that about half of those sharing needles gave as reasons the need to inject drugs with no clean needle being available and needle-sharing was done only with a close friend or relative. Thus a needle that is shared is most likely to have been used by someone in the same group. Since the pattern of development of the AIDS epidemic in IVDUs is similar initially to the pattern for homosexual men in NYC and SF, it is assumed that the distribution of the number of needle- sharing partners is similar to that for homosexual men. Thus, it is assumed that 5% or 10% are in the very active class and that they have ten times as many needle-sharing partners as those in the active class. The sensitivity of the results to these parameter choices is checked.

IVDUs may inject several times a day, but usually share needles less often. Although some needle-sharing occurs in shooting galleries with many people, it usually occurs with a few acquaintances. Although partnerships formed with unknown individuals in shooting galleries are of short duration and involve one needle-sharing, the partnerships with acquaintances can be of long duration and involve many needle sharings. No estimates have been found for the probability of transmission per needle-sharing partnership; however, the probability of transmission from one needle-sharing partner may be similar to the probability of transmission from one homosexual partner. In the NYC model it is assumed that the probability of transmission QHD per new needle-sharing partner is 0.05.

It is not clear whether the needle-sharing partnership rate has changed with time. Selwyn et al. (1987) found that some IVDUs reported that they had either stopped needlesharing or ceased being an IVDU. DesJarlais et al. (1987, 1988, 1989) found in a drug treatment center that 54% of IVDUs in 1985, 75% in 1986 and 85% in 1987 reported some reduction in behavior that could lead to AIDS, but this reporting could be biased. Thus in the NYC model, the reduction factor per year in the average number of needlesharing partners might be near 1 in contrast to the expected range of 0.4 to 0.7 for homosexual men. Since the AIDS incidence of homosexual men in NYC is about a year ahead of the incidence in SF, the starting date of the epidemic in homosexual men should be at least a year earlier than the starting date of July 1976 in SF. It is likely that the epidemic started in the IVDUs and in homosexual men at about the same time.

6.5 Modified Fit Criteria for the New York City Model.

Because of the significant number of HIV-related deaths described in Section 5, the fitting criteria for the NYC model are changed slightly from those described in Section 4. The parameter ALP is the rate constant for HIV-related deaths in the symptomatic stages (4, 5, and 6) for IVDUs and is adjusted so that these deaths in 1982 to 1986 are close to the observed value of 2520 given in Section 5. The initial guesses for the IVDU parameters are that PASD is about half of PASH and RDND is one. If the 42 HIV-related deaths per month (2520 in 5 years) occurred in a population of 10,000 pre-AIDS IVDUs, then the death rate would be 0.0042 so that this is taken as an initial estimate for ALP. The fit to the AIDS incidence data in the homosexual-IVDU population is obtained by adjusting the population size NSIZEB which is initially assumed to be 10,000. The HIV-related death rate constant ALP now joins the list of optimization parameters. The expression to be minimized in the fitting procedure is now changed to

$$CHISQH + CHISQB + CHISQD + 0.01(DTH26 - 2520)^2$$

which is the sum of the chi-square values for the homosexual men, homosexual-IVDUs and IVDUs plus a measure of how close the HIV-related deaths in symptomatic IVDUs are to the observed value of 2520. The coefficient 0.01 has been found by trial and error to give a reasonable balance between the last term and the chi-square terms.

7. Fitting in the New York City Population of Homosexual Men

The model for homosexual men is given in Section 3. The best fit for the NYC homosexual men is shown in Table 7.1. The parameter values are quite similar to those for the best fit in SF except that the population size in Table 7.1 is 100,000 instead of 56,000 in SF and the starting date in the NYC epidemic is May 1974 instead of October 1975 in SF. In Table 7.1 the average number of partners per month is 0.49 before July 1982 and the yearly reduction factor is 0.41 until December 1984. In the best fitting parameter set for the SF homosexual men, the average number of sexual partners per month was 0.75 before August 1981 and the yearly reduction factor was 0.61. The external mixing fraction η in the simulation of the epidemic in NYC homosexual men is 0.58, while η was 0.82 for the baseline simulation in SF. Some other parameter sets also give reasonable fits, so it is not possible to conclude much about the partners per month and changes in sexual behavior other than the general conclusion that the average number of partners per month was approximately constant until mid-1982 and then it decreased rapidly. Note that it was not possible to get an adequate fit using a parameter set without any change in sexual behavior. For all parameter sets which satisfy the fit criteria, the pattern is similar to the pattern in Table 7.1. Namely, the yearly HIV incidence peaks in about 1980, the HIV prevalence peaks at in about 1983, the AIDS incidence peaks in 1988 or 1989 and the AIDS deaths peak in about 1989 or 1990. Note that the peak AIDS incidence occurs about 8 or 9 years after the peak HIV incidence and about 5 years after the peak HIV prevalence.

Note in Table 7.1 that in the very active class the HIV prevalence rises rapidly until 93% are infected in 1981-82, and then the HIV prevalence decreases as infected very-active people either die from AIDS, migrate out of NYC, or move into the active class. The prevalence in the active class rises more slowly and reaches a peak of 26% infected in 1983 and then declines slowly. Note that the HIV fractional prevalence peaks in the very active class in 1981-82, and peaks in the total population and in the active class in 1983. Since very sexually active men have more partnerships and hence are more likely to be infected, it is reasonable that the HIV fractional prevalence should have a peak in the very active class before the peak in the active class. As expected, nearly everyone with AIDS in the early years is in the very active class, but only 25% are in the very active class when

Table 7.1. Simulation results for the best fit to the AIDS incidence data for NYC homosexual men with a population size of 100,000.

```
THE POPULATION SIZE IS         100000, THE VERY ACTIVE FRACTION IS
  1.000000E-01 AND THE ACTIVITY RATIO IS          10.000000
THE NATURAL MORTALITY RATE XMU IS    5.320000E-04
THE INTERCHANGE RATE   FROM THE VERY ACTIVE CLASS TO THE ACTIVE CLASS IS
   4.166667E-03   AND THE TURNOVER RATE IS DLT =      4.166667E-03
THE NUMBER OF INFECTIOUS STAGES IS  M =            7
THE G PARAMETERS FOR THE TRANSFER BETWEEN STAGES ARE      7.355444E-02
   6.433708E-02      4.867545E-02     4.199281E-02      3.997889E-02
   5.152515E-02      5.398798E-02
THE WEIGHTS OF TRANSMISSION PER INFECTIOUS PARTNER TIMES THE FRACTION STILL
SEXUALLY ACTIVE FOR THE STAGES ARE WRH(I) =          2.000000          1.000000
       1.000000          1.500000          1.500000          1.500000
       7.500000
THE PROBABILITY OF TRANSMISSION IS QH =      5.000000E-02
THE EXTERNAL MIXING FRACTION IS ETA =      5.750000E-01
THE AVERAGE NUMBER OF PARTNERS PER MONTH IS      4.923000E-01 BEFORE         1982
          7, THEN IT IS REDUCED EACH YEAR BY A FACTOR OF      4.088000E-01UNTIL
DEC,        1984
THE STARTING YEAR AND MONTH ARE              1974             5
THE STARTING NUMBER OF VERY ACTIVE INFECTIVES IS          1.000000

          *************************************************
```

YEAR	HIV INC SIM	HIV PREV	FRACTNAL_PREV ALL	V_A	ACT	YR AIDS INC DATA	SIM	AIDS(SIMULATION) PREV	DTHS	OUTSF
1974	4.	4.	.00	.00	.00	*****	0.	0.	0.	0.
1975	24.	28.	.00	.00	.00	*****	0.	0.	0.	0.
1976	132.	156.	.00	.01	.00	*****	0.	0.	0.	0.
1977	709.	843.	.01	.06	.00	*****	0.	0.	0.	0.
1978	3148.	3883.	.04	.26	.01	*****	1.	1.	0.	0.
1979	7699.	11189.	.11	.65	.05	5.	5.	4.	1.	1.
1980	8612.	18956.	.19	.87	.11	23.	24.	22.	7.	3.
1981	7745.	25432.	.25	.93	.18	95.	93.	85.	29.	14.
1982	6788.	30544.	.31	.93	.24	272.	265.	252.	98.	49.
1983	3277.	31809.	.32	.88	.26	572.	578.	577.	253.	126.
1984	1489.	31023.	.31	.82	.25	1017.	1018.	1076.	518.	263.
1985	1100.	29564.	.30	.75	.25	1463.	1520.	1708.	888.	459.
1986	1232.	27921.	.28	.68	.23	2068.	1987.	2376.	1319.	693.
1987	1336.	26091.	.26	.62	.22	2321.	2328.	2965.	1738.	930.
1988	1399.	24123.	.24	.57	.20	2489.	2494.	3383.	2076.	1133.
1989	1417.	22102.	.22	.52	.19	2451.	2490.	3587.	2286.	1273.
1990	1398.	20121.	.20	.49	.17	2378.	2355.	3586.	2356.	1340.

```
CHISQ =          7.490914
```

the AIDS incidence peaks in 1988-89. Graphs of the HIV prevalence and yearly AIDS incidences are given in Figure 7.1.

A sensitivity analysis for the simulation for homosexual men in SF has been presented in Hethcote, Van Ark, and Karon (1991). The relative sensitivities to the parameters found there would also apply here to the simulations for homosexual men in NYC. The peak HIV prevalence of about 32,000 in homosexual men in NYC is not too surprising since the AIDS incidence in homosexual men in NYC is similar to that in SF and the peak HIV prevalence there was about 20,000. If the AIDS incidence is uniformly underreported by 10% or 20%, then the HIV prevalence would increase by approximately these percentages. If all AIDS incidences in

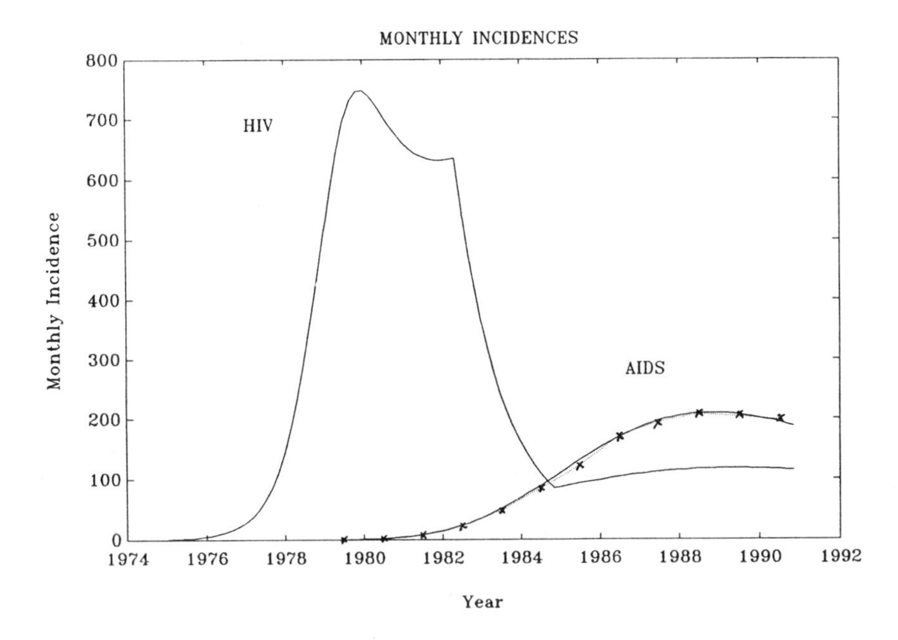

Figure 7.1. The best-fitting simulations for HIV and AIDS incidences for NYC homosexual men corresponding to Table 7.1. The AIDS incidence data (x symbols) correspond to the data in Table 5.1.

homosexual men were scaled up by 15% as done in the NYC Department of Health calculations, then the peak HIV prevalence in our model would be approximately 37,000. The HIV prevalence in this model is at the bottom of the range of 33,015 to 75,998 estimated for homosexual men in NYC in the NYC Department of Health report (NYCDOH, 1989). Note that the estimate in the dynamic model here is closest to their back-calculation estimate of 33,015 (see Section 5). Unless people develop AIDS more slowly than the current data indicates, the HIV prevalence cannot be higher and still lead to the given AIDS incidence data.

8. Fitting in the New York City Population of IVDUs

Here the AIDS incidence data for the IVDU population is fit using the submodel obtained by ignoring the homosexual and homosexual-IVDU populations. In Section 9, all three risk groups are fit simultaneously. The best fitting simulation is given in Table 8.1 and shown in Figure 8.1. Note that 10% of the population of 150,000 is ten times as active and the external

Table 8.1. Simulation results for the best fit to the AIDS incidence data for NYC IVDUs.

```
THE IVDU POPULATION SIZE IS        150000
THE VERY ACTIVE FRACTION IS     1.000000E-01
THE ACTIVITY RATIO IS        10.000000
THE NATURAL MORTALITY RATE XMU IS    5.320000E-04
THE INTERCHANGE RATE  FROM THE VERY ACTIVE CLASS TO THE ACTIVE CLASS IS
   4.166667E-03  AND THE TURNOVER RATE IS DLT =     4.166667E-03
THE HIV-RELATED DEATH RATE CONSTANT IS     4.865000E-03
THE NUMBER OF INFECTIOUS STAGES IS  M =              7
THE G PARAMETERS FOR THE TRANSFER BETWEEN ADULT STAGES ARE     7.355444E-02
   6.433708E-02     4.867545E-02     4.199281E-02     3.997889E-02
   5.152515E-02     5.398798E-02
THE WEIGHTS OF TRANSMISSION PER INFECTIOUS PARTNER TIMES THE FRACTION STILL
SEXUALLY ACTIVE FOR THE STAGES ARE WRH(I) =         2.000000         1.000000
       1.000000         1.500000         1.500000         1.500000
       7.500000
THE PROBABILITY OF TRANSMISSION IS QH =     5.000000E-02
THE EXTERNAL MIXING FRACTION IS ETA =    4.734000E-01
THE AVERAGE NUMBER OF NEEDLE-SHARING PARTNERS PER MONTH IS     3.753000E-01
BEFORE        2000            1, THEN IT IS REDUCED EACH YEAR BY A FACTOR OF
      1.000000 UNTIL DEC,        2000
THE STARTING YEAR AND MONTH ARE          1974            1
THE STARTING NUMBER OF VERY ACTIVE INFECTIVES IS          1.000000
****************************************************
```

YEAR	HIV INC	HIV PREV	HIV DTHS	FRACTNAL_PREV ALL	V_A	ACT	YR AIDS DATA	INC SIM	AIDS(SIMULATION) PREV	DTHS	OUTSF
1974	5.	5.	0.	.00	.00	.00	****	0.	0.	0.	0.
1975	18.	22.	0.	.00	.00	.00	****	0.	0.	0.	0.
1976	68.	87.	0.	.00	.00	.00	****	0.	0.	0.	0.
1977	258.	335.	0.	.00	.02	.00	****	0.	0.	0.	0.
1978	949.	1245.	1.	.01	.06	.00	0.	1.	1.	0.	0.
1979	3062.	4170.	5.	.03	.20	.01	0.	2.	2.	1.	0.
1980	6972.	10733.	18.	.07	.48	.03	5.	9.	8.	3.	1.
1981	9179.	19022.	59.	.13	.74	.06	21.	31.	29.	10.	5.
1982	8546.	26121.	151.	.17	.86	.10	115.	97.	92.	34.	17.
1983	7997.	32088.	304.	.21	.88	.14	276.	250.	243.	99.	48.
1984	8078.	37493.	495.	.25	.88	.18	503.	521.	527.	236.	116.
1985	8432.	42539.	694.	.28	.85	.22	871.	900.	960.	467.	232.
1986	8815.	47205.	877.	.31	.83	.26	1314.	1343.	1514.	789.	396.
1987	9104.	51389.	1035.	.34	.79	.29	1754.	1795.	2134.	1174.	597.
1988	9254.	54986.	1168.	.37	.75	.32	2326.	2216.	2765.	1586.	816.
1989	9263.	57922.	1279.	.39	.72	.35	2542.	2586.	3361.	1990.	1034.
1990	9155.	60168.	1370.	.40	.68	.37	2895.	2901.	3898.	2363.	1241.

```
CHISQ =        22.860970
DTH26 =      2520.323000
```

mixing fraction is 0.47. In Table 8.1 the epidemic starts in January of 1974, and the average number of needle-sharing partners is 0.38. Note that this best fitting parameter set does not have any reduction in the needle-sharing partnership rate. This is significantly different from the best fit in Section 7 for homosexual men.

The pattern in Table 8.1 is that the HIV incidence peaks is approximately level after 1981, but both the HIV prevalence and AIDS incidence increase steadily. The HIV incidence of approximately 9000 per year is consistent with the HIV incidence of 10,000 cases per annum used in Pagano et al. (1991). The HIV-related deaths in the simulation match the estimated deaths of 2520 in the years 1982 to 1986. In the simulation, the HIV-related

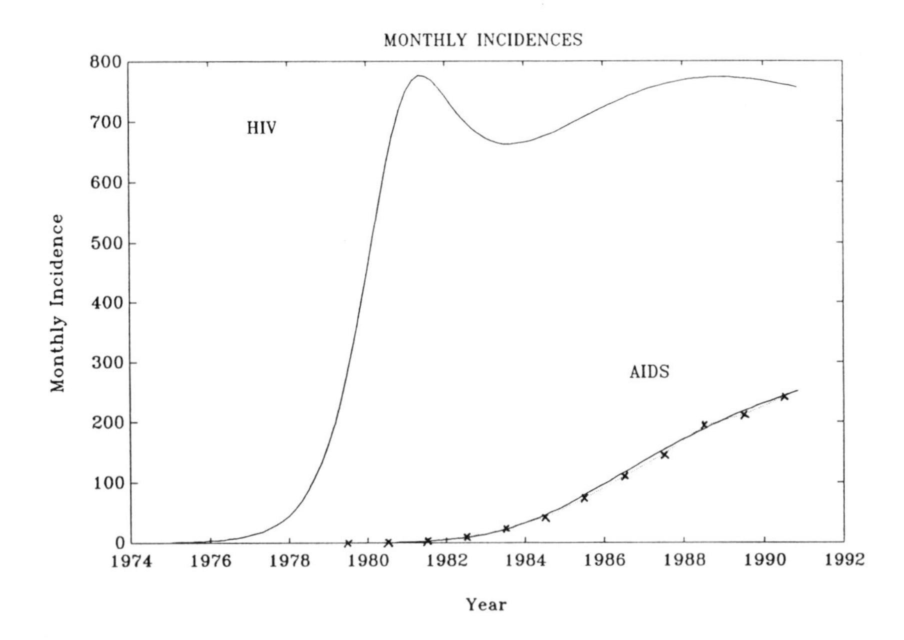

Figure 8.1. The best fitting simulations for HIV and AIDS incidences in NYC IVDUs corresponding to Table 8.1. The AIDS incidence data (x symbols) correspond to the data in Table 5.1.

deaths are about 1000 to 1400 per year in 1987 to 1990. The simulation in Table 8.1 and Figure 8.1 is not intended to be used for forecasting; however, it does show that good fits to the AIDS data through 1990 are obtained without any reduction in needle-sharing partnership rates. There may have been changes in the needle-sharing behavior of IVDUs in NYC in recent years since these changes would have almost no influence on the fit to the AIDS data through 1990.

The report (NYCDOH, 1989) of the Department of Health in NYC estimated that the HIV prevalence in IVDUs is 60,000 to 90,000 men and 20,000 to 30,000 women for a total of 80,000 to 120,000 (40% to 60%) out of their estimated IVDU population of 200,000. Their estimates of 40% to 60% HIV positivity are based on IVDUs in treatment centers in Manhattan and may be too high for NYC since the percentages are probably lower in the other boroughs. In Table 8.1 the simulated value is about 43,000 HIV positive IVDUs (non-homosexual) in 1985. This is lower than their estimated range and is 29% of the 150,000 needle-sharing IVDUs in the NYC model. In Table 8.1 the simulated HIV prevalence increases up to about 60,000 in 1990, which is 40% of the NYC needle-sharing IVDUs.

9. Fitting in the Three New York City Risk Groups

In the previous sections the best fits were found for the populations of homosexual men and IVDUs. Here three risk groups are fit simultaneously by using the modified fitting procedure outlined in Section 6, which is the sum of the chi-squares and the weighted square of the deviation from the 2520 HIV-related deaths in 1982-86. Table 9.1 gives the parameter set and the computer simulation output which satisfies this modified fit criteria. Graphs of monthly HIV and AIDS incidences for the three risk groups are given in Figure 9.1.

The fits of the model simulations to the AIDS incidence data are quite good as shown in Figure 9.1 or as measured by the chi-square values at the bottom of Table 9.1. The largest chi-square value occurs for the homosexual-IVDUs and this is primarily because the 1988-1990 AIDS incidence values are low compared to a trend curve through the previous years. For the other risk groups the largest deviations also seem to occur in 1988.

For the homosexual men the peak HIV incidence in Table 9.1 occurs in 1980, the peak HIV prevalence occurs in 1983 and the peak AIDS incidence occurs in 1988-89. This pattern is essentially the same as that in Table 7.1 where the population of homosexual men is fit separately. Essentially the same means that the peaks are within 5% of the previous peaks and they occur in the same year or within one year of the previous peaks. The starting date of the epidemic in homosexual men in Table 9.1 is May 1974, which is the same as in Table 7.1. The activity structure of 10% being ten times as active is like that in Table 7.1. The average number of homosexual partners per month before reduction and the external mixing fraction are slightly lower in Table 9.1, while the yearly reduction factor is slightly higher. The sexual activity reduction starting and stopping dates are the same in Tables 9.1 and 7.1. Thus the homosexual men part of the simultaneous fit in Table 9.1 is very similar to the separate fit for homosexual men.

For the IVDU population in Table 9.1 , the HIV incidence is approximately level after 1981, but both the HIV prevalence and the AIDS incidence increase steadily. This pattern for the IVDUs in the simultaneous fitting in Table 9.1 is very close to the pattern in Table 8.1 where the IVDUs are fit separately. In Table 9.1 compared to Table 8.1, the average number of needle-sharing partnerships per month is slightly lower, the yearly reduction factor is still one and the external mixing factor is slightly higher. The decrease in the initial average number of needle-sharing partnerships per month is not surprising, since the IVDUs now also have some

Table 9.1. Simulation results for the best fit to the AIDS incidence data for NYC homosexual men, homosexual IVDUs and IVDUs.

```
THE SIZE OF THE HOMO POPULATION IS      100000
THE SIZE OF THE HOMO-IVDU POPULATION IS         6500
THE SIZE OF THE IVDU POPULATION IS      150000
THE VERY ACTIVE FRACTIONS ARE    1.000000E-01 FOR HOMOSEXUALS
, AND    1.000000E-01 FOR IVDUs, AND THE ACTIVITY RATIO IS       10.000000
THE HIV-RELATED DEATH RATE CONSTANT FOR IVDUs IS    4.887000E-03
THE STARTING YEARS AND MONTHS ARE         1974            5
FOR HOMOSEXUALS, AND        1974            1 FOR IVDUs.
THE NATURAL MORTALITY RATE XMU IS    5.320000E-04
THE INTERCHANGE RATE  FROM THE VERY ACTIVE CLASS TO THE ACTIVE CLASS IS
   4.166667E-03  AND THE TURNOVER RATE IS DLT =    4.166667E-03
THE WEIGHTS OF TRANSMISSION PER INFECTIOUS PARTNER TIMES THE FRACTION STILL
SEXUALLY ACTIVE FOR THE STAGES ARE WRH(I) =       2.000000         1.000000
       1.000000         1.500000         1.500000         1.500000
       7.500000
THE PROBABILITY OF TRANSMISSION IS QH =     5.000000E-02
THE EXTERNAL MIXING FRACTIONS ARE ETAH, ETAD =     5.419000E-01     5.171000E-01
THE AVERAGE NUMBER OF HOMOSEXUAL PARTNERSHIPS PER MONTH IS     4.865000E-01 BEFO
RE        1982            7 AND IS REDUCED EACH YEAR BY A FACTOR OF
   4.191000E-01 UNTIL DEC,         1984
THE AVERAGE NUMBER OF NEEDLE-SHARING PARTNERS PER MONTH IS     3.445000E-01
BEFORE         2000            1, THEN IT IS REDUCED EACH YEAR BY A FACTOR OF
      1.000000 UNTIL DEC,         2000
*****************************************************
```

CLASS	HIV INC	HIV PREV	HIV DTHS	FRACTNAL_PREV ALL	V_A	ACT	YR AIDS DATA	INC SIM	AIDS(SIMULATION) PREV	DTHS	OUTSF
--1970--											
HOMO	0.	0.	0.	.00	.00	.00	****	0.	0.	0.	0.
HMDU	0.	0.	0.	.00	.00	.00	****	0.	0.	0.	0.
IVDU	0.	0.	0.	.00	.00	.00	****	0.	0.	0.	0.
--1971--											
HOMO	0.	0.	0.	.00	.00	.00	****	0.	0.	0.	0.
HMDU	0.	0.	0.	.00	.00	.00	****	0.	0.	0.	0.
IVDU	0.	0.	0.	.00	.00	.00	****	0.	0.	0.	0.
--1972--											
HOMO	0.	0.	0.	.00	.00	.00	****	0.	0.	0.	0.
HMDU	0.	0.	0.	.00	.00	.00	****	0.	0.	0.	0.
IVDU	0.	0.	0.	.00	.00	.00	****	0.	0.	0.	0.
--1973--											
HOMO	0.	0.	0.	.00	.00	.00	****	0.	0.	0.	0.
HMDU	0.	0.	0.	.00	.00	.00	****	0.	0.	0.	0.
IVDU	0.	0.	0.	.00	.00	.00	****	0.	0.	0.	0.
--1974--											
HOMO	4.	4.	0.	.00	.00	.00	****	0.	0.	0.	0.
HMDU	0.	0.	0.	.00	.00	.00	****	0.	0.	0.	0.
IVDU	4.	5.	0.	.00	.00	.00	****	0.	0.	0.	0.
--1975--											
HOMO	25.	29.	0.	.00	.00	.00	****	0.	0.	0.	0.
HMDU	2.	3.	0.	.00	.00	.00	****	0.	0.	0.	0.
IVDU	14.	18.	0.	.00	.00	.00	****	0.	0.	0.	0.
--1976--											
HOMO	146.	171.	0.	.00	.01	.00	****	0.	0.	0.	0.
HMDU	12.	14.	0.	.00	.02	.00	****	0.	0.	0.	0.
IVDU	55.	71.	0.	.00	.00	.00	****	0.	0.	0.	0.
--1977--											
HOMO	807.	954.	0.	.01	.07	.00	****	0.	0.	0.	0.
HMDU	62.	74.	0.	.01	.08	.00	****	0.	0.	0.	0.
IVDU	231.	293.	0.	.00	.01	.00	****	0.	0.	0.	0.
--1978--											
HOMO	3545.	4377.	0.	.04	.29	.02	0.	1.	1.	0.	0.
HMDU	262.	327.	0.	.05	.34	.02	0.	0.	0.	0.	0.
IVDU	977.	1234.	1.	.01	.06	.00	0.	0.	0.	0.	0.
--1979--											
HOMO	7928.	11874.	0.	.12	.69	.06	5.	5.	5.	1.	1.
HMDU	571.	866.	0.	.13	.75	.06	1.	0.	0.	0.	0.
IVDU	3310.	4402.	5.	.03	.20	.01	0.	2.	2.	1.	0.
--1980--											
HOMO	8202.	19202.	0.	.19	.89	.11	23.	27.	24.	7.	4.
HMDU	615.	1417.	0.	.22	.93	.14	3.	2.	2.	1.	0.
IVDU	6957.	10935.	18.	.07	.47	.03	5.	8.	7.	2.	1.
--1981--											
HOMO	7398.	25324.	0.	.25	.93	.18	95.	102.	94.	33.	16.
HMDU	614.	1935.	0.	.30	.96	.22	9.	8.	7.	2.	1.
IVDU	8808.	18850.	61.	.13	.71	.06	21.	31.	28.	10.	5.

--1982--											
HOMO	6605.	30255.	0.	.30	.93	.23	272.	285.	272.	107.	53.
HMDU	588.	2393.	0.	.37	.95	.30	45.	21.	20.	8.	4.
IVDU	8433.	25846.	155.	.17	.83	.10	115.	99.	93.	34.	17.
--1983--											
HOMO	3291.	31535.	0.	.32	.88	.25	572.	605.	608.	269.	135.
HMDU	405.	2637.	0.	.41	.93	.35	73.	45.	45.	20.	10.
IVDU	7971.	31798.	307.	.21	.87	.14	276.	254.	247.	101.	49.
--1984--											
HOMO	1545.	30798.	0.	.31	.82	.25	1017.	1044.	1112.	540.	275.
HMDU	324.	2770.	0.	.43	.90	.37	82.	78.	83.	40.	20.
IVDU	7983.	37124.	495.	.25	.87	.18	503.	525.	532.	239.	118.
--1985--											
HOMO	1161.	29392.	0.	.29	.75	.24	1463.	1537.	1738.	911.	471.
HMDU	320.	2866.	0.	.44	.87	.39	142.	117.	132.	68.	35.
IVDU	8255.	42017.	691.	.28	.85	.22	871.	899.	962.	470.	233.
--1986--											
HOMO	1303.	27814.	0.	.28	.68	.23	2068.	1990.	2393.	1335.	702.
HMDU	337.	2943.	0.	.45	.84	.41	167.	156.	185.	102.	54.
IVDU	8574.	46483.	872.	.31	.82	.25	1314.	1335.	1509.	788.	396.
--1987--											
HOMO	1414.	26061.	0.	.26	.63	.22	2321.	2317.	2965.	1744.	935.
HMDU	348.	2995.	0.	.46	.80	.42	206.	188.	237.	137.	73.
IVDU	8817.	50439.	1028.	.34	.79	.29	1754.	1779.	2120.	1168.	594.
--1988--											
HOMO	1482.	24181.	0.	.24	.58	.20	2489.	2475.	3368.	2072.	1132.
HMDU	354.	3021.	0.	.46	.76	.43	174.	212.	280.	168.	91.
IVDU	8935.	53800.	1157.	.36	.75	.32	2326.	2192.	2739.	1573.	809.
--1989--											
HOMO	1505.	22254.	0.	.22	.53	.19	2451.	2468.	3562.	2273.	1268.
HMDU	354.	3023.	0.	.47	.73	.44	180.	225.	312.	193.	107.
IVDU	8925.	56506.	1263.	.38	.71	.34	2542.	2553.	3322.	1969.	1024.
--1990--											
HOMO	1491.	20371.	0.	.20	.50	.17	2378.	2336.	3559.	2339.	1332.
HMDU	350.	3007.	0.	.46	.69	.44	158.	231.	332.	211.	118.
IVDU	8810.	58541.	1350.	.39	.68	.36	2895.	2856.	3845.	2334.	1225.

```
CHISQH =        12.757770
CHISQB =        93.055450
CHISQD =        22.162120
DTH26 =       2520.463000
```

needle-sharing partnerships per month is slightly lower, the yearly reduction factor is still one and the external mixing factor is slightly higher. The decrease in the initial average number of needle-sharing partnerships per month is not surprising, since the IVDUs now also have some needle-sharing partnerships with homosexual IVDUs. The dates for the start of the IVDU epidemic and the starting and stopping of reduction in partnerships per month are the same in Tables 9.1 and 8.1. Thus the IVDU part of the simultaneous fit in Table 9.1 is also very similar to the separate fit of the IVDUs in Table 8.1.

For the homosexual-IVDU population in Table 9.1, the HIV incidence peaks in 1980-81, and then decreases before it levels off at about half the peak value. The HIV prevalence increases up to 1983 and then is approximately level. The simulated AIDS incidence increases steadily. These behaviors are roughly between the corresponding behaviors for homosexual men and IVDUs. This is expected since the homosexual IVDUs are linked to the HIV epidemics in both other groups. The population size of 6500 homosexual-IVDUs is only 6.5% of the population size of 100,000 for

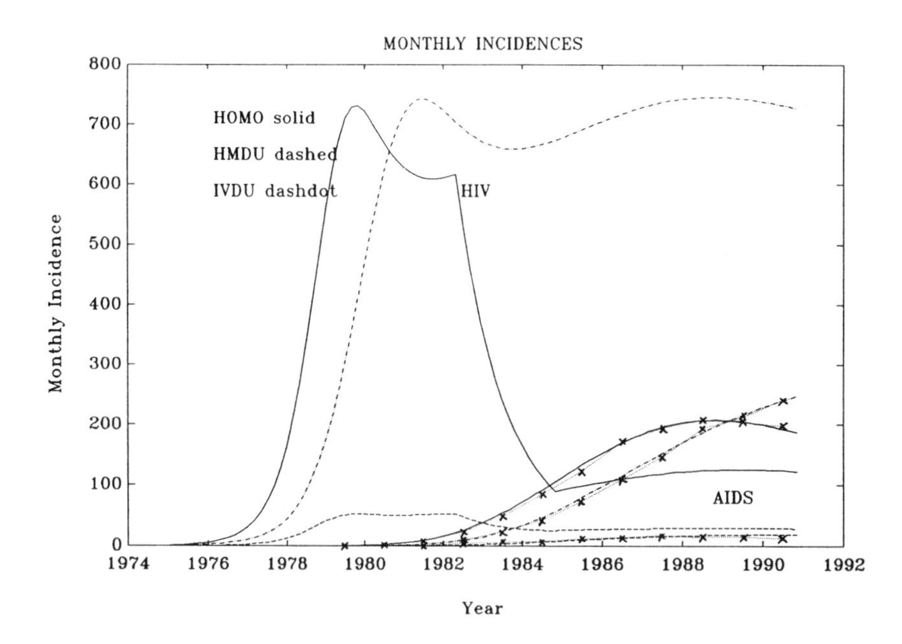

Figure 9.1. The best fitting simulations for HIV and AIDS incidences for homosexual men, homosexual IVDUs and IVDUs in NYC corresponding to Table 9.1. The AIDS incidences (x symbols) correspond to the data in Table 5.1.

homosexual men and only 4.3% of the population size of 150,000 for IVDUs. Thus the homosexual-IVDUs seem to be small in number compared to the other two groups. Although the homosexual-IVDUs do have some influence on the other two risk groups, this influence does not appear to be a crucial connection between the HIV epidemics in the two other risk groups.

From the simultaneous fitting of the three risk groups and the separate fittings of the homosexual men and IVDUs, one observes that the essential patterns are the same. Thus for these two groups the simultaneous fitting does not really change their patterns and the HIV epidemics in these two groups seem to be proceeding almost independently. This near independence is useful in subsequent modeling.

10. Discussion

In both the separate fitting of the AIDS incidence in homosexual men in Section 7 and the simultaneous fitting in Section 9, the peak HIV incidence in homosexual men occurs in 1980, the peak HIV prevalence at about 32% occurs in 1983 and the peak AIDS incidence occurs in 1988-89. In Tables 7.1 and 9.1 the fractional HIV prevalence peaks at 93% in 1981-82 in the very active class and peaks at 25-26% in 1983 in the active class. Thus the general patterns of HIV and AIDS incidences and prevalences are the same for the separate fitting of homosexual men in Table 7.1 and the simultaneous fitting of the three risk groups in Table 9.1. In Table 9.1 the average number PASH of sexual partners per month, the yearly reduction RDNH in sexual partners and the external mixing fraction ETAH are very close to those in Table 7.1. The dates for the start of the epidemic and the starting and stopping of partnership reduction are chosen to be the same in Table 9.1 as in Table 7.1. Thus the parameter values in the simultaneous fitting are close to those for the separate fitting of homosexual men. The patterns described above occur for a variety of parameter sets which satisfy the fit criteria. For example, they persist when the population size is doubled.

The pattern for the best fitting parameter sets for IVDUs in Tables 8.1 and 9.1 is that the HIV incidence levels off around 1981, but both the HIV prevalence and the AIDS incidence are increasing. Thus the general patterns of HIV and AIDS incidences and prevalences are the same whether IVDUs are fit separately or simultaneously with homosexual men and homosexual-IVDUs. Moreover, the parameter values for the IVDU fit in Table 9.1 are the same as or similar to those in Table 8.1. Hence it seems that the simultaneous fitting of the three risk groups does not have much effect on the IVDU pattern and parameter values. This observation is consistent with the theory that the linkage provided by the homosexual-IVDUs is weak enough to be considered negligible.

In the fit of the data for the homosexual-IVDUs in Section 9, it is interesting to note that the best population size is 6500 which is 6.5% of the size of the non-IVDU homosexual men. It is plausible that a homosexual-IVDU population which is 6.5% of the population of homosexual men could have an AIDS incidence which is 7-9% of the AIDS incidence in homosexual men since homosexual-IVDUs can also be infected through needle-sharing. The pattern in the homosexual-IVDUs is that the HIV prevalence rises rapidly until it is about half of the population size and then remains approximately level. The fractional prevalence near 50% is high in homosexual-IVDUs since they are infected by both homosexual and needle-sharing partnerships. The early rise in HIV prevalence in homosexual-IVDUs seems to be due to infections from the homosexual men and then the HIV prevalence is maintained by infections from the IVDUs. Thus the pattern in homosexual-IVDUs is that their HIV epidemic follows and is sustained by the HIV epidemics in homosexual men and IVDUs. The HIV epidemic in homosexual-IVDUs does not seem to be a mechanism by which one of the HIV epidemics in homosexual men or IVDUs supports or sustains the other.

Another argument supports the concept that the HIV epidemics in homosexual men and IVDUs are essentially independent. If one HIV epidemic were feeding another HIV epidemic, then there would be a delay of about 4 to 6 years between the start (or peak) in the feeder epidemic and the start (or peak) in the sustained epidemic. In simulations of HIV epidemics in IVDUs and their heterosexual partners, delays of about five years are observed between the starts of the HIV epidemics, the peaks of the HIV epidemics, the starts of the AIDS incidences and the peaks of the AIDS incidences (Hethcote and Van Ark, 1991). Similar delays are also observed for female IVDUs and perinatal cases in their children and for female heterosexual partners and perinatal cases in their children. A simplified explanation is that the delays of approximately five years occur because the average time of infecting someone is in the middle of the ten year infectious period. Since these delays do not occur between the HIV epidemics or between the AIDS incidence curves for homosexual men and IVDUs in NYC, this strongly suggests that neither of these epidemics is sustaining the other.

Forecasting future yearly AIDS incidences is difficult. The AIDS incidence data for homosexual men peaked in 1988-89 and declined slightly in 1990. This data and the best fitting simulations to this data suggest that a possible forecast is that the yearly AIDS incidence in NYC homosexual men has leveled off and may decline in the future. However, this forecast may be incorrect if the model is not realistic or if the data are incorrect for any reason. Possible data problems are recent increases in underreporting or recent changes in reporting delay patterns or a temporary leveling off of AIDS cases due to effects of the treatment of some pre-AIDS people with zidovudine (AZT) and aerosol pentamidine.

It is interesting to compare the HIV/AIDS epidemics in homosexual men in NYC and SF. In SF homosexual men the AIDS incidence data in Table 5.1 appeared to be leveling off in 1987-89 and then it jumped up again in 1990. Thus the AIDS incidence in 1990 would probably not be consistent with a forecast based on data up through 1989. Simulations of the HIV/AIDS epidemic in SF homosexual men suggested that therapy may not have had much effect on the AIDS incidence in homosexual men there. Although saturation in the very active homosexual men did occur in the simulations of homosexual men in SF, a reduction in sexual partners per month was essential in fitting the data there (Hethcote, Van Ark and Karon, 1991).

The simulations in Tables 8.1 for NYC IVDUs suggest that there may not have been significant change in needle-sharing behavior in IVDUs in NYC. Thus HIV incidence remains high in Figure 8.1 and AIDS incidence continues to increase. This forecast without any change in behavior may be a "worst case" prediction but it is consistent with the AIDS data so far. Blower et al. (1990) also modeled IVDUs in NYC and also found that their simulation scenario was able to fit the AIDS incidence data in NYC IVDUs without any change in needle-sharing behavior.

Acknowledgements

Research supported by Centers for Disease Control, contract 200-87-0515. Support services provided by The University of Iowa Center for Advanced Studies. We are grateful for valuable data, discussions and suggestions from James Fordyce and Rand Stoneburner (New York City Department of Health), James Curran, William Darrow, Timothy Green, Debra Hansen and John Karon (Division of HIV/AIDS, Centers for Disease Control) and Michael Aldrich (California AIDS Intervention Training Center, San Francisco).

References

Bacchetti, P. and Moss, A.R. (1989). Incubation period of AIDS in San Francisco. *Nature* **338**, 251-53.

Battjes, R. J., Pickens, R. W., Amsel, Z. (1989). Introduction of HIV infection among intravenous drug abusers in low prevalence areas. *J. AIDS* **2**, 533–539.

Black, J.L., Dolan, M.P. and DeFord, H.A., et al. (1986). Sharing of needles among users of iv drugs. *New England Journal of Medicine* **314**, 446-447.

Blower, S.M., Hartel, D., Dowlatabadi, H., et al. (1991). Drugs, sex and HIV: A mathematical model for New York City. *Phil Trans R Soc Lond B* **321**, 171-187.

Blythe, S.P. and Anderson, R.M. (1988). Heterogeneous sexual activity model of HIV transmission in male homosexual populations. *IMA Journal of Math App Med Biol* **5**, 237 - 260.

Blythe, S.P. and Castillo-Chavez, C. (1989). Like with like preference and sexual mixing models. *Math Biosci* **96**, 221-238.

Burke, D.S., Redfield, R.R., Fowler, A., Oster, C. (1989). Increased "viral burden" in late stages of HIV infection. *Abstract Th.A.P.93, V International Conference on AIDS*, Montreal, Canada.

Castillo-Chavez, C., Cooke, K.L., Huang, W., and Levin, S.A. (1989). On the role of long incubation periods in the dynamics of AIDS Part 2: Multiple group models, Math and Stat Approaches to AIDS Epidemiology, In *Lecture Note in Biomathematics 83*, C Castillo-Chavez (eds). Springer- Verlag, New York, Berlin, Heidelberg, pp. 200-217.

Cates, W., Jr. and Handsfield, H.H. (1988). HIV counseling and testing: does it work? *AJPH*, **78**, 1533–34.

Centers for Disease Control. (1989). Update: Acquired Immunodeficiency Syndrome-United States. *MMWR*, No. 5, **39**, 81-86.

Centers for Disease Control. (1990b). Update: HIV prevalence estimates and AIDS case projections for the United States: Report based on a workshop. MMWR, No. RR-16, **39**, 1-31.

Coates, T.J., Morin, S.F., McKusick, L. (1987). Behavioral consequences of AIDS antibody testing among gay men. *JAMA* **258**, 1889.

Curran, J.W., Jaffe, H.W., Hardy, A.M., Morgan, W.M., Selik, R.M., Dondero, T.J. (1988). Epidemiology of HIV infection and AIDS in the United States. *Science* **239**, 610-16.

Darrow, W.W., Echenberg, D.F., Jaffe, H.W., O'Malley, P.M., Byers, R.H., Getchell, J.P., Curran, J.W. (1987). Risk factors for human immunodeficiency virus infection in homosexual men. *AJPH* **77**, 479-83.

De Gruttola, V. and Mayer, K.H. (1987). Assessing and modeling heterosexual spread of the human immunodeficiency virus in the United States. *Rev Inf Dis* **10**, 138-50.

Des Jarlais, D.C. and Friedman, S.R. (Ed. review). (1987). HIV infection among I.V. drug users: epidemiology and risk reduction. *AIDS* **1**, 67-76.

Des Jarlais, D.C., Friedman, S.R., Marmor, M., et al. (1987). Development of AIDS, HIV seroconversion, and potential cofactors for T4 cell loss in a cohort of I.V. drug users. *AIDS* **1**, 105-111.

Des Jarlais, D.C., Friedman, S.R., Novick, D.M., et al. (1989). HIV-1 infection among intravenous drug users entering treatment in Manhatten, New York City, 1978-1987. *JAMA* **261**, 1008-1012.

Des Jarlais, D.C., Friedman, S.R., and Stoneburner, R.L. (1988). HIV infection and intravenous drug use: critical issues in transmission dynamics, infection outcomes, and prevention. *Reviews of Infectious Diseases* **10**, 151-158.

Dietz, K. and Schenzle, D. (1985). Mathematical models for infectious disease statistics. In *A Celebration of Statistics*, A. C. Atkinson and S. E. Fienberg (eds.). New York, Springer-Verlag, pp. 167-204.

Dolan, M. P., Black, J. L., Deford, H. A., et al. (1987). Characteristics of drug abusers that discriminate needle-sharers, Public Health Reports, July-August, 395–398.

Drucker, E. (1986). AIDS and addiction in New York City. *Amer. J. Drug Alcohol Abuse* **12**, 165-181.

Drucker, E. and Vermund, S.E. (1989). Estimating population prevalence of human immunodeficiency virus infection in urban areas with high rates of intravenous drug use: A model of the Bronx in 1988. *Am J Epi* **130**, 133-142.

Friedland, G.H. and Klein, R.S. (1987). Transmission of the human immunodeficiency virus, *New Eng J Med* **317**, 1125-1135.

Goedert, J.J., Eyster, M.E., Biggar, R.J., Blattner, W.A. (1987). Heterosexual transmission of human immunodeficiency virus: association with severe depletion of T-helper lymphocytes in men with hemophilia. *AIDS Res Human Retrov* **3**, 355-61.

Goedert, J.J., Kessler, C.M., Aledort, L.M. et al. (1989). A prospective study of human immunodeficiency virus type 1 infection and the development of AIDS in subjects with hemophilia. *New England J Med* **321**, 1141-48.

Hessol, N.A., O'Malley, P., Lifson, A., et al. (1989). Incidence and prevalence of HIV infection among homosexual and bisexual men, 1978 - 1988. *Abstract M.A.O. 27, V International Conference on AIDS.* Montreal, Canada.

Hethcote, H.W. (1987). AIDS modeling work in the United States. In: *Future Trends in AIDS*, London: Her Majesty's Stationary Office, pp. 35- 46.

Hethcote, H.W. and Van Ark, J.W. (1987). Epidemiological models for heterogeneous populations: proportionate mixing, parameter estimation, and immunization programs. *Math Biosci* **84**, 85-118.

Hethcote, H. W. and Van Ark, J. W. (1991). *Modeling HIV Transmission and AIDS in the United States*, (in preparation).

Hethcote, H.W., Van Ark, J.W., and Karon, J.M. (1991). A simulation model of AIDS in San Francisco: II. simulations, therapy, and sensitivity analysis. *Math Biosci* **106**, 223-247.

Hethcote, H.W., Van Ark, J.W., and Longini, I.M., Jr. (1991). A simulation model of AIDS in San Francisco: I. Model formulation and parameter estimation. *Math Biosci* **106**, 203-222.

Hethcote, H.W. and Yorke, J.A. (1984). *Gonorrhea Transmission Dynamics and Control.* Lecture Notes in Biomathematics 56, Heidelberg, Springer- Verlag.

Hethcote, H.W., Yorke, J.A., Nold A. (1982). Gonorrhea modeling: a comparison of control methods. *Math Biosci* **58**, 93-109.

Hyman, J.M. and Stanley, E.A. (1988). Using mathematical models to understand the AIDS epidemic. *Math Biosci* **90**, 415-73.

Jacquez, J.A., Simon, C.P., Koopman, J., Sattenspiel, L., Perry, T. (1988). Modeling and the analysis of HIV transmission: the effect of contact patterns. *Math Biosci* **92**, 119-99.

Kaplan, E.H. and Lee, Y.S. (1990). How bad can it get? Bounding worst case epidemic heterogeneous mixing models of HIV/AIDS. *Math Biosci* **99**, 157 - 180.

Kozel, N.J. and Adams, E.H. (1986). Epidemiology of drug abuse: an overview. *Science* **34**, 970-974.

Lambert, B. (1988). Halving of estimate on AIDS is raising doubts in New York. New York Times (July 20), 1-28.

Lemp, G.F., Payne, S.F., Rutherford, G.W. et al. (1990). Projections of AIDS morbidity and mortality in San Francisco. *JAMA* **263**, 1497-1501.

Lifson, A.R., Hessol, N.A., Rutherford, G..W et al. (1990). The natural history of HIV infection in a cohort of homosexual and bisexual men: clinical and immunological outcomes, 1977 - 1990. *Abstract Th.C. 33, VI International Conference on AIDS*, San Francisco, Calif.

Longini, I.M., Clark, W.S., Byers, R.H., et al. (1989). Statistical analysis of the stages of HIV infections using a Markov model. *Stat in Med* **8**, 831-43.

Longini, I.M., Clark, W.S., Gardner, L.I., Brundage, J.F. (1991). The dynamics of $CD4^+$ T-lymphocyte decline in HIV-infected individuals: A Markov modeling approach. *J AIDS*, in press.

Longini, I.M., Clark, W.S., Haber, M., et al. (1990). The stages of HIV infection: Waiting times and infection transmission probabilities. In Castillo-Chavez C, ed., *Mathematical and Statistical Approaches to AIDS epidemiology*. Lecture Notes in Biomathematics 83, New York, Springer- Verlag, pp. 111-137.

Machado, S.G., Gail, M.H., Ellenberg, S.S. (1990). On the use of laboratory markers as surrogates for clinical endpoints in the evaluation of treatment for HIV infection. *J AIDS* **3**, 1065-1073.

May, R.M. (1988). HIV infection in heterosexuals. *Nature* **331**, 655-56.

Mulleady, G. and Green, J. (1985). Syringe sharing among London drug abusers. *Lancet* **8469**, 1425.

New York City Department of Health. (1989). Report of the expert panel on HIV seroprevalence estimates and AIDS case projection methodologies, 1-33.

Nold, A. (1980). Heterogeneity in disease transmission modeling. *Math Biosci* **52**, 227-40.

Osmund, D., Bacchetti, P., Chaisson, R.E., Kelly, T., Stempel, R., Carlson, J., Moss, A.R. (1988). Time of exposure and risk of HIV infection in homosexual partners of men with AIDS. *AJPH* **78**, 944-48.

Payne, S.F., Lemp, G.F., Rutherford, G.W., et al. (1989). Effect of multiple disease manifestations on length of survival for AIDS patients in San Francisco, Abstract W.A.P.80, V International Conference on AIDS, Montreal, Canada, June 1989.

Padian, N.S. (1987). Heterosexual transmission of AIDS: International perspectives and national projections. *Rev Inf Dis* **9**, 947-960.

Pagano, M., DeGruttola, V., MaWhinney, S., Tu, X.M. (1991). The HIV epidemic in New York City: Statistical methods for projecting AIDS incidence and prevalence. In *AIDS Epidemiology: Methodological Issues*, N. Jewell, K. Dietz and V. Farewell (eds.), Boston: Birkhäuser-Boston.

Pickering, J., Wiley, J.A., Padian, N.S., Lieb, L.E., Echenberg, D.F., Walker, J. (1986). Modeling the incidence of A.I.D.S. in San Francisco, Los Angeles, and New York. *Math Modeling* **7**, 661-88.

Redfield, R.R., Wright, D.C., Tramont, E.C. (1986). The Walter Reed staging classification for HTLV-III/LAV infection. *N Eng J Med* **314**, 131-2.

Schuster, C.R. (1988). Intravenous drug use and AIDS prevention, *Public Health Reports* **103**, 1125-1135.

Seligmann, M., Pinching, A.J., Rosen, F.S. et al. (1987). Immunology of human immunodeficiency virus and the acquired immune deficiency syndrome. *Ann Int Med* **107**, 234-42.

Selwyn, P.A., Feiner, C., Cox, C.P., et al. (1987). Knowledge about AIDS and high-risk behavior among intravenous drug users in New York City. *AIDS* **1**, 247-254.

Steinbrook, R. (1988). AIDS slowdown in 3 key cities seen. Los Angeles Times, December 6, pp. 1-26.

Stoneburner, R.L., Des Jarlais, D.C., Benezra, D., et al. (1988). A larger spectrum of severe HIV-1-related disease in intravenous drug users in New York City. *Science* **242**, 916-919.

Department of Mathematics
University of Iowa
Iowa City, IA 52242

Section 3
Statistical Approaches to Markers of HIV Disease Progression

MARKER MODELS IN SURVIVAL ANALYSIS AND APPLICATIONS TO ISSUES ASSOCIATED WITH AIDS

Nicholas P. Jewell and John D. Kalbfleisch

ABSTRACT: Jewell and Kalbfleisch (1992) consider the use of marker processes for applications related to estimation of the survival distribution of time to failure. Marker processes were assumed to be stochastic processes which, at a given point in time, provide information about the current hazard and consequently on the remaining time to failure. Particular attention was paid to calculations based on a simple additive model for the relationship between the hazard function at time t and the history of the marker process up until time t. Specific applications to the analysis of AIDS data included the use of markers as surrogate responses for onset of AIDS with censored data and as predictors of the time elapsed since infection in prevalent individuals. Here we review recent work on the use of marker data to tackle these kinds of problems with AIDS data. The Poisson marker process with an additive model, introduced in Jewell and Kalbfleisch (1992) may be a useful "test" example for comparison of various procedures.

1. INTRODUCTION

In studying the natural history of HIV disease and AIDS, great attention has been placed on the role of immunological marker variables and their progression as individuals move from infection, through an asymptomatic period, to the onset of symptoms and diagnosis of disease. The use of markers of disease progression is clearly of great value in tracking individuals' disease status in time and is related to a wide variety of related but different applications. Examples of such uses include (i) the use of markers to assist in the construction of staging models, (ii) the understanding of the etiologic process underlying disease development, (iii) the use of markers in providing prognostic information of clinical relevance including guidance for the use of therapies, (iv) using markers to evaluate the impact of therapies, and (v) linking the levels of markers to other natural history parameters such as infectivity. Specific applications which have already been studied in some depth involve using marker information to predict the time of subsequent onset of

AIDS, and to predict the time of infection. The first of these has potential value in (i) improving the use of censored individuals in follow-up studies with regard to estimation of properties of the incubation distribution and related quantities, (ii) suggesting the use of markers as surrogate responses for the onset of AIDS in comparative trials, and (iii) providing clinical prognostic information. The second application, predicting the time of infection, is of interest for the analysis of data from prevalent cohorts where the lack of knowledge of infection times is a common technical problem, and for consideration of the use of marker values at recruitment as a method of adjustment for the effects of onset confounding (Brookmeyer and Gail, 1987).

While CD4 cell counts are often promoted as the most useful prototypical marker, there are many other immunological variables that have been studied as markers of disease progression. A good review of some of these variables and their role in assessing the advancement of disease can be found in Moss and Bacchetti (1989). In addition to basic immunological markers, in many applications it may also be helpful to view certain time related variables (such as time since infection itself, or time since recruitment, time on treatment, etc.) as "structural" markers.

In this article, we consider a marker process to be a stochastic process generated by an individual under study that measures in some way the state or "health" of the individual. That is, the path of the marker process provides information regarding progression towards failure. It is difficult to give specific conditions which identify marker processes. This is partly because there is a variety of covariates which we wish to cover under the general rubric of marker processes. Thus, the past sample path and/or current value of the marker process may be predictive of the residual life of the individual. Conversely, the future sample path and/or current value may be predictive of the individual's "age" or time elapsed since the onset of the survival process. In many cases, a marker process may be related to both residual life and age.

Here we briefly review the general setting surrounding the modelling of marker processes and their relation to the onset of AIDS with particular attention given to the use of marker information to improve estimation of time to AIDS distributions in follow-up studies or with prevalent cohorts.

2. GENERAL BACKGROUND AND RELATED LITERATURE

Suppose that each individual under study at time t admits measurement of a stochastic process $X(t) \geq 0$ for all $t>0$. The process $\{X(t)\}$ is modeled as a nonnegative stochastic process with left continuous sample paths. Note that the nonnegativity condition on X is not a restriction since negative valued processes can always be transformed by exponentiating for example. Suppose also that current and past values of $X(\cdot)$ affect the failure rate at time t. We will then refer to $X(\cdot)$ as a marker process. In this paper, we consider statistical models for the joint distribution of $\{X(t): t>0\}$ and the positive random variable, T, which denotes the time to failure of the individual. Loosely, we will refer to this as the joint distribution of $X(\cdot)$ and T. In many cases all that can be identified is the joint distribution of $\{X(t): 0<t<T\}$ and T, since the marker may be unobservable after failure.

Throughout most of the article, the time origin refers to infection with the HIV virus and failure indicates the onset (i.e. diagnosis) of AIDS. Failure is here considered to be the diagnosis of AIDS. Of course, the same ideas will apply for other kinds of origin and failure definitions such as diagnosis of AIDS (origin) and death from AIDS (failure).

In attempting to understand the joint distribution of $X(\cdot)$ and T it may be useful to consider various components separately as suggested by the schematic illustration shown in Figure 1. Note the three fundamental components of the system:

(i) the relationship or link between the realization of the marker process and the risk or hazard of onset of AIDS;

(ii) the relationship between other factors and the risk of onset of AIDS;

(iii) the influence of background factors on the stochastic properties of the marker process.

We envisage background factors including either fixed or time-dependent cofactors which are *unmeasured*, as against (fixed or time-dependent) covariates which are observed together with the marker process and information on AIDS status. Further, one may generalize the modelling by allowing the outcome, onset of AIDS, to be a multi-state process which allows for individuals to move between various stages of disease progression.

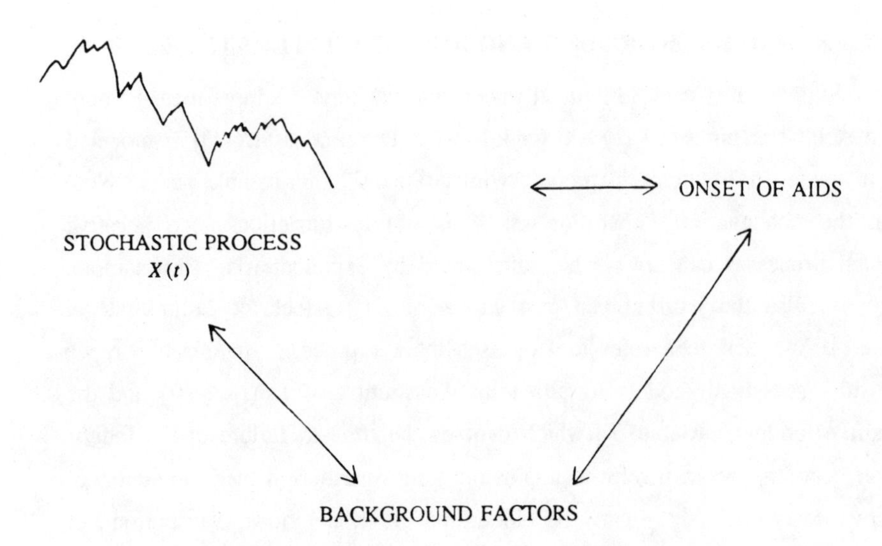

Figure 1. Schematic illustration of marker process and its relationship to other factors and onset of AIDS.

Covariates may modify the system in a variety of ways. For example, in treatment studies where a principal covariate of interest is treatment regimen (which may be fixed or time-dependent), it may be possible that treatment (i) alters the risk of AIDS onset, independent of its effect on a marker, (ii) influences the stochastic development of the marker, (iii) modifies the levels of background factors. In addition to these "main effects" of treatment, "interactive" effects may also be present. That is, treatment may modify the relationships (i)-(iii) above between the marker process, background factors and the risk of AIDS. In the next two subsections we consider models that have been investigated for the two principal components of interest, the relationship between the marker and the risk of AIDS, and the stochastic structure of the marker process. In addition to their role in understanding the joint distribution of $X(\cdot)$ and T, these models are of independent value.

2.1. The hazard of AIDS given marker history

The relationship between $\{X(t): 0 < t < s\}$ and the hazard of failure at time t is specified via the link function,

$$h(t \mid X(s): 0 \le s \le t) \equiv \lim_{\Delta t \to 0} pr\{T \in [t, t+\Delta t) \mid T \ge t, X(s): 0 \le s \le t\} / \Delta t \ . \quad (1)$$

There are several possibilities for parametric or semi-parametric models for the link function h. In follow-up studies, a familiar semiparametric model is the proportional hazards model:

$$h(t \mid X(s): 0 \le t \le s) \equiv h_0(t)\exp\{\beta X(t)\}. \tag{2}$$

The unknown parameters β and h_0 can be estimated using standard proportional hazards software that accommodates time-dependent covariates.

Jewell and Kalbfleisch (1992) pay special attention to the following additive model

$$h(t \mid X(s): 0 \le t \le s) \equiv h_0(t) + \beta X(t) \tag{3}$$

where $\beta \ge 0$. The appeal of this model is that it allows mathematical analysis of the marginal properties of the survival distribution as will be discussed below. Note that Self (1992) considers a somewhat similar model in which the right-hand side of (3) is replaced by $h_0(t)[1 + \beta X(t)]$.

In either case, the function $h_0(t)$ is a background hazard function that describes a component of the failure rate that is unrelated to the marker. The parameter β describes the manner in which the marker process modifies the hazard and more general models which allow β to depend on t or on $X(t)$ could also be considered, but will not be pursued here. The model (3) is a slight generalization of one considered by Puri (1966). For multivariate marker processes $\mathbf{X}(t)$, the above models can be easily extended by allowing β to be a vector and replacing $\beta X(t)$ with $\beta'\mathbf{X}(t)$. In a sense, (3) already describes a special case of such a multivariate marker model if we view the variable t as a (deterministic) marker process in its own right. Also, related models may be developed which replace $X(t)$ in either (2) or (3) by various derived functions of the history of X, for example, $X(t-a)$, a lagged version of X, or $\int_0^t X(u)du$. With a multivariate marker model, several kinds of these terms can be incorporated in a model simultaneously.

Fully nonparametric models for h have been studied by Fusaro, Neilsen and Scheike (1992) and Neilsen (1992). In particular, these authors consider:

$$h(t \mid X(s): 0 \le t \le s) \equiv h(X(t)). \tag{4}$$

When $X(\cdot)$ is multivariate, the function h is allowed to be multivariate. In high dimensions, it would be of interest to introduce some form of additive structure by writing, for example,

$$h(t \mid \mathbf{X}(s): 0 \le t \le s) \equiv h_1(X_1(t)) \cdots h_m(X_m(t)) \tag{5}$$

where $\mathbf{X}(t) = \{X_1(t),...,X_m(t)\}$ is a vector-valued stochastic process.

The definition (1) is heuristic since we have not explicitly defined what is meant by the hazard function conditional on the past sample path of a stochastic process. The necessary formulation for a mathematically precise definition and justification of the following development (in particular, (6) below) can be found in Segall and Kailath (1975). See also a brief discussion of this issue in Jewell and Kalbfleisch (1992).

Using model (3) for illustration, it is straightforward to demonstrate differing effects of a fixed covariate $\mathbf{z}$ on the system as discussed above. For example, we indicate three simple ways in which covariates might be introduced to (3):

(i) $h_0(t;\mathbf{z})$ can be substituted for $h_0(t)$.

(ii) $\beta(\mathbf{z})$ can be substituted for β. In this model, the covariate modifies the way in which the marker affects the failure rate.

(iii) The probability laws governing $\{X(t)\}$ can be allowed to depend on $\mathbf{z}$. In this model, the covariates affect directly the evolution of the marker process, and through the effect on that process alter the failure rate.

It is evident that a covariate could enter the model in more than one manner. For example, the level of $\mathbf{z}$ may simultaneously alter both the background hazard and the evolution of the process $\{X(t)\}$.

Before turning to some specific statistical problems involving markers, we briefly discuss the evaluation of some marginal and conditional distributions, based on model (3), that are relevant in the context of using markers as surrogate responses or as surrogates for the time scale.

The marginal distribution of the time to failure T under the model (3) is specified by the survivor function

$$S(t) = pr\{T \ge t\} = E\{\exp[-\int_0^t (h_0(u) + \beta X(u))du]\}, \tag{6}$$

where the expectation is taken with respect to the sample paths of $X(\cdot)$. The moment generating functional of the process $X(\cdot)$, with argument $\psi(\cdot)$, is

$$E\{\exp[\int_0^\infty \psi(u)X(u)du]\} = \exp\{K_X(\psi)\}, \tag{7}$$

and substitution in (6) with $\psi_t(u) = -\beta I(u < t)$ gives

$$S(t) = \exp\{-H_0(t) + K_X(\psi_t)\}, \tag{8}$$

where $H_0(t) = \int_0^t h_0(u)du$. The marginal hazard function of T is thus

$$\lambda(t) = -d \log S(t)/dt = h_0(t) - dK_X(\psi_t)/dt \quad .$$

The joint distribution of T and $X(T)$ is also of interest. To this end, let

$$p_{t,x} = E[\exp\{-H_0(t) - \beta\int_0^t X(u)du\} \mid X(t)=x]. \tag{9}$$

Note that the calculation in (9) is again basically the calculation of a moment generating functional but now with respect to the tied-down process, $X(\cdot)$ given that $X(t)=x$. It follows that

$$pr\{T \geq t, X(t) \leq x\} = \int_0^x p_{t,u}dF_{X(t)}(u) \tag{10}$$

where $F_{X(t)}$ is the marginal c.d.f. of $X(t)$. The marginal distribution of $X(T)$ can then be obtained as

$$pr\{X(T) \leq x\} = \int_0^\infty\int_0^x [h_0(t)+\beta u]\, p_{t,u}dF_{X(t)}(u)dt. \tag{11}$$

For processes that admit a simple form for the conditional moment generating functional, these calculations are straightforward.

Finally, given the current value of $X(t)$ and the fact that the item has survived to time t, the distribution of residual life is often of interest. It can be seen that

$$pr\{T \geq t+s \mid T \geq t, X(t)=x\} = E\{\exp\{-\int_t^{t+s} (h_0(u)+\beta X(u))du \mid X(t)=x\}. \tag{12}$$

In summary, we note that simple expressions for the moment generating functionals of both the unconstrained stochastic process $\{X(\cdot)\}$ and the tied-down version of $X(\cdot)$ are the requirements for pursuing further analytic development. As alluded to earlier, the additive relationship in (3) facilitates these calculations; the alternative and more standard multiplicative relationship between the hazard and the covariate $X(t)$ given in (2) is less amenable to analytic investigation. Note that, whatever model is used to describe the relationship between the marker history and the current hazard for AIDS, it is necessary to describe the stochastic properties of the marker process in order to derive marginal properties of the time to failure distribution.

We finish this subsection by pointing out a somewhat different class of models that incorporate marker information. These models are related to shock or wear models in the reliability literature which model the development of shocks or wear with failure occurring when the "amount" of wear or stress exceeds a certain threshold. For an introduction to such models in the context of the analysis of AIDS data, see Doksum (1992) and the references therein.

2.2. The stochastic properties of the marker process $X(\cdot)$

Several investigators have studied the longitudinal behavior of various markers of HIV disease progression with particular attention to CD4 cell counts. For example, DeGruttola, et al. (1991) use a linear random effects model applied to data from the San Francisco Men's Health Study, a prevalent cohort. Berman (1990) assumed that serial measurements of CD4 can be explained on the logarithmic scale by a stationary Gaussian process with a deterministic exponential drift after seroconversion. Mũnoz, et al (1988) consider a simple autoregressive model. Longini, et al. (1989, 1991) and Longini (1990) consider multistage Markov models. See also Taylor and Cumberland (1991). For models that are related to attempts to describe the immune system more directly see, for example, Bremermann and Anderson (1990a,b) and Perelson (1987).

Several problems complicate the fitting of even the simplest of models to serial measurements of CD4 data. First, in dealing with data from prevalent cohorts, the times of infection of individuals are usually unknown so that the natural time scale is unavailable (but see Vittinghoff and Jewell, 1992). Second, the number of repeated observations on any given individual is usually small and may cover only a short part of their overall incubation period. Finally, the available cohorts often are subject to various kinds of selection bias potentially associated with the nature of their CD4 measurements. For example, individuals previously diagnosed with AIDS are usually ineligible for recruitment into a prevalent cohort so that those persons with unusually rapid CD4 decline may be selectively removed from the sample. Also, prevalent individuals who develop symptoms or are diagnosed with AIDS may be at greater risk of loss to follow up so that the number of repeated observations available is associated with the rate of decline of CD4. Attempts to incorporate these selection issues into the analysis of the data will necessarily involve the modelling of the link between CD4 sample paths and the risk of onset of AIDS so that the investigator is forced into modeling the joint distribution of the marker and time to AIDS simultaneously. Of course, the longitudinal modelling of CD4 counts including the above issues is complicated by the inherent high natural variability (noise), and the need to accommodate other time-varying covariates.

3. POISSON MARKER PROCESSES

Jewell and Kalbfleisch (1992) developed a marker process model based on a Poisson process representation for the marker process, coupled with the additive model discussed above. Here we briefly describe some of the properties of this model to facilitate use as an example in further sections.

Suppose that $X(t)$ is a Poisson process with intensity function $\mu(t)$ and assume the marker model (3). It is easily seen that the marginal survivor function (8) of T is

$$S(t) = \exp\{-H_0(t) - \int_0^t \mu(s)ds + \int_0^t \mu(s)e^{-\beta(t-s)}ds\}. \tag{13}$$

The marginal hazard function is then

$$\lambda(t) = h_0(t) + \beta e^{-\beta t}\int_0^t \mu(s)e^{\beta s}\,ds. \tag{14}$$

The special case where $\mu(t) = \mu$ so that the process $X(t)$ is homogeneous is of some interest. Here, the marginal hazard function is $\lambda(t) = h_0(t) + \mu(1-e^{-\beta t})$. If, for example, $h_0(t) = h_0$ is constant, the marginal hazard increases from h_0 at $t=0$ to the finite asymptote $h_0 + \mu$ as $t \to \infty$. The rate of increase is governed by the parameter β.

It is also straightforward to calculate the moment generating functional of the tied-down process, $X(\cdot)$ given that $X(t) = m$. For example, if $w_1, \ldots, w_m$ denote the jump points of $X(\cdot)$, it follows from (9) that

$$pr\{T \geq t, X(t) = m\} = E\{\exp[-H_0(t) - \sum_{j=1}^{m} \beta \int_{w_j}^{t} ds]\} pr\{X(t)=m\}$$

where the expectation is over the joint distribution of $w_1,\ldots,w_m$ given $X(t) = m$. Then

$$pr\{T \geq t, X(t) = m\} = \exp\{-H_0(t) - \int_0^t \mu(s)ds\} A^m / m! \qquad (15)$$

where $A = \int_0^t \mu(s) e^{-\beta(t-s)} ds$. The summation of this expression over m reproduces the marginal survivor function of T, (13). The marginal p.d.f. of $X(T)$, i.e., the value of the marker process at failure, can be derived by multiplying by $h_0(t)+\beta m$ and then integrating over t. For example, with $\mu(t) = \mu$ and $h_0(t) = h_0$, we have

$$pr\{T \geq t, X(t) = m\} = (\frac{\mu}{\beta})^m (1-e^{-\beta t})^m e^{-(h_0+\mu)t} / m! \ , \qquad (16)$$

and

$$pr\{X(T) = m\} = (\frac{\mu}{\beta})^m ((h_0/\beta)+m) / [(B+m)(B+m-1) \cdots B] \qquad (17)$$

where $B = (h_0+\mu)/\beta$.

Using (12), it is easy to see that at time t, given that $T \geq t$ and $X(t)=m$, the residual life S follows a marginal survival distribution with associated hazard function given by

$$\lambda^*(s) = h_0(s) + \beta X(t) + \mu(1-e^{-\beta s}) .$$

Thus, the "covariate" $X(t)$ has an additive effect on the hazard for residual life. Specifically, the regression relationship between residual life at time t, denoted by S_t, and the status of the marker at time t, $X(t)$, is given by $S_t = \min(T_1, T_2)$ where T_1 and T_2 are independent; the random variable T_1 has a standard distribution (in fact, given by the marginal distribution of T described above), and T_2 is exponential with hazard $\beta X(t)$.

Finally, returning to the general case (13), we describe a useful regression model. Suppose $h_0(t) \equiv 0$ and that a covariate vector $\mathbf{z}$ modifies the marker model solely through the intensity function $\mu(\cdot)$; in particular, let

$$\mu(t \mid \mathbf{z}) = \mu(t) e^{\gamma \cdot \mathbf{z}} \quad . \tag{18}$$

Then, from (14), we have

$$\begin{aligned} \lambda(t \mid \mathbf{z}) &= \beta e^{-\beta t} \int_0^t \mu(s) e^{\gamma \cdot \mathbf{z}} e^{\beta s} ds \\ &= \lambda_0(t) e^{\gamma \cdot \mathbf{z}} \end{aligned} \tag{19}$$

where $\lambda_0(t) = \beta e^{-\beta t} \int_0^t \mu(s) e^{\beta s} ds$. Thus, marginally the failure times and covariates follow a proportional hazards model.

4. MARKERS AS A PROXY FOR RESIDUAL LIFE

In this section we consider using observation of present and/or past values of a marker process at time t as a predictor of the residual life of the individual beyond time t. The principal statistical application of such calculations is to supplement information on failure time for individuals who are not observed beyond time t. Censored data is a familiar component of most lifetime data structures where, for individuals censored at time t, the only information used in standard methodology is that $T > t$. With observation of $X(u)$ for $0 \leq u \leq t$, and the assumption of a relationship between $X(\cdot)$ and the risk of failure of the kind described by (2) or (3), there is clearly additional information available.

For simplicity consider a simple situation. Suppose the lifetimes of n individuals are observed subject to right censoring. For each observation, the data available are $(y_i, \delta_i, \mathbf{z}_i)$ where y_i is the observed follow-up time, δ_i is a binary indicator of survival status at time y_i (i.e., $\delta_i = 1$ represents failure at time y_i, $\delta_i = 0$ represents a censored observation), and $\mathbf{z}_i$ is a vector of covariates for the ith individual. Methodology has been extensively developed (e.g. Kalbfleisch and Prentice, 1980; Cox and Oakes, 1984) for the purpose of estimation of the survival distribution in the single group situation, either parametrically or nonparametrically, and for estimation of the relationship between the survival distribution and the covariate $\mathbf{z}$ based on a variety of regression models. Now, suppose that, in addition to $(y_i, \delta_i, \mathbf{z}_i)$, data are available in the form of $\{X_i(u): 0 \leq u \leq y_i\}$, individual sample paths of the marker process up until time y_i. One can now consider extending the current methodology by developing inference procedures based on the likelihood of the complete data $(y_i, \delta_i, \mathbf{z}_i, X_i(u): 0 \leq u \leq y_i)$. Two forms of inference are now possible: in the first, inferences are based on the marginal information provided by (y_i, δ_i) ignoring the information on $X_i(u)$. In the second, the full data are used. Jewell and Kalbfleisch (1992) provide efficiency comparisons between these two approaches for Poisson markers within the regression model (18).

For the reasons discussed in Section 2 it is unlikely that there is sufficient a priori knowledge or available data to carefully model the joint distribution of $X(\cdot)$ and T in the manner needed to use the full likelihood of $(y_i, \delta_i, \mathbf{z}_i, X_i(u): 0 \leq u \leq y_i)$ (but see Self, 1992). Further, the likelihood is additionally complicated by the fact that $\{X_i(u): u = u_1, \ldots, u_{k_i}\}$ is usually observed rather than $\{X_i(u): 0 \leq u \leq y_i\}$, where $u_1, \ldots, u_{k_i}$ are a finite set of observation times for the ith individual. For these reasons various ad-hoc approaches have been suggested to incorporate the additional available marker data in estimation of either a single sample incubation distribution or covariate effects.

Taylor, et al. (1990) use an imputation scheme based on an assumed regression model for residual lifetimes:

$$\log T_t = a + bX(t) + \varepsilon \tag{20}$$

for any $t>0$ with $T \geq t$, where T_t is the residual time to AIDS at time t and ε is a random variable whose distribution function belongs to a specified parametric family (e.g., Gaussian). However, as Neilsen and Jewell (1992) show, models such as (20) impose very strong conditions on the behavior of the stochastic process X. In particular, it is impossible for the residual life distribution at time t to follow a log normal (or Weibull) distribution *for all* t, however we modify the parameters of the lognormal (or Weibull) at differing t's.

Robins (1992) suggests a quite different approach to the incorporation of marker information into estimation of covariate effects. First, he assumes a model for the *marginal* relationship between T and the covariate $\mathbf{z}$, in particular, the accelerated failure time model

$$\log T_i = \beta . \mathbf{z}_i + \varepsilon_i \tag{21}$$

where the error variable ε_i is independent of $\mathbf{z}_i$. For a given $\mathbf{b}$, define $\varepsilon_i(\mathbf{b}) = \log T_i - \mathbf{b} . \mathbf{z}_i$ and $D_i(\mathbf{b}) = R_i(\mathbf{b})[g(\mathbf{z}_i) - E(g(\mathbf{z}_i))]$ with $R_i(\mathbf{b}) = r(\varepsilon_i(\mathbf{b}))$; r and g are known smooth deterministic functions. Let $S(\mathbf{b}) = \sum_{i=1}^{n} D_i(\mathbf{b})$. In the absence of censoring, and under suitable regularity conditions, it is known that $n^{-1/2} S(\beta)$ is asymptotically Gaussian with mean 0, and that a solution of $\hat{\beta}$ to $S(\mathbf{b}) = 0$ yields a consistent estimator of β. The optimal choice for $r(\cdot)$ is the derivative of $\log f_{\varepsilon}(\cdot)$ where f_{ε} is the density of ε and the optimal choice for g is $g(\mathbf{z}) = \mathbf{z}$.

To accommodate censored observations and use the available marker information, Robins assumes that the cause-specific hazard function for *censoring* is independent of ε given the history of the marker, i.e.,

$$h_C(u \mid Y_i \geq u, H_{X_i}(u), \varepsilon) \equiv \lim_{h \to \infty} \frac{1}{h} Pr\{u \leq Y_i \leq u+h, \delta_i=0 \mid Y_i \geq u, H_{X_i}(u), \varepsilon_i\}$$

$$= \lim_{h \to \infty} \frac{1}{h} Pr\{u \leq Y_i \leq u+h, \delta_i=0 \mid Y_i \geq u, H_{X_i}(u)\}$$

$$\equiv h_C(u \mid H_{X_i}(u))$$

where $H_{X_i}(u) = \{X_i(t): 0 \leq t \leq u; \mathbf{z}_i\}$. Then, in the above, $D_i(\mathbf{b})$ is replaced by $\delta_i D_i(\mathbf{b})/K_i(y_i)$ where $K_i(y) = \exp[-\int_0^y h_C(u \mid H_{X_i}(u))du$. The key observation is that, with these assumptions and definitions,

$$E[S^*(\beta)] \equiv E[\sum_{i=1}^{n} \delta_i D_i(\beta)/K_i(Y_i)] = 0 \ ,$$

suggesting the solution of $S^*(\mathbf{b}) = 0$ as an estimator for $\boldsymbol{\beta}$. In order to implement this procedure, one must estimate $K_i(y_i)$ for each y_i and thus $h_C(\cdot \mid H_{X_i}(\cdot))$. Robins suggests the use of a stratified proportional hazards model

$$h_C(u \mid H_{X_i}(u)) = h_{J_i}(u)\exp(\boldsymbol{\gamma} . \mathbf{W}_i(u)] \tag{22}$$

where J_i is a stratum indicator that is a function of $\mathbf{z}_i$, $\boldsymbol{\gamma} = (\gamma_1,...,\gamma_k)$ is a k-vector of parameters to be estimated and $\mathbf{W}_i(u) = (W_{1i}(u),...,W_{ki}(u))$ is a k-vector of functions of $H_{X_i}(u)$. The parameter $\boldsymbol{\gamma}$ can, of course, be estimated using standard proportional hazards model fits that accommodate time-dependent covariates.

The advantage of Robins' approach is that it avoids the need to model the relationship between residual lifetimes and the history of the marker process. It may be much simpler to model $h_C(u \mid H_{X_i}(u))$ and the possibility of misspecification of this model can be reduced by choosing high dimensional versions of both $\mathbf{W}$ and X. For fixed X (i.e., not time-dependent), this procedure corresponds to one suggested by Koul, Susarla and Van Ryzin (1981). One might consider performing a similar generalization of the method of Buckley and James (1979); however, this immediately leads to the need to model the relationship between residual lifetimes and markers.

Several interesting questions remain regarding Robins' procedure including the choice of functions, r, g and $\mathbf{W}$. It would also be of interest to consider special cases of the general approach, for example, the single sample setting (no covariate $\mathbf{z}$), and the Poisson marker regression model (18). Note that the latter model does follow an accelerated failure time model marginally if the intensity function $\mu(\cdot)$ is appropriately specified.

The role of markers as proxies for residual life has a close link to the work of Prentice (1989) on surrogate endpoints in follow-up studies. In particular, the basic model relating the marker to hazard and the various covariate models as described in Section 2 are critical in determining the effects of using a marker process as a surrogate endpoint for failure in assessing covariate effects, such as treatment efficacy, according to the operational criteria introduced by Prentice (1989). Careful consideration of these issues illustrates the difficulty in identifying a marker as a surrogate for the onset of AIDS in therapeutic trials. Further, even if a marker, say CD4, is shown to be an effective surrogate for the study of a given treatment regimen, there is no guarantee that it will remain an appropriate surrogate for a different therapy.

5. MARKERS AS A PROXY FOR PAST LIFE

In certain instances, the origin of the failure time process is not directly observed. Instead, individuals, identified for follow-up, have already been subject to the disease process for some unknown period of time. A cohort of such individuals is termed a prevalent cohort by Brookmeyer and Gail (1987). If, at the time of ascertainment, information is available on a marker or series of markers, there is potential to use this information to "predict" or estimate the time since the onset of the disease process.

One area of potential application is in the study of cohorts of HIV positive individuals. At the time of ascertainment, various markers of disease status can be measured and these provide information on the time since infection. For two ad-hoc approaches to this problem, see Berman (1990) and Mũnoz et al. (1989). As discussed by Neilsen and Jewell (1992), this problem is, in many regards, equivalent in the reversed time scale to predicting residual lifetime based on marker history. As such, the regression imputation scheme of Mũnoz et al. (1989) is analogous to the forward prediction model (20) of Taylor et al. (1990) discussed in Section 4. Again, Nielsen and Jewell (1992) indicate the difficulty of modelling time since infection against marker information consistently without specifying the joint distribution of T and $X(\cdot)$. A current area of interest to the authors is the application of the semiparametric methods of Robins (1992) introduced in Section 4 to the backwards prediction problem.

5.1. Adjustment for onset confounding

Onset confounding (Brookmeyer and Gail, 1987) refers to the bias incurred in using follow-up time to study quantities based on time since infection when studying a prevalent cohort. For example, such bias may be introduced when estimating either the incubation distribution or the effect of covariates on incubation.

Wang et al. (1992) show, however, that there is a relationship between proportional hazards models defined on the time since infection scale and the time of follow-up scale. In a simple case assume that, marginally, the proportional hazards model $\lambda(t \mid \mathbf{z}) = h_0(t)\, e^{\beta . \mathbf{z}}$ holds, where t is time since infection. Now, suppose a prevalent infected individual (who was infected at chronological time u) is identified at time τ when follow-up commences. Denoting time since beginning of follow-up by r we have

$$\lambda^*(r \mid \tau - u, \mathbf{z}) = h_0(r + (\tau - u))e^{\beta . \mathbf{z}}$$

so that $\dfrac{\lambda^*(r \mid \tau-u, \mathbf{z}_1)}{\lambda^*(r \mid \tau-u, \mathbf{z}_2)} = \exp[\beta . (\mathbf{z}_1 - \mathbf{z}_2)]$. Thus, the parameter β still has the usual interpretation with regard to the relative hazard, based on the residual failure time scale r, so long as we argue conditionally on $\tau - u$. A similar argument holds in reverse if a proportional hazards model holds on the follow-up time scale, and can be extended to include u and τ in the covariate vector. Thus, if one assumes and fits a proportional hazards model in the follow-up time scale, including u and τ as covariates as necessary, then the estimated regression parameter β still has a relative hazard interpretation on the time since infection scale, conditional on u and τ.

Of course with most HIV infected prevalent cohorts, the infection time u is unknown so that one is unable to fit models conditional on time since infection, $\tau - u$. Suppose, however, one has data on a marker process $X(\cdot)$ which provides information on time since infection. Then, one might try fitting a proportional hazards model conditional on, say, the value of $X(\cdot)$ at recruitment. We briefly examine this by considering the Poisson marker regression model (18) of Section 3. Note that, marginally, $\lambda(t \mid \mathbf{z}_i)/\lambda(t \mid \mathbf{z}_2) = \exp[\gamma . (\mathbf{z}_1 - \mathbf{z}_2)]$ by (19). Now, from (12), assuming all individuals are AIDS-free at the time of recruitment,

$$\lambda^*(r\,|X(\tau-u),\mathbf{z}) = \beta X(\tau-u) + \beta e^{-\beta t}\int_0^t \mu(s)e^{\gamma\cdot\mathbf{z}}e^{\beta s}\,ds$$

$$= \beta X(\tau-u) + \lambda_0(t)e^{\gamma\cdot\mathbf{z}} \;.$$

Therefore, $\dfrac{\lambda^*(r\,|X(\tau-u),\mathbf{z}_1)}{\lambda^*(r\,|X(\tau-u),\,\mathbf{z}_2)} = \dfrac{\beta X(\tau-u) + \lambda_0(t)e^{\gamma\cdot\mathbf{z}_1}}{\beta X(\tau-u) + \lambda_0(t)e^{\gamma\cdot\mathbf{z}_2}}$, so that the ratio of hazards in the follow-up time scale, conditional on the marker value at recruitment, is biased towards one as compared to the ratio on the time since infection scale. This example thus illustrates that conditioning on $X(\tau-u)$ at recruitment introduces additional complications to simply conditioning on time since infection, $\tau-u$.

6. DISCUSSION

The work described here is preliminary. Further development is needed to (i) extend the calculations of Jewell and Kalbfleisch (1992) to more complex marker models, (ii) allow for more complex dependence of the hazard on the past history of the marker process than that which depends solely on the current value of the marker, (iii) examine other marker-hazard models in addition to the simple additive model (2), and (iv) pursue the use of marker models for the kinds of applications described in the introduction. Furthermore, attempts to fit stochastic models for marker variables, including the link to the hazard function, based on real data would be of great interest in illuminating the values and limitations of these models and problems surrounding practical implementation.

For certain markers there is a relationship of some of the ideas discussed to the issue of the choice of time scales in certain survival settings. Specifically, if the marker process $X(t)$ always possesses increasing sample paths, the random variable $X(t)$ can be viewed as an alternative time scale to t. In this light, the model (2) can be viewed as a model which describes the dependence of the hazard on the two (or more) alternative time scales. Subsequently, one can phrase various questions of interest regarding this relationship; for example, whether the hazard depends solely on one specific time scale, or whether it may be possible to derive a single univariate time scale which incorporates the hazard dependence and combines the separate time scales. The issue of several time scales is of much interest in several applications (for example, see Farewell and Cox, 1979, and Oakes, 1988) including certain follow up studies where there may be several "natural" time origins (see, for example, Wang, Brookmeyer and Jewell, 1992).

7. ACKNOWLEDGEMENTS

This research was supported by grants from the National Institute of Allergy and Infectious Diseases (grant #AI29162) and the National Sciences and Engineering Research Council of Canada. Additional support was provided by SIMS (Societal Institute of the Mathematical Sciences) via a grant from the National Institute on Drug Abuse (grant #DA04722).

8. REFERENCES

Berman, S. M. (1990). A stochastic model for the distribution of HIV latency time based on T4 counts. *Biometrika,* **77**, 733-741.

Bremermann, H. J. and Anderson, R. W. (1990a). The HIV cytopathic effect: Potential target for therapy? *J. Acquired Immune Deficiency Syndromes*, **3**, 1119-1128.

Bremermann, H. J. and Anderson, R. W. (1990b). Mathematical models of HIV infection. I. Threshold conditions for transmission and host survival. *J. Acquired Immune Deficiency Syndromes*, **3**, 1129-1134.

Brookmeyer, R. and Gail, M. (1987). Biases in prevalent cohorts. *Biometrics*, **43**, 739-749.

Buckley, J. and James, I. (1979). Linear regression with censored data. *Biometrika*, **66**, 429-436.

Cox, D. R. and Oakes, D. (1984). *Analysis of Survival Data.* Chapman and Hall, London.

DeGruttola, V., Lange, N. and Dafni, U. (1991). Modeling the progression of HIV infection. *J. Amer. Statist. Assoc.*, **86**, 569-577.

Doksum, K. A. (1992). Degradation rate models for failure time and survival data. To appear, *Centrum voor Wiskunde en Informatica*, Amsterdam.

Farewell, V. and Cox, D. R. (1979). A note on multiple time scales in life testing. *Applied Statistics*, **28**, 73-75.

Fusaro, R. E., Nielsen, J. P. and Scheike, T. H. (1992). Marker-dependent hazard estimation: an application to AIDS. Submitted for publication.

Jewell, N. P. and Kalbfleisch, J. D. (1992). Marker processes in survival analysis. Submitted for publication.

Kalbfleisch, J. D. and Prentice, R. L. (1980). *The Statistical Analysis of Failure Time Data.* Wiley, New York.

Koul, H., Susarla, V. and Van Ryzin, J. (1981). Regression analysis with randomly right censored data. *Annals of Statistics*, **9**, 1276-1288.

Longini, I. M. (1990). Modeling the decline of $CD4^+$ T-lymphocyte counts in HIV-infected individuals. *J. Acquired Immune Deficiency Syndromes*, **3**, 930-931.

Longini, I. M., Clark, W. S., Byers, R. H. et al. (1989). Statistical analysis of the stages of HIV infection using a Markov model. *Statistics in Medicine*, **8**, 831-843.

Longini, I. M., Clark, W. S., Gardner, L. I. et al. (1991). The dynamics of $CD4^+$ T-lymphocyte decline in HIV-infected individuals: A Markov modeling approach. *J. Acquired Immune Deficiency Syndromes*, **4**, 1141-1147.

Mũnoz, A., Carey, V., Saah, A. J. et al. (1988). Predictors of decline in CD4 lymphocytes in a cohort of homosexual men infected with human immunodeficiency virus. *J. Acquired Immune Deficiency Syndromes*, **1**, 396-404.

Mũnoz, A., Wang, M.-C., Bass, S. et al. (1989). Acquired Immunodeficiency Syndrome (AIDS)-free time after Human Immunodeficiency Virus Type 1 (HIV-1) seroconversion in homosexual men. *American Journal of Epidemiology*, **130**, 530-539.

Moss, A. R. and Bacchetti, P. (1989). Natural history of HIV infection. *AIDS*, **3**, 55-61.

Nielsen, J. P. (1992). Marker dependent hazard estimation. Submitted for publication.

Nielsen, J. P. and Jewell, N. P. (1992). A framework for consistent prediction rules based on markers. Submitted for publication.

Oakes, D. (1988). An equivalency model for multiple time scales in survival analysis. University of Rochester Technical Report.

Perelson, A. S. (1987). Toward a realistic model of the immune system. In *Theoretical Immunology Part I and II, vols. 2,3*, A. S. Perelson (ed.), Redwood City, California: Addison-Wesley.

Prentice, R. L. (1989). Surrogate endpoints in clinical trials: definition and operational criteria. *Statistics in Medicine*, **8**, 431-440.

Puri, P. S. (1966). A class of stochastic models of response after infection in the absence of defense mechanism. *Proceedings of the Fifth Berkeley Symposium on Mathematical Statistics and Probability*, Berkeley and Los Angeles, University of California Press, Vol. 4, 511-536.

Robins, J. M. (1992). Estimating regression parameters in the presence of dependent censoring. Submitted for publication.

Segall, A. and Kailath, T. (1975). The modeling of randomly modulated jump processes. *IEEE Transactions on Information Theory*, **IT-21**, 135-143.

Self, S. (1992). Modeling a marker of disease progression and onset of disease. In *AIDS Epidemiology: Methodological Issues*, N. Jewell, K. Dietz and V. Farewell (eds.), Boston: Birkhäuser-Boston.

Taylor, J. M. G., Mũnoz, A., Bass, S. M. et al. (1990). Estimating the distribution of times from HIV seroconversion to AIDS using multiple imputation. *Statistics in Medicine*, **9**, 505-514.

Taylor, J. M. G. and Cumberland, W. G. (1991). A stochastic model for analysis of longitudinal data. Preprint.

Vittinghoff, E. and Jewell, N. P. (1992). Estimating patterns of $CD4^+$ lymphocyte decline using data from a prevalent cohort of HIV infected individuals. Submitted for publication.

Wang, M-C., Brookmeyer, R. and Jewell, N. P. (1992). Statistical models for prevalent cohort data. *Biometrics*, to appear.

Nicholas P. Jewell
Group in Biostatistics
University of California
Berkeley, CA 94720 USA

John D. Kalbfleisch
Department of Statistics & Actuarial Science
University of Waterloo
Waterloo, Ontario N2L 3G1 Canada

Modeling a Marker of Disease Progression and Onset of Disease

Steve Self and Yudi Pawitan

Abstract

We consider the problem of developing joint models for a periodically observed marker of underlying disease progression and its relationship to either onset of disease or occurrence of a disease-related endpoint. We use the framework of relative risk regression models with time-dependent covariates to specify the relationship between marker and disease onset and use a mixed linear model to describe the evolution of the marker process. The construction of partial likelihood is discussed and a two step procedure is described for estimation of parameters in the model. For a special case a heuristic development of a large sample distribution theory for the proposed estimators is presented which suggests variance estimators. The method is illustrated by applying it to an analysis of periodic measurements of T4 and T8 cells and time from seroconversion to AIDS diagnosis.

1 Introduction

There is a large literature on models and associated statistical methods for the analysis of the progression of disease. Two different approaches have been followed in this literature. In the first approach, periodic observations of a variable thought to reflect underlying progression of disease are available on each of a number of individuals. The focus of the modeling effort in this approach is characterization of the underlying stochastic process generating these observations. For example, DeGruttola et, al. (1991) analyzes progression of human immunodeficiency virus (HIV) infection by modeling short time-series of T-helper lymphocyte counts observed on each individual in a cohort of

490 HIV-infected men. In this analysis, DeGruttola uses multivariate normal linear models with patterned covariance matrices and likelihood-based statistical methods.

In the second approach to modeling disease progression, information is available on time of disease onset and the focus of the modeling effort is to characterize the distribution of time of disease onset. This characterization typically involves description of the relationship between covariates measured at baseline and subsequent risk of disease. Relative risk regression models and the associated partial likelihood-based statistical methods have been the primary analytic tools used in this approach.

In some situations, time-series of marker variables and time of disease onset are both of interest. Such is the case for many follow-up studies of HIV-infected individuals in which periodic measurements of hematologic variables reflecting immune status are made. In epidemiologic studies, the disease-related endpoint of interest might be diagnosis of AIDS; in clinical studies of patients already diagnosed with AIDS, the endpoint might be onset of a particular opportunistic infection or death. In either case, a complete and consistent description of disease progression requires a joint model for the marker time-series and time to occurrence of the disease endpoint. In addition to providing a more complete description of the natural history of the disease process, such joint models can also form the basis of evaluation of the marker process as an alternative endpoint in the context of randomized clinical trials.

In our work, we consider the problem of developing joint models for a periodically measured marker of disease progression and occurrence of a disease-related endpoint. We note that almost all of the previous work on this problem has addressed the case of categorical marker processes under the heading of multistate survival analyses. In this work, levels of the marker variable are combined with disease status to form a collection of mutually exclusive "states". Markov or semi-Markov models are then used to describe the rates with which individuals move from one state to another over time. The main distinction between our work and the multistate survival literature is the required intensity of observation of the marker process. Most multistate survival methods require observation of transition times from one state another for each individual. This requirement is tantamount to continuous observation of the marker process which, as noted by Andersen (1986), is likely to limit the usefulness of the approach. In contrast, we will assume that the marker process is only observed periodically during the follow-up of each individual.

Our work is motivated by the analysis of clinical or epidemiologic cohort studies of HIV-infected individuals where the marker processes are various measures of immune function and the endpoints are death or diagnosis with AIDS. For ease of exposition, we will describe our model and statistical methods in relation to the specific problem of modeling measurements of ratios of T4 cells to T8 cells (denoted by T4/T8) and time from seroconversion to diagnosis with AIDS. In Section 2, models for the time-series of T4/T8 measurements and risk of AIDS are described. Construction of partial likelihoods will be presented in Section 3 and the potential for using these likelihoods for inference will be discussed. In Section 4, a two step estimation procedure is described and an outline of a large sample distribution theory is given for a special case. The method is applied to an analysis of T4 and T8 cell counts and time to seroconversion to AIDS diagnosis in Section 5.

2 A Model for Disease Progression

2.1 A Model for the Marker Process

Let $Z_{io}(t)$ denote the T4/T8 ratio for individual i at time t and let $(s_{i1}, \ldots, s_{ik_i})$ be the times at which Z_{io} is observed. We will assume that $Z_{io}(t) = Z_i(t) + \epsilon_i(t)$ with

$$Z_i(t) = W_i^T(t)\alpha + X^T(t)\phi_i \tag{1}$$

where $X(t)$ is a known p-vector valued function of t, $W_i(t)$ is a known q-vector valued function of t, α_1 is an unknown regression parameter, $\epsilon_i(t)$ is "white noise" with variance σ_ϵ^2 and the

ϕ_i's are unknown random p-vector valued regression parameters with mean E_ϕ and variance/covariance matrix V_ϕ. In this formulation, the $\epsilon_i(t)$'s represent measurement errors and the $W_i(t)$'s represent functions of covariates observed at baseline and t. The $W_i(t)$'s may also include time-dependent covariates that are observed over time but whose evolution will not be modeled.

The term $X^T(t)\phi_i$ is meant to reflect the underlying fluctuations in T4/T8 ratios within an individual over time after accounting for the effects of $W_i(t)$. Choice of $X(t)$ should reflect prior information about the nature of these fluctuations although one would expect $X^T(t)\phi_i$ to be a fairly smooth function of time for most reasonable marker processes.

One attractive choice for the components of $X^T(t)$ is B-spline basis functions (deBoor, 1978) associated with a fixed set of knot points selected by the data analyst. With an appropriate selection of knot points, this choice would provide a rich class of shapes with which to model T4/T8 fluctuations making the assumption of independence of $\epsilon_i(t)$ and $\epsilon_i(s)$ palatable. In addition, such basis functions have local support which results in an attractive feature. For each individual, only the components of ϕ_i that are associated with elements of $X(t)$ whose support overlaps the actual follow-up period of follow-up are required to describe that individual's data. Thus, features of the model pertaining to times that are remote to the actual follow-up of an individual need never be considered for that individual.

2.2 A Model for Disease Onset

It will be convenient to formulate the model for disease onset in terms of multivariate counting processes (Anderson and Borgan, 1985). Using the notation of Andersen and Gill (1982), let $N_i(t)$ and $Y_i(t)$ denote the counting process for disease onset and the "at risk" process for individual i, respectively. Let $\{\mathcal{G}_t : t \geq 0\}$ represent a filtration such that all variables observed prior to time t are $\mathcal{G}_t$-measurable with the ϕ_i's, W_i's and measurement errors ϵ_i's all $\mathcal{G}_0$-measurable. We assume that the intensity of N_i at time t with respect to the filtration $\mathcal{G}_t$, denoted by $d\Lambda_i^{\mathcal{G}}(t)$, is specified by the relative risk regression model of the form

$$Y_i(t)exp\{W_i^T(t)\gamma\}\{1+\sum_{j=1}^{m}(\mathcal{L}_{j;t}X^T\phi_i)\beta_j\}d\Lambda_0(t) \qquad (2)$$

where Y_i is a predictable function, $\mathcal{L}_{j;t}f$ represents a linear functional of $f(s)$ over the interval $[0,t]$, $\Lambda_0(t)$ is a fixed but arbitrary "baseline" cumulative intensity function and the β_j's are unknown regression coefficients. Note that, as in Prentice's formulation of measurement errors (1982), the assumption that the ϵ_i's carry no information about risk of disease conditional on the ϕ_i's is implicit in model (2).

Model (2) is somewhat different than the usual form of a relative risk regression model in that the relative risk function is not represented as $r(\eta_{it})$ where $r(\cdot)$ is a non-decreasing function scaled so that $r(0) = 1$ and η_{it} is a linear combination of possibly time-dependent covariates. In model (2) the effects of all covariates except for those associated with the marker process are multiplicative with each multiplicative term having an exponential form. This is the most commonly used form of relative risk function. However, the multiplicative term representing the effect of the marker process uses a linear relative risk form. As noted by Prentice (1982), the additive relative risk form requires fewer distributional assumptions regarding random terms in the model such as the ϕ_i's.

The use of linear functionals in (2) is simply a convenient device to allow risk of disease onset to depend in a flexible and fairly general way on the history of T4/T8 ratios at time t $\{Z_i(s) : s \leq t\}$. For example, covariates represented by $\mathcal{L}_{j;t}X^T\phi_i$ might be the current T4/T8 ratio, the initial T4/T8 ratio or the integrated average T4/T8 ratio over the year preceeding time t. Model (2) can be rewritten as

$$Y_i(t)exp\{W_i^T(t)\gamma\}\{1+\sum_{j=1}^{m}\beta_jX_j^T(t)\phi_i\}d\Lambda_0(t) \qquad (3)$$

where $X_j(t) = \mathcal{L}_{j;t}X.$

Because model (3) depends on the unobserved ϕ_i's, it is not directly estimable. However, as in Prentice's analysis of measurement error models (1982), an estimable intensity can be induced by use of the Innovation Theorem (Aalen, 1978). Let $\{\mathcal{F}_t : t \geq 0\}$ represent a filtration for which all variables observed prior to time t are $\mathcal{F}_t$-measurable. Thus, $\mathcal{F}_t$ represents information prior to t about disease onset, measurement times of T4/T8 ratios and the observed values of T4/T8 ratios at those times, baseline-covariates, time-dependent covariates other than T4/T8 ratios and times at which individuals enter and leave follow-up. However $\mathcal{F}_t$ does not represent the ϕ_i's and ϵ_i's. The intensity of N_i at time t with respect to the filtration $\mathcal{F}_t$, denoted by $d\Lambda_i^{\mathcal{F}}(t)$, is given by

$$Y_i(t)exp\{W_i^T(t)\gamma\}\{1+\sum_{j=1}^{m}\beta_j X_j^T(t)E[\phi_i|\mathcal{F}_t]\}d\Lambda_0(t) \quad (4)$$

where the expectation is taken over the distribution of ϕ_i conditional on all data observed prior to time t. More precise construction of filtrations analogous to $\mathcal{F}_t$ and $\mathcal{G}_t$ is given by Nielsen et. al. (1991).

3 Construction of Partial Likelihoods

There are several approaches that one might consider in constructing a partial likelihood that would be useful for estimation of parameters in the model described in Section 2. The first approach would proceed with a factorization of the likelihood function that is marginal with respect to the ϕ_i's. Using the informal approach as in Kalbfleisch and Prentice (1980) such a factorization would proceed by making the following definitions: $\mathcal{H}_t$ represents the history of all observable variables prior to time t, $\mathcal{S}_t$ represents all times at which T4/T8 ratios were measured prior to time t, $\mathcal{M}_t$ represents values of observed T4/T8 ratios measured prior to time t (i.e., $\mathcal{M}_t$ includes $\mathcal{S}_t$ and values of Z_{io} at all exam times prior to time t for each individual), $\mathcal{D}_t$ represents all observed disease onset times prior to time t, and $\mathcal{Y}_t$ represents all times prior to time t that individuals either entered or left follow-up (i.e., history of the "at risk" processes).

Letting $\mathcal{P}_{t\geq 0}$ denote product integral, the likelihood function is written as $P(\mathcal{H}_0)\mathcal{P}_{t\geq 0}P(\mathcal{H}_{t+dt}|\mathcal{H}_t)$ where $P(\mathcal{H}_{t+dt}|\mathcal{H}_t)$ is further factored as

$$\begin{aligned} &P(\mathcal{D}_{t+dt}|\mathcal{H}_t) \times \\ &P(\mathcal{Y}_{t+dt}|\mathcal{H}_t, \mathcal{D}_{t+dt}) \times \\ &P(\mathcal{S}_{t+dt}|\mathcal{H}_t, \mathcal{D}_{t+dt}, \mathcal{Y}_{t+dt}) \times \\ &P(\mathcal{M}_{t+dt}|\mathcal{H}_t, \mathcal{D}_{t+dt}, \mathcal{Y}_{t+dt}, \mathcal{S}_{t+dt}). \end{aligned} \tag{5}$$

The first and fourth factors in this expression represent the terms that are informative about parameters in the model. Extracting these two terms and making an assumption of independence among individuals gives the partial likelihood

$$\begin{aligned} \mathcal{PL} \;=\; &\mathcal{P}_{i,t\geq 0}[d\Lambda_i^{\mathcal{F}}(t)]^{dN_i(t)}[1 - d\Lambda_i^{\mathcal{F}}(t)]^{1-dN_i(t)} \times \\ &\mathcal{P}_{i,t\geq 0}[dP_{Z_{io}(t)|\mathcal{H}_t,\mathcal{D}_{t+dt},\mathcal{Y}_{t+dt},\mathcal{S}_{t+dt}}]^{dS_i(t)} \end{aligned} \tag{6}$$

where S_i represents the counting process that jumps each time a T4/T8 ratio is measured on individual i.

The partial likelihood (6) is not useful in its current form. The terms associated with disease onset involve the quantities $E[\phi_i|\mathcal{F}_t]$ which are complicated functions depending on Λ_0 and the censoring process as well as T4/T8 ratios measured prior to t. The likelihood elements in (6) associated with observed T4/T8 ratios suffer from a similar problem in that they depend on the distribution of the ϕ_i's conditional on $\mathcal{F}_t$. Thus, partial likelihood (6) not only has a very complicated form, it also fails to separate parameters of interest from those parts of the larger model that one would like to avoid having to model.

A second approach to the construction of a partial likelihood is to factor the likelihood that treats the ϕ_i's as observable and then integrate the resulting partial likelihood over the ϕ_i's. Assuming independence among individuals, the resulting function is the product over i of terms

$$\int_{\Re^p} \mathcal{P}_{t\geq 0}[d\Lambda_i^{\mathcal{G}}(t)]^{dN_i(t)}[1 - d\Lambda_i^{\mathcal{G}}(t)]^{1-dN_i(t)}[f_\epsilon(r_{i;t})]^{dS_{it}}dP_\phi(\phi_i) \tag{7}$$

where $r_{i;t} = Z_{io}(t) - W_i^T(t)\alpha - X^T\phi_i$. Under the assumption that the censoring mechanism and the mechanism generating the times of the T4/T8 ratio measurements are independent of the ϕ_i's, Gill (1991) has noted that this "marginal partial likelihood" is also a partial likelihood. This provides the justification for the use of (7) provided parametric models are specified for Λ_0 and for the distributions of the ϕ_i's and ϵ_i's. In addition, if the censoring and exam-time distributions are non-informative (Kalbfleisch and Prentice, 1980), then use of (7) will result in fully efficient estimation.

One drawback to the use of (7) is the challenging computational problem of its maximization. It is tempting to consider use of the EM algorithm in this problem because of the simplicity of the M-step. However, the conditional distributions required in the E-step are precisely of the form that made partial likelihood (6) so unpalatable. Thus it appears that the computational challenge of maximizing the partial likelihood (7) is best met head-on.

Another drawback to the use of (7) is the requirement of specifying fully parametric models for Λ_0 and for the distributions of the ϕ_i's and ϵ_i's. Although there is no theoretical justification, it is tempting to consider the use of (7) as the basis for estimation in a semi-parametric setting with an arbitrary Λ_0. In this approach, the estimation procedure alternates between computation of a non-parametric estimate of Λ_0 given values of other parameters and maximization of the partial likelihood evaluated at the current estimate of Λ_0. Similar programs have been examined in the context of frailty models by Clayton and Cuzick (1985), Self and Prentice (1986) and Nielsen et. al. (1991) and, in spite of their computational complexity, have behaved in a fairly stable manner. However, a rigorous large sample distribution theory for such procedures is not yet available.

A third approach to the construction of a partial likelihood is to treat the ϕ_i's as unknown parameters to be estimated. Under the assumption of a Gaussian distribution for the ϵ_i's, the estimators of the ϕ_i's will be very close to the least squares estimators. In fact, if one considers the partial likelihood consisting only of fourth terms in (5), then the estimators of the ϕ_i's (and α_1) will be the least squares estimators. Although these estimators of the individual ϕ_i's might not be the most efficient in terms of mean square error, they might form the basis of good estimators of aggregate properties of the ϕ_i's. The main virtue of this approach is that conditioning on the ϕ_i's eliminates complications in the analysis of the T4/T8 measurements due to the informative nature of the censoring of the T4/T8 time-series by disease onset and loss-to-followup (Wu and Carroll, 1988). The biggest drawback to this approach is in the estimation of the parameters in the model for disease onset. Insertion of the least squares estimator of ϕ_i into the relative risk function introduces a variability that is likely to ruin the distributional properties of the estimators of γ and β. This situation will not improve with large samples except in the unrealistic case in which more and more observations are made on T4/T8 ratios for each individual.

4 A Two-Step Estimation Procedure

In this section, we propose a two-step estimation procedure that first analyzes the T4/T8 time-series conditional on the ϕ_i's by least squares. This analysis requires that all but a negligible number of individuals have sufficient numbers of observations in their T4/T8 time-series to produce a unique estimate of ϕ_i. The second step of the analysis produces estimates of parameters in the disease onset model and is performed marginally to the ϕ_i's. In this step, the least squares estimators of the ϕ_i's are pooled and, together with T4/T8 measurements observed on individual i prior to time t, are used to estimate $E[\phi_i|\mathcal{F}_t]$. An estimated partial likelihood is then computed which is maximized for the estimation of γ and β.

Let $Z_{io;t}^T = (Z_{io}(s_{i1}), \ldots, Z_{io}(s_{ik(i,t)}))$ where $s_{ik(i,t)}$ is greatest observation time for Z_{io} prior to time t. Also define $X_{i;t}$ and $W_{i;t}$ to be the matrices with j^{th} column $X_i(s_{ij})$ and $W_i(s_{ij})$, respectively, for $j = 1, \ldots, k(i,t)$. Now we assume that; 1) $E[\phi_i|\mathcal{F}_t]$ depends only on $Z_{io;t}$ and the fact that $Y_i(t) = 1$, and 2) $E[\phi_i|\mathcal{F}_t]$

is linear in $Z_{io;t}$. Under these assumptions,

$$E[\phi_i|\mathcal{F}_t] = E_\phi(t) + M_{i;t}(Z_{io;t} - W_{i;t}\alpha_1 - X_{i;t}^T E_\phi(t)) \tag{8}$$

and

$$Var[\phi_i|\mathcal{F}_t] = [I - M_i X_{i;t}^T]V_\phi(t) \tag{9}$$

where $E_\phi(t)$ denotes $E[\phi|Y(t) = 1]$, $V_\phi(t)$ denotes $Var[\phi|Y(t) = 1]$, $M_{i;t} = V_\phi(t)X_{i;t}[X_{i;t}^T V_\phi(t)X_{i;t} + \sigma_\epsilon^2 I_{i;t}]^{-1}$ and $I_{i;t}$ represents the $k(i,t) \times k(i,t)$ identity matrix. This representation of $E[\phi_i|\mathcal{F}_t]$ separates information about ϕ_i that is available at time t into two sources; "individual-level" information represented by $Z_{io;t}$, and "group level" information represented by $E_\phi(t)$ and $V_\phi(t)$. This separation provides the opportunity to borrow strength across individuals for estimation of $E_\phi(t)$ and $V_\phi(t)$.

Let $\hat{\phi}_i$ denote the least squares estimator of ϕ_i using all of the T4/T8 time-series data from all individuals and let $\hat{\sigma}_\epsilon^2$ denote the estimator of the error variance based on the least squares analysis. Our estimators of $E_\phi(t)$ and $V_\phi(t)$ are given by

$$\hat{E}_\phi(t) = \sum_i Y_i(t)\hat{\phi}_i / \sum_i Y_i(t) \tag{10}$$

and

$$\begin{aligned}\hat{V}_\phi(t) \quad = \quad & \sum_i Y_i(t)[\hat{\phi}_i - \hat{E}_\phi(t)]^{\otimes 2} / (\sum_i Y_i(t) - 1) - \\ & \hat{\sigma}_\epsilon^2 \sum_i Y_i(t)C_{ii} / \sum_i Y_i(t) + \\ & \hat{\sigma}_\epsilon^2 \sum_{i \neq j} Y_i(t)Y_j(t)C_{ij} / [\sum_i Y_i(t)(\sum_i Y_i(t) - 1)].\end{aligned} \tag{11}$$

where $\sigma_\epsilon^2 C_{ij}$ represents the $(i,j)^{th}$ submatrix of the variance/covariance matrix of the $\hat{\phi}_i$'s. $\hat{E}_\phi(t)$ may be recognized as a moment estimator of $E_\phi(t)$. Unbiasedness of $\hat{E}_\phi(t)$ and $\hat{V}_\phi(t)$ follows from simple calculations.

Under the above modeling assumptions, if $E_\phi(t)$ and $V_\phi(t)$ were known, estimation of γ and β would proceed by maximization over γ and β of the partial likelihood

$$\mathcal{P}_{i,t \geq 0}\{Y_i(t)r_{it}(\gamma,\beta) / \sum_j Y_j(t)r_{jt}(\gamma,\beta)\}^{dN_i(t)} \tag{12}$$

where $r_{it}(\gamma, \beta)$ is given by $exp\{W_i^T(t)\gamma\}\{1+\sum_{j=1}^m \beta_j X_j^T(t)\ E[\phi_i \mid \mathcal{F}_t]\}$ and the form of $E[\phi_i|\mathcal{F}_t]$ is given by (8). Evaluating the partial likelihood (12) at $\hat{E}_\phi(t)$ and $\hat{V}_\phi(t)$ yields a "pseudo partial likelihood" in the sense of Gong and Samaniego (1981) which is then maximized in order to obtain estimates of γ and β.

The variance of the estimators of $\hat{\gamma}$ and $\hat{\beta}$ that are obtained by maximization of the estimated version of (12) will not be consistently estimated by the inverse of the information matrix based on (12) because of the variation in $\hat{E}_\phi(t)$ and $\hat{V}_\phi(t)$. Thus, a large sample theory for $\hat{\gamma}$ and $\hat{\beta}$ that incorporates this variation must be developed along the lines of Gong and Samaniego (1981). We will sketch a large sample distribution theory here with the goals of identifying a likely candidate for a variance estimator of $\hat{\gamma}$ and $\hat{\beta}$ and indicating what arguments might be useful in developing such a theory. We do not intend this sketch to be comprehensive. We will only consider the effect of variability of $\hat{E}_\phi(t)$ on the distribution of $\hat{\beta}$ and presume $V_\phi(t)$ to be fixed and known. We also will only consider the case in which no additional covariates $W_i(t)$ are included in the model for disease onset and risk of disease onset depends only a single linear functional of $X^T(t)\phi_i$. This sketch is also not intended to be technically rigorous. A more comprehensive, and hopefully rigorous, development of a large sample distribution theory will be presented elsewhere.

Let $S_{n;\beta,E_{\phi t}}$ represent the partial likelihood score function based on (12) for β viewed as a function of β and $E_{\phi t}$ $(= E_\phi(\cdot))$ so that $\hat{\beta}_n$ is the solution to the equation $0 = S_{n;\hat{\beta},\hat{E}_{\phi t}}$. Now assume that $n^{1/2}(\hat{\beta}_n - \beta)$ can be represented as $o_p(1)$ plus $(n^{-1}I_{n;\beta,\beta})^{-1}$ times

$$n^{-1/2}S_{n;\beta,E_{\phi t}} + n^{-1}dS_{n;\beta,E_{\phi t}}(n^{1/2}[\hat{E}_{\phi t} - E_{\phi t}]) \tag{13}$$

where $I_{n;\beta,\beta}$ is the observed information about β and $dS_{n;\beta,E_{\phi t}}(f)$ represents the derivative of $S_{n;\beta,E_{\phi t}}$ with respect to the function $E_{\phi t}$ evaluated at the function $f(\cdot)$. Now write the matrix transpose of $n^{-1}dS_{n;\beta,E_{\phi t}}(n^{1/2}[\hat{E}_{\phi t} - E_{\phi t}])$ as

$$\int n^{1/2}[\hat{E}_\phi(t) - E_\phi(t)]n^{-1}\sum_i dS_{ni}(t)dN_i(t) \tag{14}$$

where $dS_{ni}(t)$ represents the derivative of the contribution by individual i to $S_{n;\beta,E_{\phi t}}$ with respect to $E_\phi(t)$. Note that the integrand in (14) is predictable when considering the filtration $\mathcal{G}_t$. In particular, $n^{1/2}[\hat{E}_\phi(t) - E_\phi(t)]$ is predictable as it depends only on the ϕ_i's and ϵ_i's. Therefore, assuming $n^{1/2}[\hat{E}_\phi(t) - E_\phi(t)]$ is $O_p(1)$, martingale convergence properties can be used to prove the asymptotic equivalence of (14) and

$$\int n^{1/2}[\hat{E}_\phi(t) - E_\phi(t)]A_n(t)d\Lambda_0(t). \tag{15}$$

where $A_n(t) = n^{-1}\sum_i Y_i(t)dS_{ni}(t)\{1 + X^T(t)\phi_i\beta\}$. Convergence of $A_n(t)$ to a fixed function and writing $n^{1/2}[\hat{E}_\phi(t) - E_\phi(t)]$ as the sum of independent random variables results in a representation of $n^{-1}dS_{n;\beta,E_{\phi t}}(n^{1/2}[\hat{E}_{\phi t} - E_{\phi t}])$ as the sum of independent random variables $U_{2,i}$. We note that the partial likelihood score for β can also be represented as the sum of independent random variables $U_{1,i}$ (Lin and Wei, 1989; Wei et al., 1989) so that (13) can be written as

$$n^{-1/2}\sum_i (U_{1,i} + U_{2,i}). \tag{16}$$

Estimates of the $U_{1,i}$'s have been shown to be useful for variance estimation by using the empirical variance of the $\hat{U}_{1,i}$'s (Lin and Wei, 1989; Wei et al., 1989). We propose using a similar strategy with the $U_{2,i}$'s although a bit more care is required in the estimation the $U_{2,i}$'s because of their dependence on the unobserved ϕ_i's. In particular, it must be verified that $\hat{A}_n(t) = n^{-1}\sum_i Y_i(t)dS_{ni}(t)\{1 + X^T(t)\hat{E}[\phi_i|\mathcal{F}_\infty]\beta\}$ is asymptotically equivalent to $A_n(t)$. Expression (16) suggests the "sandwich" estimator of variance of $\hat{\beta}_n$ of

$$(I_{n;\beta,\beta})^{-1}(\sum_i [\hat{U}_{1,i} + \hat{U}_{2,i})^{\otimes 2}](I_{n;\beta,\beta})^{-1}. \tag{17}$$

where the form of $\hat{U}_{1,i}$ is described in Wei et al. (1989) and $\hat{U}_{2,i}$ is given by

$$\int [Y_i(t)/\overline{Y}(t)][\hat{\phi}_i - \hat{E}_\phi(t)]\hat{A}_n(t)d\hat{\Lambda}_0(t) \tag{18}$$

with $\hat{\Lambda}_0$ representing the Nelsen-Aalen estimator of Λ_0 and $\overline{Y}(t) = n^{-1}\sum_i Y_i(t)$.

5 An Application

In this section, we apply the two-step method of estimation described above to the analysis of periodic measurements of T4 and T8 cells and the relationship of the ratio of T4 to T8 cells to time from seroconversion to diagnosis with AIDS. We will use a sample of 159 men participating in the Toronto Cohort Study (Coates, et al. 1990) who were either seropositive at the time of entry into the study or were observed to seroconvert during followup. Of these, 39 were diagnosed with AIDS during followup. Clinical exams were scheduled every three months during followup of each individual in the cohort and measurements of T4 cells, T8 cells and HIV antibody status were obtained at these exams. For those individuals who were seronegative for HIB antibody at entry and seroconverted during followup, we will assume that seroconversion occurred at the midpoint between their last seronegative and first seropositive exam. A time of seroconversion was imputed for individuals who were seropositive for HIV antibody at entry with the imputation based on an interview about time of first and last contact with their HIV infected partner. The imputed seroconversion time is taken to be the mid-point between the first and last contact date. Additional details about data collection and the imputation of seroconversion dates may be found in Coates et al. (1986) and Coates et al. (1990).

The ratio of T4 cells to T8 cells was obtained at each clinical exam. These values were multiplied by 100 and log-transformed to stabilize the variance. A plot of these measurements for a random sample of 20 individuals is given in Figure 1. A model for the expected log-T4T8 ratio for each individual was assumed which is linear in time from seroconversion with an individual-specific slope and intercept. This model was fit in the first step of the two-step procedure and an estimated error variance of 0.0744 on 1337 degrees of freedom was obtained. Estimates of the individual-specific slopes and intercepts were then used to compute $\hat{E}_\phi(t)$ and $\hat{V}_\phi(t)$ for each time corresponding to an observed time of diagnosis with AIDS. Plots of these estimates are

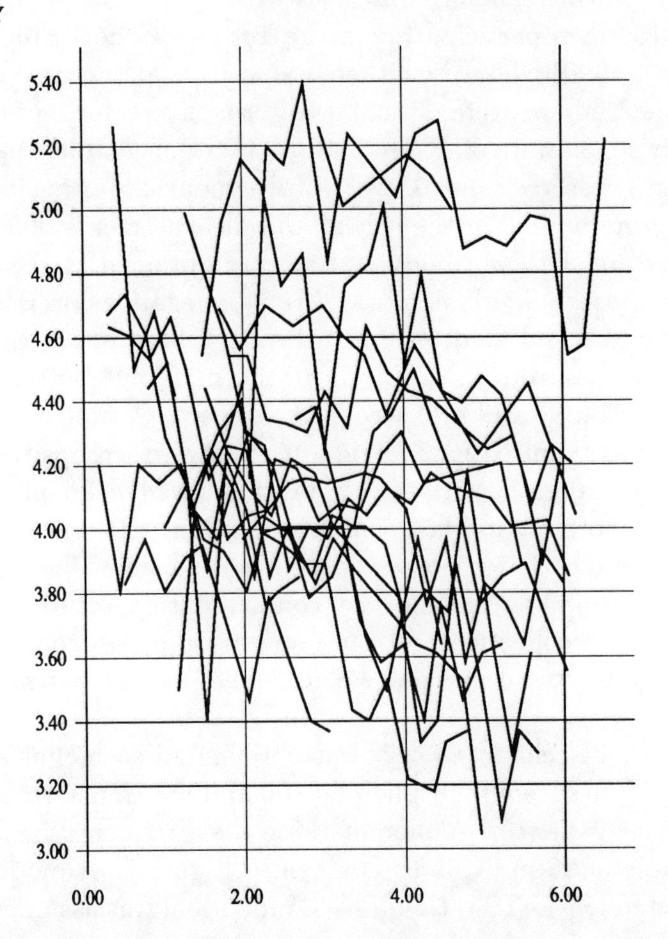

Figure 1: Observed log-T4T8 Ratio Trajectories for 20 Individuals

given in Figure 2 through Figure 5. As can be seen from these figures, the expected slope and its variance is fairly stable as a function of time. However the expected intercept and its variance increases greatly as a function of time from seroconversion.

A simple model for the risk of AIDS diagnosis was assumed in which risk at time t from seroconversion depends on the history of T4T8 ratios only through the current value. To be specific, the relative risk of diagnosis with AIDS at time t is given by $1 + [4 - Z_i(t)]\beta$ where $Z(t)$ represents the value of (transformed) T4T8 ratio for individual i at time t. The covariate in the model is taken to be $4 - Z_i(t)$ rather than $Z_i(t)$ to avoid positivity constraints. Figure 6 is a plot of estimated values of (transformed) T4T8 ratios ($Z_i(t)$) for each individual at risk at each risk set time t. Values of $Z_i(t)$ associated with the individual diagnoses with AIDS at each risk set are indicated with a large "dot". As can be seen from this plot, individuals who are diagnosed with AIDS at each time t tend to have much lower T4T8 ratios than do those individuals who are AIDS-free at that time. The estimated partial likelihood is maximized at a value of 7.37 for β. Thus, the risk of AIDS diagnosis for an individual with current $\log(100 \times T4T8)$ of 3 is estimated to be 8.37 times that for an individual with a current $\log(100 \times T4T8)$ of 4. The estimated variance of $\hat{\beta}$ based on the observed information is 2.42 while the robust variance estimator (Lin and Wei, 1989) which does not account for the additional variation due to the first-step of the procedure is 2.28. The proposed variance estimator that takes into account the variability of $\hat{E}_\phi(t)$ is 3.84. Thus, the estimation performed in the first step of the procedure appears to contribute significantly to the variability of the relative risk parameter estimators.

Although the functions $E_\phi(t)$ and $V_\phi(t)$ are not the primary quantities of interest in this analysis, they can provide some interesting and useful insights into the data. For example, some insight into the the imputation strategy for seroconversion times is gained by considering interpretation of the increases in expected value and variance of the random intercept of T4T8 ratios. In this data set, the later risk sets are composed primarily

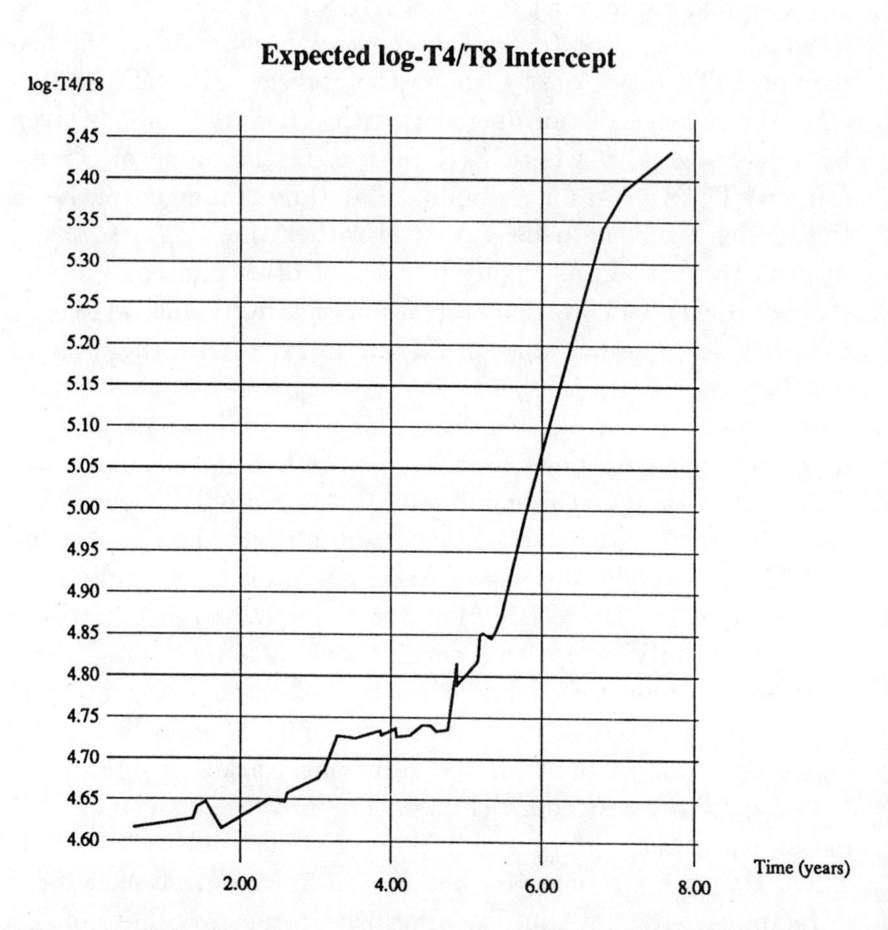

Figure 2: Expected Intercept given AIDS-free at Time t from Seroconversion

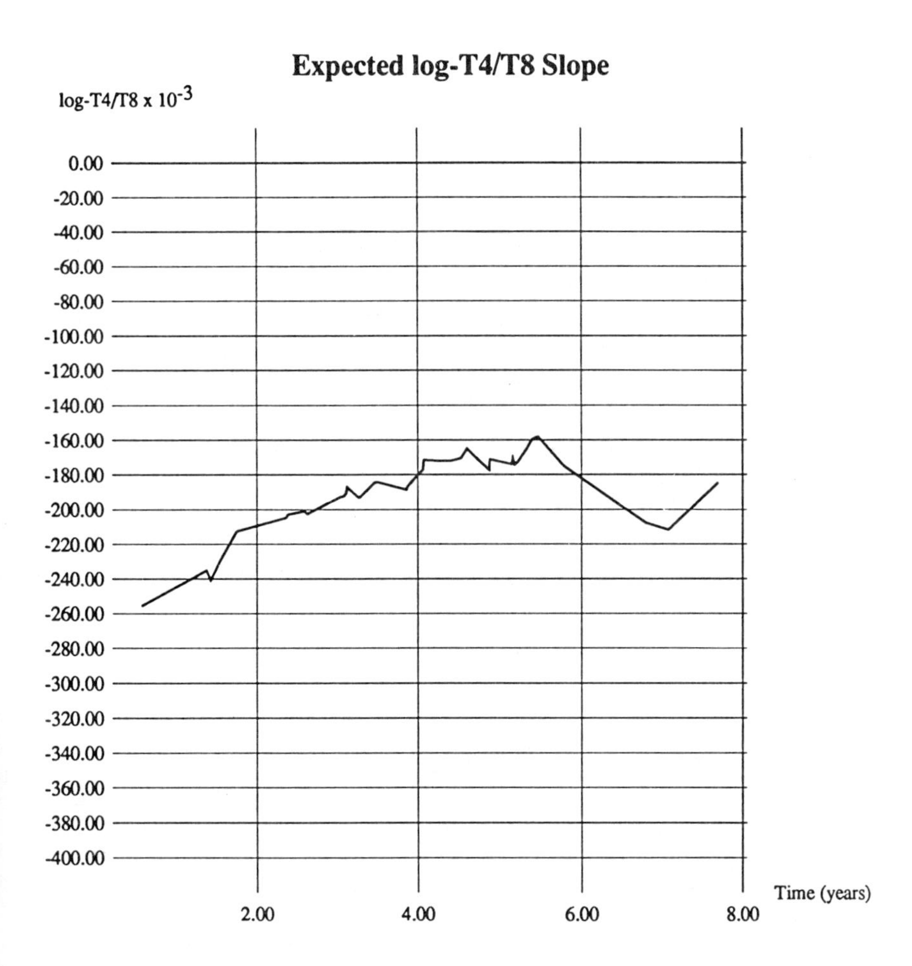

Figure 3: Expected Slope given AIDS-free at Time t from Seroconversion

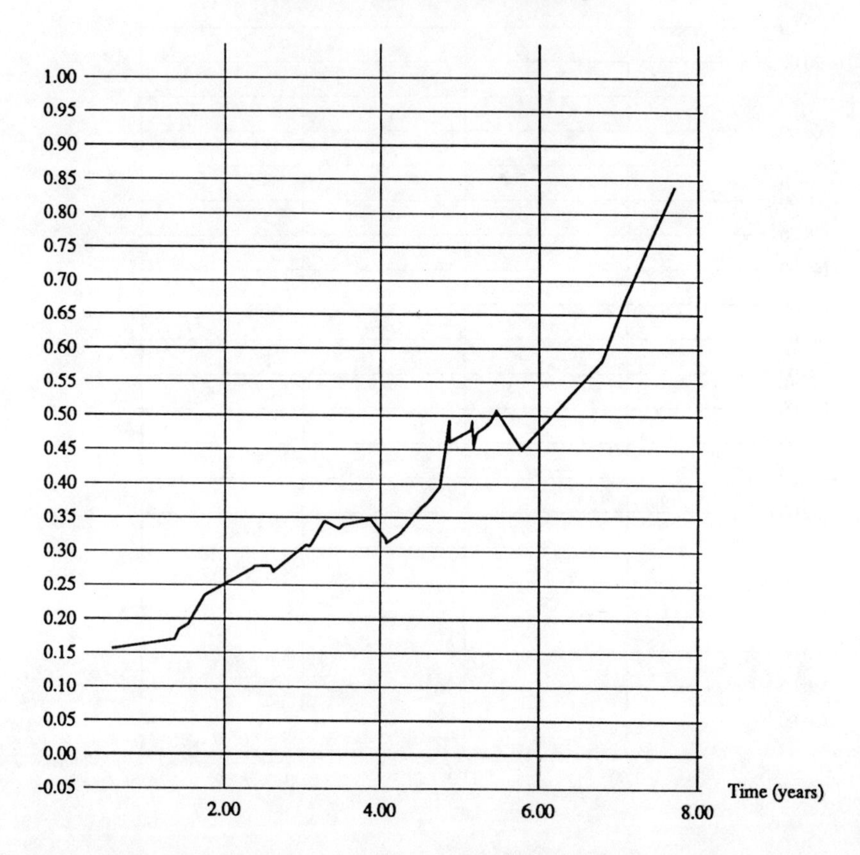

Figure 4: Variance of Intercept given AIDS-free at Time t from Seroconversion

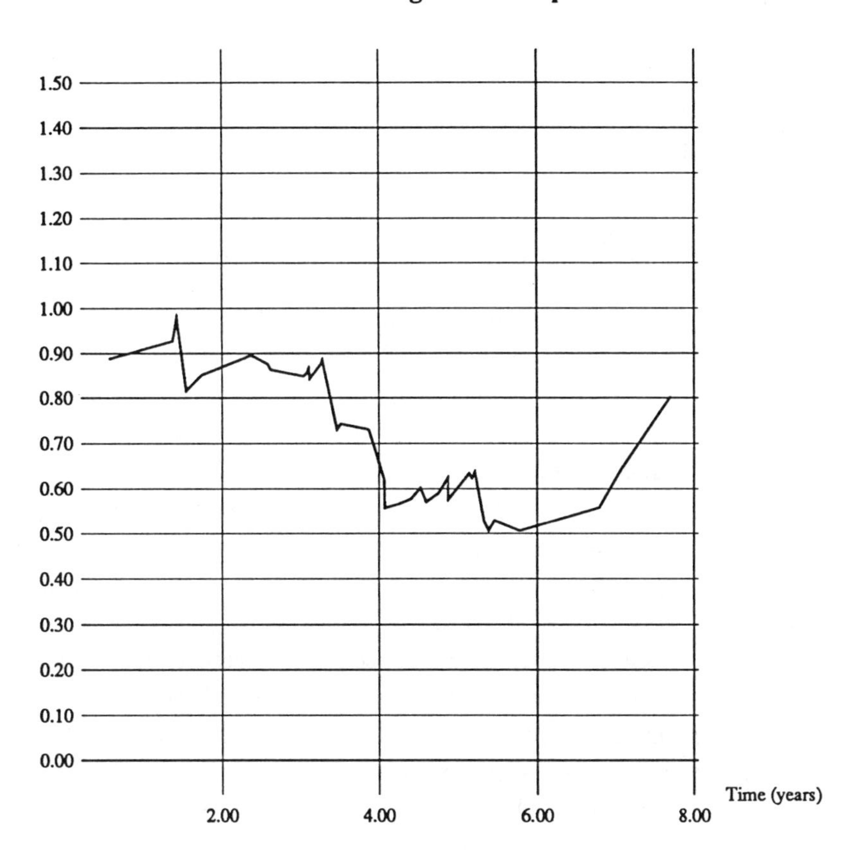

Figure 5: Variance of Slope given AIDS-free at Time t from Seroconversion

of individuals who were seropositive for HIV antibody at entry and, therefore, have seroconversion times imputed on the basis of interview data at time of entry. The schematic drawing in Figure 7 indicates how variation of the imputed seroconversion times about the true times would have the effect of increasing the variance of the T4T8 intercept parameter. In addition, the increase in expected T4T8 intercept can be interpreted as the result of a systematic bias in the seroconversion time imputations. In particular, an increase over time in expected T4T8 intercept of the magnitude exhibited in Figure 2 would imply that the imputed seroconversion times are up to three years earlier than the true seroconversion times.

6 Discussion

Although this work has been motivated by problems in which models for the marker process and endpoint occurrence are both of primary interest, the models and methods we present can also be useful for analyses with time-dependent covariates in which the primary goal is inference about relative risk regression parameters. Time-dependent covariates in such analyses are typically defined conceptually as functions of the underlying marker process such as the "current value" of the marker process. Rarely, however, is the current value available for each individual at each event time. Instead, a surrogate for the current value is used in evaluating the relative risk function. Such surrogates for the value of the marker at time t might be the last recorded value observed prior to time t (Gail, 1989) provided that an observation of the marker process was made within a relatively recent time prior to t. If no such recent observation is made, the covariate at time t for that individual might be considered as missing and the individual dropped from the likelihood calculations at time t. No adjustment is typically made in the variance of the resulting estimator of regression coefficients for the fact that the "true" covariate was not available. In addition, there is typically no recognition of the fact that the estimator of regression coefficients may be biased due to the use of surrogate

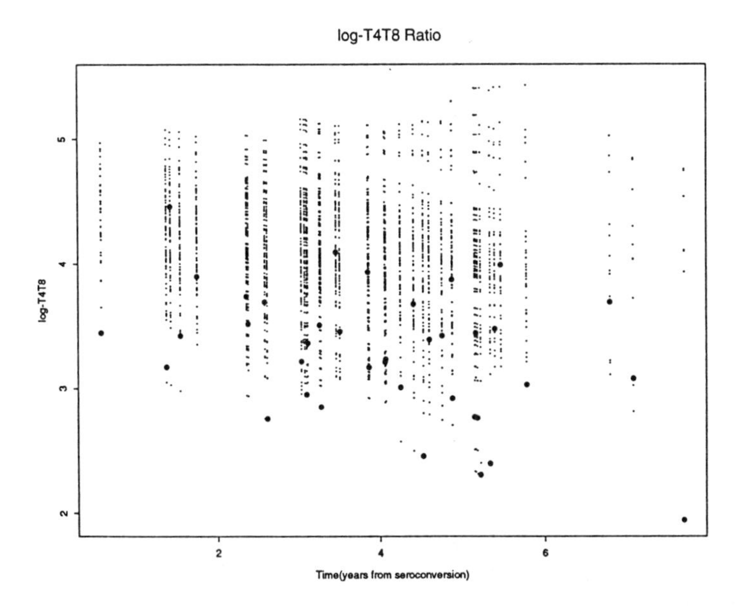

Figure 6: Smoothed log-T4T8 Ratios at Times of AIDS Diagnoses

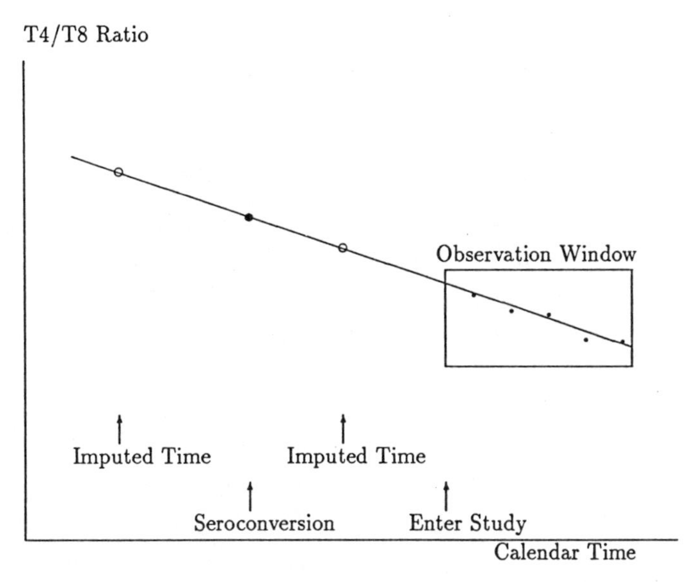

Figure 7: Schematic Drawing Illustrating Variance and Possible Bias of Imputed Seroconversion Times

covariate values. Thus, there is no feedback to the data analyst to indicate just how well the chosen surrogate is performing and choice of how recent an observation must be in order to be used as a surrogate is left to the analyst's speculation and conscience. The models and statistical methods described in this work can provide a framework within which to evaluate potential bias and under-estimation of variance.

In the first step of the two-stage estimation procedure described in Section 4, we assume that sufficient observations are made on the marker process from all but a negligible number of individuals to allow least square estimates of each p-vector ϕ_i to be computed. In addition, we require that there be sufficient degrees of freedom left over from these least squares fits to stably estimate the measurement error variance σ_ϵ^2. At first glance, this would seem to require at least p observations made on the marker process for each individual. Clearly, if the marker process exhibits considerable fluctuations over time that can not be attributed to measurement errors (so that p is not small), then observations must be made on the marker process frequently enough to characterize these fluctuations. However, even if observations are made frequently enough on the marker process, some individuals with a short followup periods will not have p marker measurements taken. Some relief from this data requirement can be obtained by use of B-spline basis functions as components of $X(t)$ as mentioned in Section 2.1. Because of the local support property of these functions, only those components of ϕ_i associated with functions whose support overlaps the actual followup period of individual i need be estimated. Thus, least squares estimates of the required components of ϕ_i can potentially be obtained with fewer than p marker measurements. For example, in an epidemiologic cohort study for which participants were scheduled for quarterly exams to obtain hematologic data, we have used linear splines with knot points one year apart to model T4/T8 ratio trajectories. In this situation, least squares estimates of the required parameters are computable provided there is at at least one marker measurement made within each inter-knot interval during which the individual is at risk and at least one inter-knot interval which has more than one marker observation. The vast majority of individuals in the data set satisfied these requirements even though there were many with fewer than p marker measurements.

Although we have not pursued methods that are strictly likelihood-based in this work, the partial likelihood (7) could be quite useful. Unlike the two-step method described in this work, (7) could be generalized in a reasonably straightforward manner to accommodate the problems of left-censoring and truncation that occur in many epidemiologic cohort studies.

Acknowledgments: The authors would like to gratefully acknowledge Dr. R. A. Coates for allowing us to use his data. We also would like to express our appreciation to Dr. V. Farewell, Dr. R. Gentleman and Dr. J. Raboud for sharing their insights into the problems of collection and modeling of AIDS data. This work was supported in part by NIH Grants CA 53996-14 and AI 29168-03.

References

Aalen, O. (1978). Nonparametric inference for a family of counting processes. *Annals of Statistics* **6**: 701-726.

Andersen, P.K. and Gill, R.D. (1982). Cox's regression model for counting processes: a large sample study. *Annals of Statistics* **10**: 1100-1120.

Andersen, P.K. and Borgan, O. (1985). Counting process models for life history data: a review (with discussion). *Scand. J. Statistics* **7**: 161-171.

Andersen, P.K. (1986). Time-dependent covariates and Markov processes. In, *Modern Statistical Methods in Chronic Disease Epidemiology*, (eds., Moolgavkar, S.H. and Prentice, R.L.). John Wiley and Sons, New York.

Clayton, D.G. and Cuzick, J. (1985). Multivariate generalizations of the proportional hazards model (with discussion). *J. Roy. Statist. Soc. A* **148**: 82-117.

Coates, R.A., Soskolne, C.L., Read, S.T., et. al. (1986). A prospective study of male sexual contacts of men with AIDS-related conditions (ARC) or AIDS: HTLV III antibody, clinical, and immune functions status at induction. *Can. J. Public Health* **77**(Suppl 1): 26-32.

Coates, R.A., Farewell, V.T., Raboud, J., Read, S.T., MacFadden, D.K., Calzavara, L.M., Johnson, J.K., Shepherd, F.A., Fanning, M.M. (1990). Cofactors of progression to acquired immunodeficiency syndrome in a cohort of male sexual contacts of men with human immunodeficiency virus disease. *American J. Epidemiology* **132**: 717-722.

deBoor, C. (1978). *A Practical Guide to Splines.* Springer-Verlag, New York.

DeGruttola, V., Lange,N. and Dafni, U. (1991). Modeling the progression of HIV infection. *J. Amer. Statistical Assoc.* **86**: 569-577.

Gail, M.H. (1981). Evaluating serial cancer marker studies in patients at risk of recurrent disease. *Biometrics* **37**: 67-78.

Gill, R.D. (1991). Marginal partial likelihood. Preprint 644, Department of Mathematics, University of Utrecht.

Gong, G. and Samaniego, F.J. (1981). Pseudo maximum likelihood estimation: Theory and applications. *Annals of Statistics* **9**: 861-869.

Kalbfleisch, J.D. and Prentice, R.L. (1980). *The Statistical Analysis of Failure Time Data.* John Wiley and Sons, New York.

Lin, D.Y. and Wei, L.J. (1989). The robust inference for the Cox proportional hazards model. *J. Amer. Statist. Assoc.* **84**: 1074-1078.

Nielsen, G.G., Andersen, P.K., Gill, R.D. and Sørensen, T.I.A. (1991). A counting process approach to maximum likelihood estimation in frailty models. Preprint 646, Department of Mathematics, University of Utrecht.

Prentice, R.L. (1982). Covariate measurement errors and parameter estimation in a failure time regression model. *Biometrika* **69**: 331-342.

Self, S.G. and Prentice, R.L. (1986). Incorporating random effects into multivariate relative risk regression models. In, *Modern Statistical Methods in Chronic Disease Epidemiology*, (eds., Moolgavkar, S.H. and Prentice, R.L.). John Wiley and Sons, New York.

Wei. L.J., Lin, D.Y. and Weissfeld, L. (1989). Regression analysis of multivariate incomplete failure time data by modeling marginal distributions. *J. Amer. Statist. Assoc.* **84**: 1065-1073.

Wu,. M.C. and Carroll, R.J. (1988). Estimation and comparison of changes in the presence of informative right censoring by modelling the censoring process. *Biometrics* **44**: 175-188.

S. Self, Fred Hutchinson Cancer Research Center,
1124 Columbia St., Seattle, WA 98104
and
Y. Pawitan, University of Washington, Seattle, WA.

The Relationship of CD4 Counts over Time to Survival in Patients with AIDS: Is CD4 a Good Surrogate Marker?

Anastasios A. Tsiatis   Urania Dafni
Victor DeGruttola   Kathleen J. Propert
Robert L. Strawderman   Michael Wulfsohn

Abstract

Methods are developed to analyze the relationship of survival to time dependent covariates that are measured longitudinally with possible measurement error using a two stage approach. In the first stage, the longitudinal time dependent data are modelled using repeated measures random components models. In the second stage methods are developed for estimating the parameters in a Cox proportional hazards model when the time dependent data is of this form. These methods are applied to CD4 data from a randomized clinical trial of AIDS patients where half the patients received AZT and the other half received placebo. Although a strong corellation between CD4 counts and survival is demonstrated, we also show that CD4 may not serve as a useful surrogate marker for assessing treatments for this population of patients.

1 Introduction

Randomized clinical trials are often used to evaluate new therapies in patients with HIV virus. Generally, most HIV trials use clinical progression as the primary outcome. A surrogate marker of clinical outcome would permit clinical trials to be completed in a shorter period of time and with a much smaller sample size. An acceptable surrogate marker would be one that responds rapidly to treatment and whose response implies a benefit regarding clinical outcome. Because of its observed rapid response to some anti-retroviral therapy and observed correlation with clinical outcome measures, the number of CD4–lymphocytes has been proposed as such a marker for HIV trials. However, before CD4–lymphocyte measurements can be widely substituted for clinical endpoints in HIV clinical trials, the relationship between the CD4 count response to therapy and clinical outcome needs to be more clearly established.

In this paper, we examine the degree to which survival benefits of the anti-retroviral agent ZDV are explained by increases in CD4 counts. Our results are based on a completed double-blind placebo controlled trial conducted by Burrough-Wellcome which treated 282 patients with advanced HIV disease. In this study, CD4 counts were determined prior to treatment and approximately every four weeks while on therapy. The median duration of follow-up was 120–127 days. Nineteen placebo recipients and one ZDV recipient died during the study. At the termination of the study, all patients actively participating in the study were offered ZDV and subsequently followed for clinical outcomes.

We used Cox's proportional hazards regression model to study the relationship between CD4 counts over time and survival. In order to apply such models, knowledge of the entire CD4 time dependent covariate history is necessary. However, in clinical trials, CD4 counts are measured only periodically and with a substantial amount of variability with 50% coefficient of variation not being unusual. This variability arises from measurement error, true biologic differences among individuals, and changes over time. Changes over time may be short term, such as diurnal fluctuations, or longer term, reflecting the progressive decline in CD4 counts with increasing viral replication.

The variability of CD4 counts, together with the infrequency of individual measurements, creates certain difficulties in the survival analysis. These issues are discussed in Section 2. In Sections 3 and 4 we discuss methods for analysis that will account for these difficulties. These methods are applied to the Burroughs-Wellcome data in Sections 5 and 6 with two specific aims. The first goal is to better understand the relationship between the hazard rate of dying and an individual's CD4 count history. The second aim was to study whether CD4 may serve as a useful surrogate marker in assessing treatment, that is, to establish whether the beneficial effect of ZDV on survival is mediated entirely through its effect on CD4 counts.

1.1 The Model and Notation

Let $Z^*(t)$ denote the true value of CD4 count at time t and let $\bar{Z}^*(t)$ denote history up to time t, $\{Z^*(u), u \leq t\}$. The primary interest is to estimate the relationship between survival and the CD4 count history. This relationship will be described through the hazard function. If we denote by T the survival time of an individual, then the hazard function is defined as,

$$\lambda\left(t|\bar{Z}^*(t)\right) = \lim_{h\to 0} \frac{1}{h}\left\{pr\left(t \leq T < t+h | T \geq t, \bar{Z}^*(t)\right)\right\}.$$

As in most clinical trials, the survival data is subject to right censoring, hence we observe $X = \min(T, C)$ where C corresponds to a potential censoring time. Also, let Δ denote failure indicator, which is equal to 1 if the individual is observed to fail $(T \leq C)$, and 0 otherwise. In such a case, we observe the cause specific hazard, namely,

$$\lim_{h\to 0} \frac{1}{h}\left\{pr\left(t \leq X < t+h, \Delta = 1 | X \geq t, \bar{Z}^*(t)\right)\right\}. \quad (1.1)$$

It is assumed that censoring is non-informative, in which case, the cause specific hazard given by (1.1) is equal to the hazard of interest $\lambda(t|\bar{Z}^*(t))$.

A class of models which are useful for modeling the relationship of hazard to time dependent covariates are the proportional hazards model introduced by Cox (1972). Namely

$$\lambda\left(t|\bar{Z}^*(t)\right) = \lambda_0(t) f\left(\bar{Z}^*(t), \beta\right),$$

where $f(Z^*(t), \beta)$ is a function of the covariate history specified up to an unknown parameter $\boldsymbol{\beta}$ (possibly vector valued). If the underlying hazard $\lambda_0(t)$ is left unspecified, then the parameter β

is estimated by maximizing the partial likelihood given by Cox (1975). Namely,

$$\prod_{i=1}^{n}\left[f(\bar{Z}_i^*(X_i),\beta)/\sum_{j=1}^{n}f(\bar{Z}_j^*(X_i),\beta)Y_j(X_i)\right]^{\Delta_i}, \qquad (1.2)$$

where $Y_j(v)$ is the indicator of being at risk at time v, namely, $I(X_j \geq v)$.

In order to apply this methodology, one needs the knowledge of $Z^*(t)$ for all values $t \leq X$. This is generally not the case. For example, the CD4 counts are only measured periodically and those measurements are made with substantial laboratory measurement error. That is, the observable data is given by the vector $\{Z(t_1), \cdots, Z(t_m)\}$, $t_m \leq X$, where $Z(t)$ is the observed laboratory measured CD4 count at time t. Therefore, modeling the hazard directly of the observed CD4 counts $Z(t)$ would lead to biased estimates of the true hazard relationship. Biases in the Cox-model due to measurement error have been discussed by Prentice (1982).

2 The Effect of Measurement Error

To describe the effect of measurement error, we consider the problem as follows. The observed CD4 count $Z(t)$ is equal to the true CD4 count $Z^*(t)$ plus measurement error $e(t)$. That is,

$$Z(t) = Z^*(t) + e(t). \qquad (2.1)$$

We shall assume that $e(t)$ is random noise so that $E(e(t)) = 0$, $\mathrm{Var(e(t))} = \sigma^2$ and $\mathrm{Cov(e(s), e(t))} = 0,\ \mathrm{s} \neq \mathrm{t}$.

Denote by $\bar{Z}(t)$ the history of observed CD4 counts up to time t, that is, $\bar{Z}(t) = \{Z(t_1), \cdots, Z(t_j);\ t_j \leq t\}$. In such a case, the observable hazard is $\lambda\left(t|\bar{Z}(t)\right)$. A simple application of the law of conditional probability yields,

$$\lambda\left(t|\bar{Z}(t)\right) = \int \lambda\left(t|\bar{Z}(t), \bar{Z}^*(t)\right)\, dP\left(\bar{Z}^*(t)|\bar{Z}(t), X \geq t\right).$$

If it is additionally assumed that neither measurement error nor the timing of the visits prior to time t are prognostic, then

$$\lambda\left(t|\bar{Z}(t),\ \bar{Z}^*(t)\right) = \lambda\left(t|\bar{Z}^*(t)\right) = \lambda_0(t) f\left(\bar{Z}^*(t), \beta\right).$$

In which case,

$$\lambda\left(t|\bar{Z}(t)\right) = \lambda_0(t) E\left[f\left(\bar{Z}^*(t), \beta\right)|Z\left(t_1\right), \cdots, Z\left(t_j\right), X \geq t\right]. \tag{2.2}$$

If the conditional expectation in (2.2), which will be referred to by $E(t, \beta)$, is known, then this is also a proportional hazards relationship. Therefore, β can be estimated by maximizing the partial likelihood,

$$\prod_{i=1}^{n}\left[E_i\left(X_i, \beta\right) / \sum_{j=1}^{n} E_j\left(X_i, \beta\right) Y_j\left(X_i\right)\right]^{\Delta_i}. \tag{2.3}$$

The conditional expectation above, however, is generally not tractable. In the next section, we shall consider methods for approximating the conditional expectations $E_i(u, \beta)$ under various assumptions.

3 Approximating the Relationship for Conditional Expectation

For illustration, we shall consider the case only when the hazard is a function of the current value, $Z^*(t)$, rather than a functional of the entire history $\bar{Z}^*(t)$. The computations that are necessary for the latter case are very similar. Additionally, it is biologically natural when considering possible surrogate markers to assume that the hazard function is related to the current value of that marker.

3.1 The Additive Relative Risk Model

Let us first consider the case when $f(Z^*(t), \beta)$ is linear, that is, $1+\beta Z^*(t)$. This is the additive relative risk model of Prentice and Self (1983). For this model, the conditional expectation is given by,

$$E(t,\beta) = 1 + \beta E\left[Z^*(t)|\bar{Z}(t), X \geq t\right], \tag{3.1}$$

where $\bar{Z}(t) = \{Z(t_1), \cdots, Z(t_j)\}$, $t_j \leq t$.

In order to compute $E\left[Z^*(t)|\bar{Z}(t),\ X \geq t\right]$ we must be able to characterize the joint distribution of $\{Z(t_1), \cdots, Z(t_j), Z^*(t)\}$ given that $X \geq t$.

A way of looking at this problem is to think of the history of true CD4 counts up to time t for an individual i, $\bar{Z}_i^*(t)$, given that the individual is at risk at time t, i.e., $(X_i \geq t)$, as a realization of a stochastic process. If we additionally make the assumption that this process is a normal process, then it can be characterized by the structure of its first two moments. That is, for $u \leq t$,

$$\begin{aligned} E(Z^*(u)|X \geq t) &= \mu_t(u) \\ \text{and} \qquad\qquad & \\ Cov(Z^*(u), Z^*(v)|X \geq t) &= C_t(u,v). \end{aligned} \tag{3.2}$$

If the measurement error $e(u)$, given in (2.1), is also normally distributed, independent of the stochastic process $Z^*(u)$, and $X \geq t$, then the random vector $\{Z(t_1), \cdots, Z(t_j), Z^*(t)\}$ is jointly normal. The mean is given as the $j+1$ vector $\boldsymbol{\mu}_t = (\mu_t(t_1), \cdots, \mu_t(t_j), \mu_t(t))$ and the variance is the $(j+1) \times (j+1)$ matrix,

$$M_t = \begin{bmatrix} C_t(t_1,t_1), \cdots, & C_t(t_1 t_j), & C_t(t_1,t) \\ \vdots & & \\ C_t(t_j,t_1) \cdots, & C_t(t_j,t_j), & C_t(t_j,t) \\ C_t(t,t_1), \cdots, & C_t(t,t_j), & C_t(t,t) \end{bmatrix} + \begin{bmatrix} \sigma^2 & & 0 & \\ & \ddots & & \\ & 0 & \sigma^2 & \\ & & & 0 \end{bmatrix}.$$

For jointly normal random variables, the conditional expectation $E\left[Z^*(t)|\bar{Z}(t), X \geq t\right]$ is equal to

$$\mu_t(t) - \left(M_t^{22}\right)^{-1}\left(M_t^{21}\right)\left[\mathbf{Z} - \boldsymbol{\mu}_t\right], \tag{3.3}$$

where $\mathbf{Z} = (Z(t_1), \cdots, Z(t_j)),'\ \boldsymbol{\mu}_t = (\mu_t(t_1), \cdots, \mu_t(t_j))$, and M_t^{-1} can be written as the partitioned matrix,

$$\begin{bmatrix} (M_t^{11})^{j\times j} & (M_t^{12})^{j\times 1} \\ (M_t^{21})^{1\times j} & (M_t^{22})^{1\times 1} \end{bmatrix}. \tag{3.4}$$

Therefore, if we knew the mean and variance structure of the stochastic process $Z^*(u)$, $u \leq t$ among individuals at risk at time t for all $t > 0$, then β could be estimated by maximizing the partial likelihood given in (2.3) by evaluating $E(t, \beta)$ using (3.1) and (3.3). In the next section, we shall discuss methods for estimating the mean and covariance structure of $Z^*(u)$.

The methodology described for the relative additive risk model has been worked out in more detail in Self and Pawitan (1991).

3.2 Cox Proportional Hazards Model

Another relative risk formulation is that of the original Cox Model (1972), where

$$f(Z^*(t), \beta) = \exp(\beta Z^*(t)). \tag{3.5}$$

For such a model, the value $E(t, \beta)$ is given by $E[e^{\beta Z^*(t)} | \bar{Z}(t), X \geq t]$.

This is the moment generating function for the conditional distribution of $Z^*(t)$ given $\{Z(t), \cdots, Z(t_j)\}$ among the individuals at risk at time t. Under the assumption of joint normality, together with (3.3), it is well known, see Rao (1973), that the moment generating function above is given by,

$$\exp\left\{\beta\mu\left(t|\bar{Z}(t)\right) + \beta^2\sigma^2\left(t|\bar{Z}(t)\right)/2\right\}, \tag{3.6}$$

where $\mu(t|\bar{Z}(t)) = E\{Z^*(t)|\bar{Z}(t), X \geq t\}$ given by (3.3), and

$$\sigma^2(t|\bar{Z}(t)) = Var\{Z^*(t)|\bar{Z}(t), X \geq t\},$$

which is equal to (M_t^{22}) defined in (3.4). Here also the estimate of β is obtained by maximizing the partial likelihood (2.3), substituting the expression in (3.6) for $E(t, \beta)$.

A slight generalization of (3.5), is obtained by considering the relative risk,

$$f\left(Z^*(t),\beta\right) = \exp\left[\beta_1 Z^*(t) + \beta_2 \left\{Z^*(t)\right\}^2\right]. \qquad (3.7)$$

The conditional expectation, $E(t,\beta)$ for model (3.7), together with the assumption of joint normality and (3.3), is equal to

$$\frac{1}{\sqrt{2\pi\sigma^2\left(t|\bar{Z}(t)\right)}} \int_{-\infty}^{\infty} \exp\left(\beta_1 x + \beta_2 x^2\right)$$

$$exp - \left(\left[\left\{x - \mu\left(t|\bar{Z}(t)\right)\right\}^2 \sigma^2\left(t|\bar{Z}(t)\right)\right]\right) dx$$

which, after a simple exercise of completing the square, becomes

$$\left\{1 - 2\beta_2\sigma^2\left(t|\bar{Z}(t)\right)\right\}^{-1/2} \qquad (3.8)$$

$$\exp\left[\frac{\left\{\beta_1\mu\left(t|\bar{Z}(t)\right) + \beta_1^2\sigma^2\left(t|\bar{Z}(t)\right)/2 + \beta_2\mu^2\left(t|\bar{Z}(t)\right)\right\}}{\left\{1 - 2\beta_2\sigma^2\left(t|\bar{Z}(t)\right)\right\}}\right].$$

Therefore, the estimates of β_1 and β_2 in model (3.7) are obtained by maximizing the partial likelihood (2.3), using (3.9) for $E(t,\beta)$.

3.3 More General Relative Risk Functions

In the subsequent analyses of CD4 counts and survival, we used relative risk functions, $f(Z^*(t),\beta)$ which were more general than those considered so far. Therefore, simple expressions for $E(t,\beta)$ could not be obtained, even with the assumption of joint normality. For such models, we considered a simple first order approximation to $E(t,\beta)$, namely,

$$\begin{aligned} E(t,\beta) &= E\left[f\left(Z^*(t),\beta\right)|\bar{Z}(t), X \geq t)\right] \\ &\approx f\left(E\left(Z^*(t)|\bar{Z}(t), X \geq t\right),\beta\right). \end{aligned}$$

The adequacy of this approximation for general models is under study. However, when we applied this approximation to the Cox model (3.5) as well as to model (3.7), we obtained virtually the same estimates for β. As an example, if we used this approximation in the Cox model, the estimate β would be obtained by maximizing the partial likelihood,

$$\prod_{i=1}^{n}\left[\exp\left\{\beta\mu_i\left(X_i|\bar{Z}(X_i)\right)\right\} / \sum_{i=1}^{n}\exp\left\{\beta\mu_j\left(X_i|\bar{Z}(X_i)\right)\right\}\right]^{\Delta_i}.$$

This is exactly the same functional form used by the Cox model (1.2) with $\mu_j(X_i|\bar{Z}(X_i))$ substituted for $Z_j^*(X_i)$. This is useful since standard software for the Cox model can be used.

4 Describing the Stochastic Process

In order to apply the methods described in Section 3, we require some transformation of the time dependent covariate data $Z(u)$, that is approximately normal. Also, within each risk set, $X \geq t$, we must compute the mean and covariance structure of $Z(u), 0 \leq u \leq t$ conditional on $X \geq t$. In order to do this we consider a class of flexible, parsimonious models to help aid us in the choice of the mean and covariance structure.

Due to the nature of the data and also, the available software, we modeled the covariate data using linear random components models as described by Laird and Ware (1982). We found that transforming to a log scale, normalized the data. Also, the log CD4 counts declined over time in a linear fashion for patients receiving no therapy, whereas patients given ZDV, had an increase for the first eight weeks, followed by a linear decline.

In Figure 1, the log CD4 over time is depicted for the entire sample by fitting a nonparametric lowess curve to the mean of the data. In Figure 2, the longitudinal data for the first five patients on ZDV and five patients on placebo are plotted. These figures illustrate the log linear decline of CD4 after eight weeks, as well as the large degree of within patient variability due in large part to measurement error.

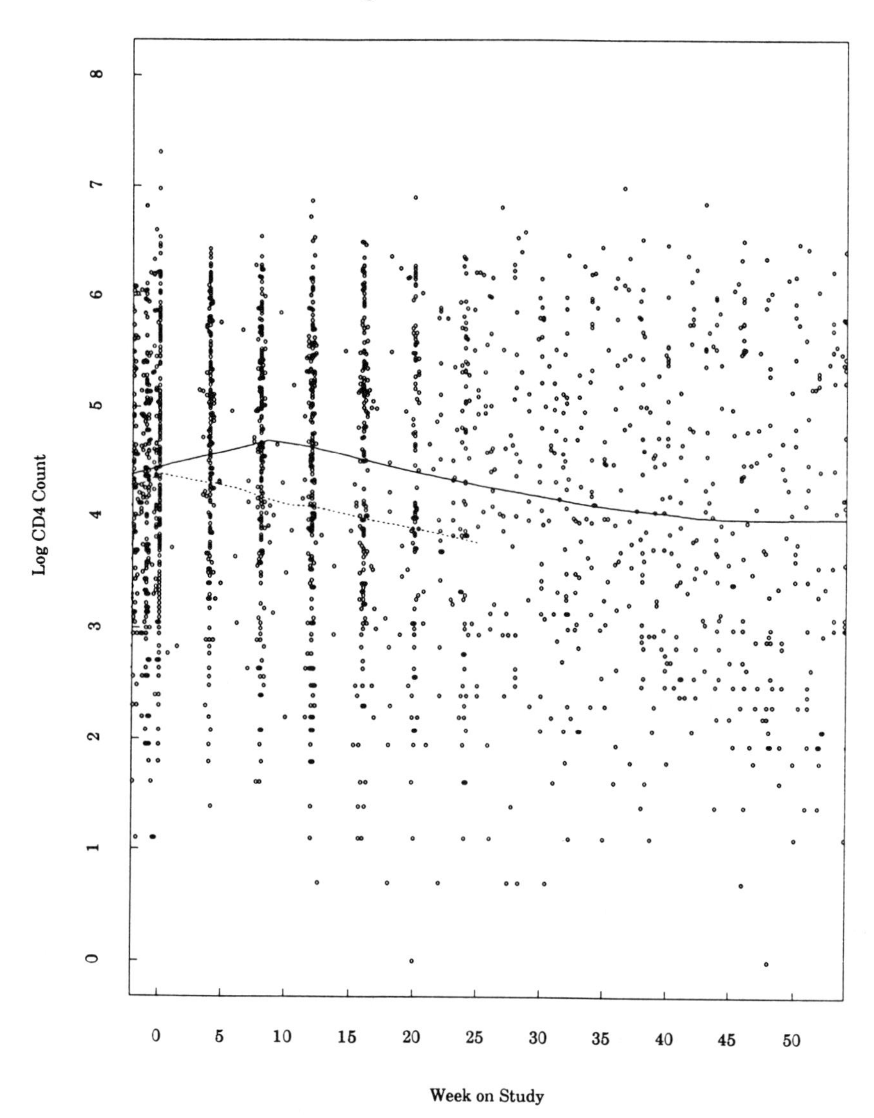
Log CD4 Counts Over Time
Log CD4 Count
0
1
2
3
4
5
6
7
8
0
5
10
15
20
25
30
35
40
45
50
Week on Study

Figure 1

Therefore, for placebo patients we used linear growth curve models in each risk set to model the log CD4 counts. That is, given $X \geq t$, it is assumed that the ith patient has log CD4 counts given by,

$$Z_i(u) = Z_i^*(u) + e_i(u), \quad u \leq t$$

where

$$Z_i^*(u) = \theta_{0i} + \theta_{1i}u$$

and $e_i(u)$ corresponds to random measurement error. In this model, it is assumed that each individual follows a linear trajectory with their own slope and intercept, θ_{i1} and θ_{01} respectively, which are themselves considered to be independent realizations of a bivariate normal random variable. That is, $(\theta_{0i}, \theta_{1i})'$ are *iid* normal bivariate vectors with mean $(\theta_0^{(t)}, \theta_1^{(t)})'$ and covariate matrix,

$$\begin{bmatrix} \sigma_{00}^{(t)} & \sigma_{01}^{(t)} \\ \sigma_{01}^{(t)} & \sigma_{11}^{(t)} \end{bmatrix}.$$

The measurement error $e_i(u)$ is also assumed to be distributed as a normal random variable with mean zero and variance σ_e^2 independent of the random vector $(\theta_{01}, \theta_{1i})$. This conceptualization yields a mean and non-stationary covariance structure in (3.3) given by,

$$\begin{aligned} \mu_t(u) &= \theta_0^{(t)} + \theta_1^{(t)}u \\ \text{and} & \\ C_t(u,v) &= \sigma_{00}^{(t)} + \sigma_{01}^{(t)}(u+v) + \sigma_{11}^{(t)}uv. \end{aligned} \tag{4.1}$$

We note that the mean and covariance structure among individuals at risk at time t are allowed to change by letting the mean and variance of the random components be a function of t.

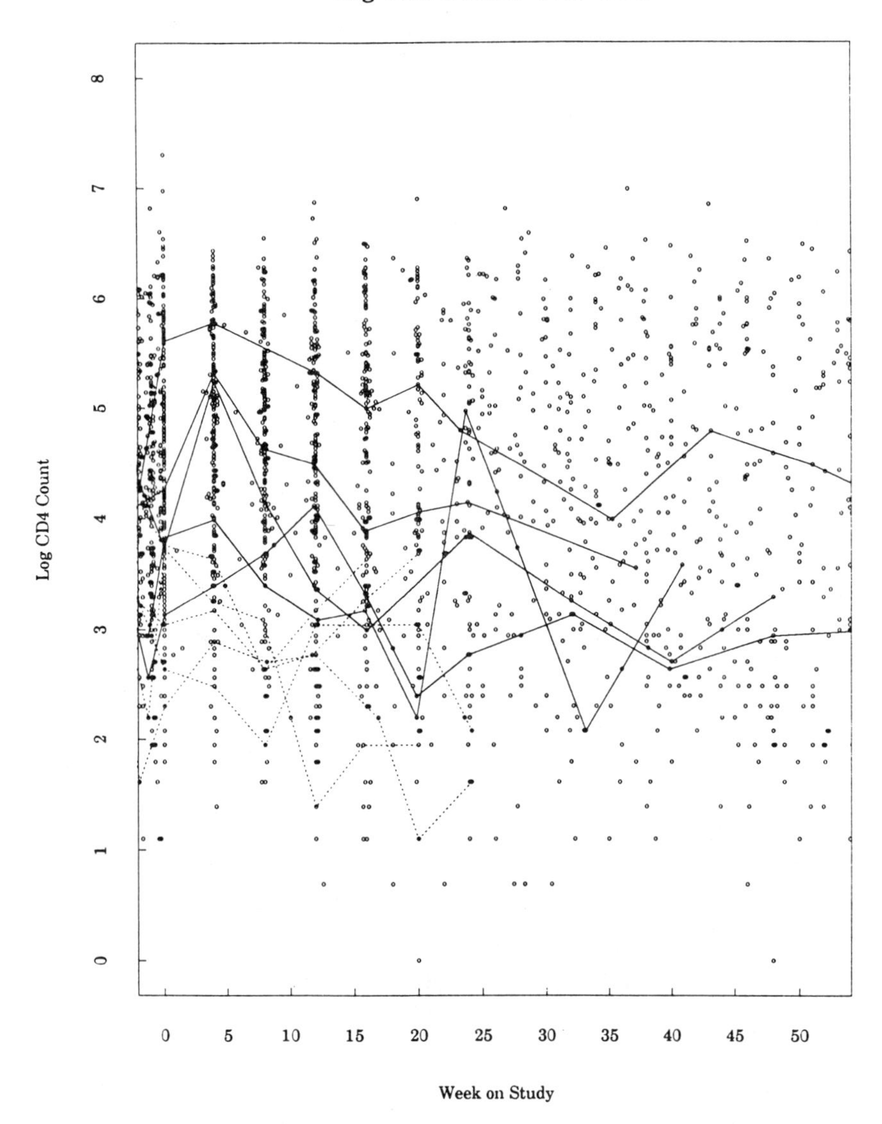
Log CD4 Counts Over Time
Log CD4 Count
0
1
2
3
4
5
6
7
8
Week on Study
0
5
10
15
20
25
30
35
40
45
50

Figure 2

For each patient receiving ZDV, we assume that $Z_i^*(u)$ is a piecewise linear spline with a knot at eight weeks to reflect the increase that occurs at that time. That is, we assume that

$$Z_i^*(u) = \theta_{oi} + \theta_{1i}u + \theta_{2i}(u-8)_+$$

where x_+ is equal to x for $x \geq 0$, and 0 for $x < 0$. Here we assume that $(\theta_{0i}, \theta_{1i}, \theta_{2i})$ are independent realizations from a normal distribution with mean $(\theta_0^{(t)}, \theta_1^{(t)}, \theta_2^{(t)})$ and

$$\text{covariance matrix} = \begin{bmatrix} \sigma_{00}^{(t)} & \sigma_{01}^{(t)} & \sigma_{02}^{(t)} \\ \sigma_{01}^{(t)} & \sigma_{11}^{(t)} & \sigma_{12}^{(t)} \\ \sigma_{02}^{(t)} & \sigma_{12}^{(t)} & \sigma_{22}^{(t)} \end{bmatrix}.$$

The methods of in Section 3 require knowledge of the mean and covariance structure at each risk set t, $\mu_t(u)$ and $C_t(u,v)$, given by (4.1). For these models, this is equivalent to knowing the population parameters $\boldsymbol{\theta}^t, \boldsymbol{\sigma}^t$, and σ_e^2. Of course, these quantities are not known and have to be estimated by the data, $\{\bar{Z}_i(t)\}$, for all i such that $\{X_i \geq t\}$. We estimated these parameters using restricted maximum likelihood, as described by Laird and Ware (1982) using software provided by Lindstrom and Bates (1988).

The values $E(t,\beta)$ in the partial likelihood of (2.3) are functions of $\boldsymbol{\theta}^t, \boldsymbol{\sigma}^t$, and σ_e^2. We therefore used $\hat{E}(t,\beta)$ which are the values of $E(t,\beta)$ with the estimates $\hat{\boldsymbol{\theta}}^t, \hat{\boldsymbol{\sigma}}^t, \hat{\sigma}_e^2$ substituted for their true value. An important question that still needs to be addressed is the impact of using $\hat{E}(t,\beta)$ instead of $E(t,\beta)$ in the partial likelihood (2.2). We suspect this will produce a second order effect which will not change the estimate of β or its standard error substantially.

The use of linear random effects models were made primarily for convenience. Any model that reasonably approximates the mean and covariance structure of $Z(u)$ among individuals at risk at time t might be used. Of course, methods for evaluating the adequacy of fit of the mean and covariance structure have to be explored as well as the effect that mismodeling might have on the estimate of β. This work is in progress.

5 Analysis of CD4 Data

The use of the growth curve random components model described in Section 4 is very useful in describing the history or trajectory of CD4 counts over time. At any point in time t, the trajectory of CD4 counts up to that time could be summarized by the vector $\boldsymbol{\theta}_i$. For example, patients not receiving drug have linear trajectories in the log CD4 which are summarized by their slope and intercept $(\theta_{1i}, \theta_{0i})$. Therefore the hazard function can be modeled to the past history of CD4 counts as follows:

$$\lambda_i(t) = \lambda_0(t) f(\boldsymbol{\theta}_i, t, \beta), \tag{5.1}$$

where $f(\boldsymbol{\theta}_i, t, \beta)$ is some function of the CD4 history up to time t (summarized by $\boldsymbol{\theta}_i$), specified as a function of unknown parameters $\boldsymbol{\beta}$ which have to be estimated. For example, a model that relates the hazard function to both the current value of CD4 as well as the slope of CD4 can be written as,

$$\lambda_i(t) = \lambda_0(t) \exp\{\beta_1(\theta_{0i} + \theta_{1i}t) + \beta_2\theta_{1i}\}. \tag{5.2}$$

As discussed in Section 3.3, the hazard function that is induced by (5.1) as a function of the observed history of CD4 counts is approximately equal to

$$\lambda\left(t|\bar{Z}_i(t)\right) = \lambda_0(t) f\left(\hat{\boldsymbol{\theta}}_i^{(t)}, t, \beta\right),$$

where

$$\hat{\boldsymbol{\theta}}_i^{(t)} = \hat{E}\left(\boldsymbol{\theta}_i|\bar{Z}_i(t), X \geq t\right).$$

The values $\hat{\theta}_i^t$ are the so called empirical Bayes estimates of the individual random effects as described by Laird and Ware (1982), evaluated at risk time t. Therefore, in order to estimate the parameters $\boldsymbol{\beta}$ in model (5.1), we first fit a separate growth curve random components model at each risk set time t. The empirical Bayes estimates $\hat{\boldsymbol{\theta}}_i^{(t)}$ were then substituted for $\boldsymbol{\theta}_i$ in the partial likelihood

$$\prod_{i=1}^{n}\left\{f\left(\hat{\boldsymbol{\theta}}_i^{(X_i)}, X_i, \beta\right) / \sum_{j=1}^{n} f\left(\hat{\boldsymbol{\theta}}_j^{(X_i)}, X_i, \beta\right) Y_j(X_i)\right\}^{\Delta_i}.$$

Using the proportional hazards model of Cox (1972), we analyzed the data from the patients receiving ZDV separately from those receiving placebo. For each treatment group, we considered different aspects of CD4 trajectory, individually and in combination, as the time dependent covariates that were included in the Cox model, similar to the example given in (5.2). For patients randomized to placebo, we considered baseline CD4 (θ_{0i}); slope of decline (θ_{1i}), and current value, ($\theta_{0i} + \theta_{1i}t$). For patients receiving ZDV, we considered baseline CD4 (θ_{0i}), slope of decline after eight weeks ($\theta_{1i} + \theta_{2i}$), initial increase ($\theta_{1i}$) and current value ($\theta_{0i} + \theta_{1i}t + \theta_{2i}(t-8)_+$).

The analysis of each treatment group separately showed similar results. Namely, that CD4 counts are significantly predictive of survival. Also, the current value of CD4 was the most predictive aspect of the trajectory; other features of the path did not add significantly to the log likelihood.

6 The Surrogate Marker Issue

In the previous section, we considered only the simple Cox regression model. In order to study the relationship of the hazard function to the current value of CD4 count more carefully, we consider models

$$\lambda_i(t) = \lambda_0(t) f\left(Z_i^*(t), \beta\right)$$

where $f(Z_i^*(t), \beta)$ were log regression splines with fixed knots. This allowed us to obtain more flexible relationships of the relative hazard ratio. That is, we assume that $f(Z_i^*(t), \beta)$ is equal to

$$\exp\left\{\beta_1 g_1\left(Z^*(t)\right) + \cdots + \beta_k g_k\left(Z^*(t)\right)\right\}, \text{where } g_1(.), \cdots, g_k(.)$$

represent the basis functions for piecewise polynomial functions which have smooth continuous derivatives at specified fixed knots. The actual fitting and knot selection procedure are described in more detail in a technical report by Strawderman and Tsiatis (1991). As described in section 3, the empirical Bayes estimates for $Z_i^*(t)$ were used in all the estimation procedures in order to account for the bias due to measurement error and incomplete CD4 histories.

The primary interest of this research was to estimate the hazard function not just the relative hazard ratio. For this reason, we also modeled the underlying hazard ratio $\lambda_0(t)$ as a log regression spline with fixed knots. That is, we assume $\lambda_0(t) = \exp\{\alpha_0 h_0(t) + \cdots + \alpha_\ell h_\ell(t)\}$ where $h_i(t)$ are the basis function of a polynomial regression spline. Therefore, we considered a fully parametric model

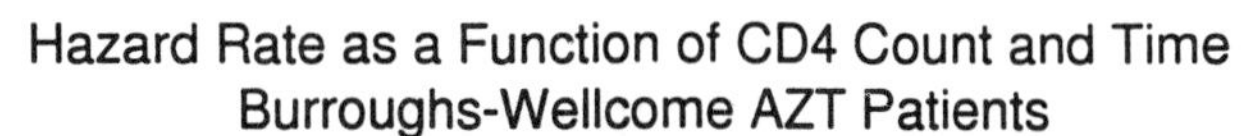

$$\lambda\left(t|\bar{Z}_i^*(t)\right) = \exp\left\{\boldsymbol{\alpha}'\boldsymbol{h}(t) + \boldsymbol{\beta}'\boldsymbol{g}\left(Z^*(t)\right)\right\}.$$

The parameters $\boldsymbol{\alpha}$, and $\boldsymbol{\beta}$ were estimated by maximizing the full likelihood with the empirical Bayes estimate $\hat{\mu}(t|\bar{Z}(t))$ substituted for $Z^*(t)$.

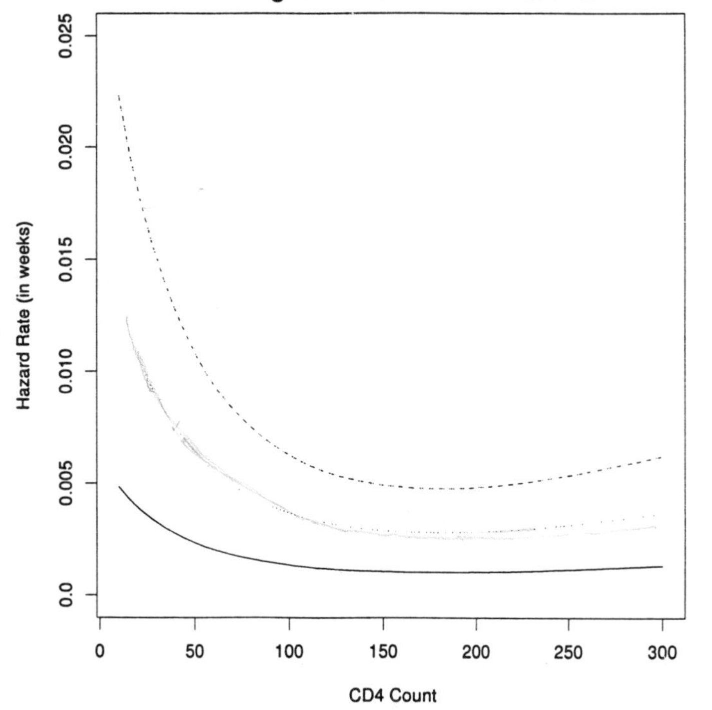

Figure 3

An alternative analysis is to estimate $\boldsymbol{\beta}$ by maximizing the partial likelihood and then estimate $\lambda_0(t)$ by smoothing the Breslow (1974) estimate. We found, however, that the estimate of $\boldsymbol{\beta}$ was virtually the same for either method. However, the estimate of $\lambda_0(t)$ was much more stable with the use of log regression splines and maximization of the full likelihood.

These data analytic techniques were applied to the data from the Burroughs-Wellcome 02 clinical trial. In Figure 3, we show the relationship of the hazard function to CD4 counts at 3, 6, 12, and 18 months after start of therapy for patients receiving ZDV. This figure clearly shows that the hazard rate increases as CD4 declines, with the greatest effect occurring for patients with CD4 counts less than 50. It also demonstrates a substantial effect of time trend, that is, the hazard rate increases as a function of time from treatment initiation even after adjusting for CD4 values.

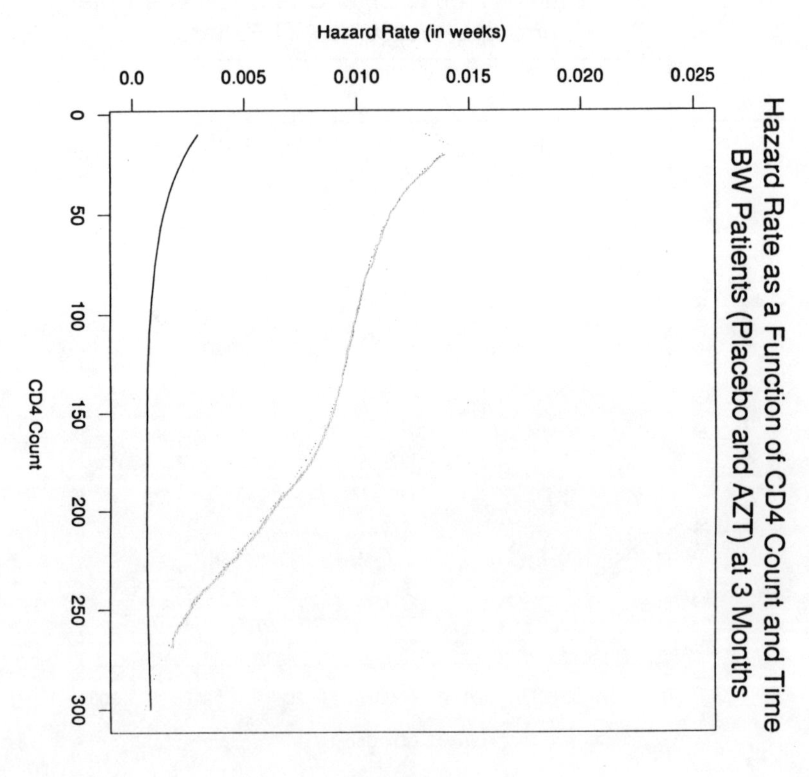

Figure 4

The relationship of the hazard rate as a function of CD4 counts for patients receiving placebo was computed at three months as is shown in Figure 4. In this clinical trial, seven months after the study opened, it was determined that ZDV significantly decreased mortality and therefore the study was closed at that point. The patients receiving placebo were then encouraged to switch to ZDV. Therefore, we could only analyze the CD4 survival relationship during that time. For comparison, we also plotted the hazard rate at three months for the patients receiving ZDV in Figure 4.

It is clear that the relationship of the hazard function to CD4 counts is very different for patients receiving ZDV versus those receiving placebo. Obviously, the beneficial effect of ZDV are not mediated only through their effect on CD4 counts. Therefore, although CD4 counts are highly predictive of survival, they might not serve as a good surrogate marker for detecting treatment difference.

References

Breslow, N. (1974). Covariance analysis of censored survival data, *Biometrics* **30**: 89-99.

Cox, D.R. (1972). Regression models and life tables, *J. Roy. Statist. Soc Ser. B* **34**: 187-220.

Cox, D.R. (1975). Partial likelihood, *Biometrika* **62**: 269-276.

Laird, N.M. and Ware, J.H. (1982). Random-effects models for longitudinal data, *Biometrics* **38**: 963-974.

Lindstrom, M.J. and Bates, D.M. (1988) Newton-Raphson and EM algorithms for linear mixed-effects models for repeated-measures data, *JASA* **83**: 1014-1022.

Prentice, L.R. (1982). Covariate measurement errors and parameter estimation in a failure time regression model, *Biometrika* **69**: 331-342.

Prentice, R.L. and Self, S.G. (1983). Asymptotic distribution theory for Cox-type regression models with general relative risk form, *Annals of Statistics* **11**: 804-813.

Rao, C.R. (1973). *Linear Statistical Inference at its Applications*, Wiley, New York.

Self, S.G. and Pawitan, Y. (1991). Modeling a marker of disease progression and onset of disease, Submitted for publication.

Strawderman, R.L. and Tsiatis, A.A. (1991). Hazard estimation in the surrogate marker problem, Submitted to *Biometrics*.

Department of Biostatistics
Harvard School of Public Health
677 Huntington Avenue
Boston, MA 02115

Modeling The Relationship Between Progression Of CD4-Lymphocyte Count And Survival Time

Victor DeGruttola and Xin Ming Tu

Abstract

In models for repeated observations of a measured response, the length of the response vector may be determined by a survival process related to the response. If the measurement error is large, and probability of death depends on the true, unobserved value of the response, then the survival process must be modelled. Wu and Carroll (1988) proposed a random effects model for a two-sample longitudinal data in the presence of informative censoring, in which the individual effects included only slopes and intercepts. We propose methods for fitting a broad class of models of this type, in which both the repeated measures and the survival time are modelled using random effects. These methods permit us to estimate parameters describing the relationship between measures of disease progression and survival time; and we apply them to results of AIDS clinical trials.

1 Introduction

This paper describes methods to investigate the relationship between the progression of CD4 lymphocyte count and survival for patients enrolled in a clinical trial of two doses of Zidovudine. The number of CD4+ T lymphocytes cells per volume of blood (hereafter referred to as CD4 lymphocyte count) decreases in HIV-infected people and leaves them vulnerable to infection with many other pathogens. This paper considers new models for repeated measures of CD4 count among AIDS patients receiving treatment with Zidovudine (ZDV). Because many such patients do not survive throughout the study period and because probability of death is related to the CD4 count, models for progression must take into account the missing CD4 counts caused by attrition. In addition, models must accommodate the high degree of measurement error and biologic variability in the CD4 count. For this type of setting, Wu and Carroll (1988) proposed a growth-curve model for two-sample longitudinal data, in which individual effects included personal slopes and intercepts. In this report, we propose a method for fitting a broad class of growth curve models by maximum likelihood,when the pattern of missingness depends on the true, unobserved response vector. This method also permits us to estimate parameters describing the relationship between characteristics of the individual progression and survival time.

Our approach models survival times as well as disease progression using normally distributed random effects. Thus we model the joint distribution of CD4 counts and survival times as multivariate normal. This approach permits estimation using a version of the EM algorithm by extending the method of Laird and Ware (1982). Section 2 presents the models for disease progression and survival, and develops the likelihood. Section 3.1 describes the estimation procedure in the case that all survival times are observed, and section 3.2 extends this technique to allow right-censored survival times. Section 4 applies these methods to data from a randomized trial of two doses of ZDV undertaken by the AIDS Clinical Trials Group (ACTG), and Section 5 discusses the implications of these results and the need for further research.

2 Modeling the Disease Progression and Survival

In this section, we introduce notation and develop the likelihood for our model for disease progression and survival time. We consider a population of n study subjects, indexed by i, each of whom has m_i observations of a marker of disease progression. Let $\mathbf{y}_i$ be a $m_i \times 1$ vector, whose elements y_{ij} are the values of the marker for the ith person on the jth occasion of measurement for $i = 1, \ldots, n; j = 1, \ldots, m_i$. Let $\tau_i = \min(x_i, c_i)$, where x_i and c_i denote the failure and censoring times for the ith subject, respectively.

We model the progression of the marker $\mathbf{y}_i$ using a random effects model (Harville, 1974; Dempster *et al.*, 1981; Laird and Ware, 1982):

$$\mathbf{y}_i = \mathbf{T}_i\boldsymbol{\alpha} + \mathbf{Z}_i\mathbf{b}_i + \boldsymbol{\epsilon}_i; \qquad i = 1, \ldots, n, \tag{1}$$

where $\boldsymbol{\alpha}$ is a $p \times 1$ vector of unknown parameters; $\mathbf{T}_i$ is a known full rank $m_i \times p$ design matrix linking $\boldsymbol{\alpha}$ to $\mathbf{y}_i$; $\mathbf{b}_i \overset{iid}{\sim} N(\mathbf{0}, \mathbf{D})$ denotes a $k \times 1$ vector of unknown individual effect; $\mathbf{Z}_i$ is a known $m_i \times k$ design matrix linking $\mathbf{b}_i$ to $\mathbf{y}_i$; $\boldsymbol{\epsilon}_i \sim N(\mathbf{0}, \sigma^2\mathbf{I}_i)$ is a vector of residuals; and $\mathbf{I}_i$ is an $m_i \times m_i$ identity matrix.

To model survival times, we assume there is a one-to-one transformation of survival time so that the transformed x (which we continue to denote by x) can be modelled as:

$$x_i = \mathbf{w}_i^{\top}\boldsymbol{\zeta} + \boldsymbol{\lambda}^{\top}\mathbf{b}_i + r_i, \tag{2}$$

where $\boldsymbol{\zeta}$ is a $q \times 1$ vector of unknown parameters; $\mathbf{w}_i$ is a $q \times 1$ design matrix linking x_i to $\boldsymbol{\zeta}$; $\boldsymbol{\lambda}$ is a $k \times 1$ vector of unknown parameters linking $\mathbf{b}_i$ to x_i; $r_i \overset{iid}{\sim} N(0, s^2)$ is the residual.

To write the log-likelihood function, we assume that all censoring of survival time is noninformative, *i.e.* the probability of being censored does not depend on the unobserved failure time. The joint log-likelihood function can now be written as:

$$\begin{aligned} L_{obs} = & \sum_{i=1}^{N^o} log \left[\int_{\mathbf{b}_i} \phi(\mathbf{y}_i|\mathbf{b}_i, \boldsymbol{\alpha}, \sigma^2)\phi(\mathbf{b}_i|\mathbf{D})\phi(x_i|\mathbf{b}_i, \boldsymbol{\zeta}, s^2)d\mathbf{b}_i \right] + \\ & \sum_{i=1}^{N^c} log \left[\int_{\mathbf{b}_i} \phi(\mathbf{y}_i|\mathbf{b}_i, \boldsymbol{\alpha}, \sigma^2)\phi(\mathbf{b}_i|\mathbf{D}) \right. \\ & \left. (1 - \Phi(c_i|\mathbf{b}_i, \ \boldsymbol{\zeta}, s^2))d\mathbf{b}_i \right] \end{aligned} \tag{3}$$

where $\Phi(c_i|\mathbf{b}_i, \boldsymbol{\zeta}, s^2) = \int_{-\infty}^{c_i} \phi(x|\mathbf{b}_i, \boldsymbol{\zeta}, s^2)dx$, and N^o and N^c denote the number of failed and censored individuals. The parameters to be estimated are $\boldsymbol{\alpha}$, $\boldsymbol{\zeta}$, $\boldsymbol{\lambda}$, σ^2, s^2 and $\mathbf{D}$, which we denote collectively by θ. In Section 3, we discuss ML estimation procedures that extend the methods of Harville (1974) and Laird and Ware (1982) for random effects models (1).

3 Estimation

3.1 Uncensored Survival Times

In the absence of right censoring of survival times, *i.e.*, $\tau_i = x_i$, the log-likelihood (3) reduces to:

$$L_{obs} = \sum_{i=1}^{n} log \left[\int_{\mathbf{b}_i} \phi(\mathbf{y}_i|\mathbf{b}_i, \boldsymbol{\alpha}, \sigma^2)\phi(\mathbf{b}_i|\mathbf{D})\phi(x_i|\mathbf{b}_i, \boldsymbol{\zeta}, s^2) d\mathbf{b}_i \right] \quad (4)$$

As in Laird and Ware (1982), estimation of the parameters makes use of an adaptation of the EM algorithm, where the E-step consists of finding the expected log-likelihood conditional on the observed data, denoted by $Y_{obs} = (\mathbf{y}_i, x_i)_{1 \leq i \leq n})$ and previous parameter estimates, and the M-step maximizes this expectation. In our setting, this is achieved by finding the conditional expectation of the sufficient statistics (E-step) and then estimating model parameters by substituting these expected values for the sufficient statistics (M-step).

The complete-data log-likelihood, *i.e.*, the likelihood that would apply if $\mathbf{b}_i$ were observed, is written as

$$L_c = \sum_{i=1}^{n} log \left[\phi(\mathbf{y}_i|\mathbf{b}_i, \boldsymbol{\alpha}, \sigma^2)\phi(\mathbf{b}_i|\mathbf{D})\phi(x_i|\mathbf{b}_i, \boldsymbol{\zeta}, s^2) \right]. \quad (5)$$

To find the conditional expectations for the sufficient statistics for the complete data likelihood, we first need an expression for the joint distribution

$$\phi(\mathbf{b}, \mathbf{y}, x|\theta),$$

which is multivariate normal under the model assumptions and is completely determined by its first and second moments. This allows us to use the properties of conditional distributions to develop expressions for the conditional expectations. The first moment, and the covariances between $\mathbf{b}$ and $\mathbf{y}$ and between $\mathbf{b}$ and x can be calculated from the model assumptions in (1) and (2). The covariance of $\mathbf{y}$ and x is complicated by the fact that the dimension of $\mathbf{y}$ is dependent on x. We address this problem by considering the vector of measurements to be of the same dimension, m, for each individual, and treating the values of the marker that occur after death as "missing data", with the pattern of missingness determined by x. In this case, the unobserved values are missing at random in the sense of Rubin (1976)–an assumption that is implicit in the likelihood (4). Since the parameter estimates depend only on the observed portions of individual responses,

$$\begin{aligned} Cov([\mathbf{y}_i, x_i]) &= E\{Cov([\mathbf{y}_i, x_i]|\mathbf{b}_i)\} + \\ &\quad Cov\{[E(\mathbf{y}_i|\mathbf{b}_i), E(x_i|\mathbf{b}_i)]\}. \end{aligned}$$

Here the brackets refer to a column vector composed of the quantities inside the brackets, *i.e.*, $[\mathbf{y}_i, x]$ is a $(m_i + 1) \times 1$ vector composed of the elements of $\mathbf{y}_i$ followed by x_i. Because $\mathbf{y}_i$ and x_i are conditionally independent, the first expectation is 0. The models for $\mathbf{y}_i$ and x_i above imply that the second term is $\mathbf{Z}_i\mathbf{D}_i\boldsymbol{\lambda}$. We can now express

$$Cov([\mathbf{b}, \mathbf{y}, x]) = \begin{pmatrix} \mathbf{D} & \mathbf{D}\mathbf{Z}^\top & \mathbf{D}\boldsymbol{\lambda} \\ \mathbf{Z}\mathbf{D} & \mathbf{Z}\mathbf{D}\mathbf{Z}^\top + \sigma^2\mathbf{I} & \mathbf{Z}\mathbf{D}\boldsymbol{\lambda} \\ \boldsymbol{\lambda}^\top\mathbf{D} & \boldsymbol{\lambda}^\top\mathbf{D}\mathbf{Z}^\top & \boldsymbol{\lambda}^\top\mathbf{D}\boldsymbol{\lambda} + s^2 \end{pmatrix}, \tag{6}$$

where the subscript i has been suppressed for clarity.

The sufficient statistics required for the M-step include:

$$\begin{aligned} &\sum_{i=1}^n \mathbf{b}_i\mathbf{b}_i^\top, \ \sum_{i=1}^n \epsilon_i^\top\epsilon_i, \ \sum_{i=1}^n r_i^2, \ \sum_{i=1}^n \mathbf{Z}_i\mathbf{b}_i, \ \sum_{i=1}^n x_i\mathbf{b}_i, \\ \textit{and} \quad &\sum_{i=1}^n w_{ji}\mathbf{b}_i, \ (1 \le j \le q) \end{aligned} \tag{7}$$

where w_{ji} refers to the jth element of $\mathbf{w}_i$. We calculate their expectations in the E-step, as shown in De Gruttola and Tu (1991). Using the results from the E-step, the M-step results from a straightforward maximization of the conditional log-likelihood. We estimate σ^2, s^2 and $\mathbf{D}$ by:

$$\widehat{\sigma^2} = (\sum_{i=1}^n m_i)^{-1} E(\sum_{i=1}^n \epsilon_i^\top \epsilon_i | Y_{obs}, \widehat{\theta}), \tag{8}$$

$$\widehat{s^2} = n^{-1}E(\sum_{i=1}^{n} r_i^2 | Y_{obs}, \widehat{\theta}), \tag{9}$$

and

$$\widehat{\mathbf{D}} = n^{-1}E(\sum_{i=1}^{n} \mathbf{b}_i \mathbf{b}_i^\top | Y_{obs}, \widehat{\theta}). \tag{10}$$

To estimate $\boldsymbol{\lambda}$, we note that if $\mathbf{b}_i$ were observed and $\boldsymbol{\zeta}$ were known, the ML estimate of $\boldsymbol{\lambda}$ would be

$$\widehat{\boldsymbol{\lambda}} = \left[\sum_{i=1}^{n} \mathbf{b}_i \mathbf{b}_i^\top\right]^{-1} \left[\sum_{i=1}^{n} (x_i - \mathbf{w}_i^\top \boldsymbol{\zeta})\mathbf{b}_i\right] \tag{11}$$

Once again, $\widehat{\boldsymbol{\lambda}}$ is estimated by replacing the sufficient statistics with their conditional expectations:

$$\widehat{\boldsymbol{\lambda}} = (n\widehat{\mathbf{D}})^{-1} \sum_{i=1}^{n} (x_i - \mathbf{w}_i^\top \widehat{\boldsymbol{\zeta}})\widehat{\mathbf{b}}_i. \tag{12}$$

The parameters $\boldsymbol{\alpha}$ and $\boldsymbol{\zeta}$ are estimated by:

$$\begin{aligned} \widehat{\boldsymbol{\alpha}} &= \left(\sum_{i=1}^{n} \mathbf{T}_i^\top \mathbf{T}_i\right)^{-1} \left[\sum_{i=1}^{n} \mathbf{T}_i^\top (\mathbf{y}_i - \mathbf{Z}_i \widehat{\mathbf{b}}_i)\right], \\ \widehat{\boldsymbol{\zeta}} &= \left(\sum_{i=1}^{n} \mathbf{w}_i \mathbf{w}_i^\top\right)^{-1} \left[\sum_{i=1}^{n} \mathbf{w}_i (x_i - \widehat{\boldsymbol{\lambda}}^\top \widehat{\mathbf{b}}_i)\right]. \end{aligned} \tag{13}$$

From the observed-data log-likelihood (4), which is multivariate normal, we estimate the covariance matrix of $[\widehat{\boldsymbol{\alpha}}, \widehat{\boldsymbol{\zeta}}]$ at convergence of the algorithm by

$$Cov\left([\widehat{\boldsymbol{\alpha}}, \widehat{\boldsymbol{\zeta}}] | Y_{obs}, \widehat{\theta}^*\right) = \left[\sum_{i=1}^{n} \mathbf{U}_i^\top \mathbf{C}_{22}^{-1}(i) \mathbf{U}_i\right]^{-1}, \tag{14}$$

where

$$\mathbf{U}_i = \begin{pmatrix} \mathbf{T}_i & \mathbf{0} \\ \mathbf{0} & \mathbf{w}_i^\top \end{pmatrix}$$

and $\widehat{\theta}^*$ is the ML estimate of θ.

Testing whether the components of $\boldsymbol{\lambda}$ are different from 0 will indicate which features of the progression of the marker are related to survival. Since the log-likelihood (4) is multivariate normal on the joint marginal of $[\mathbf{y}_i, x_i]$, the likelihood ratio test is easily performed. Obtaining closed-form expressions for the standard errors for the parameters presents more difficulty because it requires the second-order derivatives from the log-likelihood (4). These, in turn, involve differentiating variables inside a determinant. The method of Louis (1982) may be applied to simplify the computation, but it remains computationally burdensome. Numerical techniques, such as those described by Meng and Rubin (1990), may also apply.

3.2 Censored and Uncensored Survival Times

Censored survival times may be accommodated under the assumption that the censoring mechanism acts non-informatively on both the survival time and the marker response. This assumption is equivalent to the missing-at-random assumption discussed earlier and is implicit in the likelihood (3).

The EM algorithm discussed above must be modified so that the conditional expectations of the sufficient statistics include subjects with censored as well as those with observed survival times. These modifications are discussed in De Gruttola and Tu (1991). At convergence of the algorithm, the variance-covariance matrix of $[\widehat{\boldsymbol{\alpha}}, \widehat{\boldsymbol{\zeta}}]$ is computed by applying the method of Louis (1982):

$$Cov([\widehat{\boldsymbol{\alpha}}, \widehat{\boldsymbol{\zeta}}] | Y_{obs}, \widehat{\theta}^*) = \Bigg[\sum_{i=1}^{n} \mathbf{U}_i^\top \mathbf{C}_{22}^{-1}(i) \mathbf{U}_i - \sum_{i=1}^{n} \mathbf{U}_i^\top \mathbf{C}_{22}^{-1}(i) \; Cov_x\left([\mathbf{y}_i, x] | \mathbf{y}_i, \tau_i, \widehat{\theta}^* \right) \mathbf{C}_{22}^{-1}(i) \mathbf{U}_i \Bigg]^{-1}.$$

where τ_i is equal to x_i for uncensored observations and c_i for censored observations. Note that terms necessary to compute $Cov_x\left([\mathbf{y}_i, x] | \mathbf{y}_i, \tau_i, \widehat{\theta}^* \right)$ for the censored subjects have already been evaluated in maximizing the likelihood.

Analytical expressions for the observed information matrix of $\boldsymbol{\lambda}$, involve fairly tedious computations. We recommend the likelihood ratio test, which is still easily computed. To simplify computation of the second summation of the observed-data log-likelihood (3), we interchange the order of the integration and integrate out $\mathbf{b}_i$; the second term is now written

$$\sum_{i=1}^{N^c} log \left\{ \phi(\mathbf{y}_i|\widehat{\theta}^*) \left[1 - \Phi \left(c_i | \mu_{x|\mathbf{y}_i,\widehat{\theta}^*}, \sigma_{x|\mathbf{y}_i,\widehat{\theta}^*} \right) \right] \right\}.$$

where ϕ and Φ refer to normal and cumulative normal distributions. Hence, the computation of the log-likelihood only involves evaluation of the normal density and cumulative functions at the ML estimate $\widehat{\theta}^*$.

4 Results

The methods described above were applied to data from protocol 002 of the AIDS Clinical Trials Group (ACTG). This was a two-dose randomized trial of ZDV for patients with AIDS, which enrolled 560 patients between December 1986 and November, 1987 (Fischl et al., 1990). Of these, 524 evaluable patients were included in the final analysis of the study; and among these patients, 511 had at least one CD4 count. By June, 1990, 421 of the patients were known to have died. Because no difference in CD4 response by dose was detected, the two arms of the study were combined. The random effects model that best fit the data based on analysis by De Gruttola *et al.* (1991) was:

$$\begin{aligned} \log CD4_{ij} &= \alpha_1 + \alpha_2 I_{(t_{ij} \geq 8)} + \alpha_3 (t-8) I_{(t_{ij} \geq 8)} + \\ & \quad b_{1i} + b_{2i} I_{(t_{ij} \geq 8)} + b_{3i} (t-8) I_{(t_{ij} \geq 8)} + \epsilon_{ij} \end{aligned} \tag{15}$$

where $I_{(t \geq a)}$ is an indicator function, the b_i are random effects, ϵ_{ij} are residuals. The unit of time is weeks. Models were fit separately to data from 421 patients with known times of death and to the data from all 511 patients with at least one CD4 count. Since the survival times were approximately normally distributed (Figure 1), no transformation was used.

Table 1 shows the results for three different models fit to data on the 421 patients with known times of death. The first

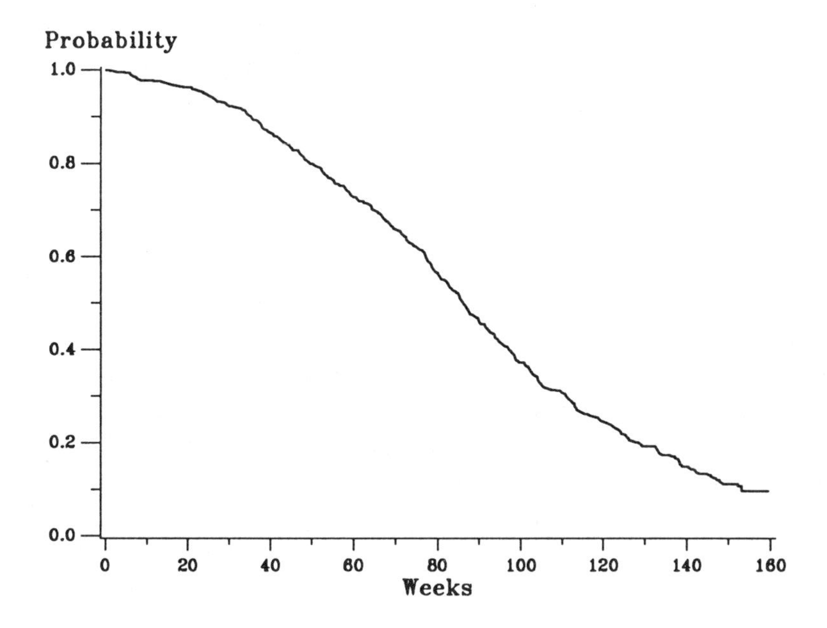

Figure 1: Survival of patients in ACTG protocol 002

was the Joint Maximization (JM) model described in section 3 with the progression of the CD4 count modeled according to (15). The other models were composed of two steps: the first step, denoted GC, fit the growth curve model (15) using Maximum Likelihood (Laird and Ware, 1982) to the data on CD4 counts; and the second step was ordinary least squares (OLS) or proportional hazards (PH) regression of the survival times on the estimated random effects from the growth curve model. The parameters λ_1, λ_2, and λ_3 are the regression coefficients corresponding to the random effects for the intercept, b_1; rise, b_2; and slope, b_3 respectively. Since the assumed distribution of the random effects is centered at 0, the intercept, λ_0 estimates the mean of the survival distribution. The estimated parameters of both models showed that ZDV induced a short term rise in CD4 count followed by a steady decline. Note that the estimates of intercept (α_1) and rise (α_2) are very similar for the

JM model and GC models, but that the slope (α_3) is steeper when estimated by the JM model. The reason for the steeper slope of the JM estimates may be that this method increases the influence of the short series of observations on people who died early. The results of the regression of survival time on the random effects for intercept, rise and slope are very similar for the three models. Although the entry level CD4 count is not related to survival, greater initial rise in CD4 and less steep decline in CD4 are associated with longer survival. The significance levels for the parameters are highest for the JM model as indicated by the smaller *p*-values; this may reflect the greater efficiency of this model. Of course, the parameter estimates, $\boldsymbol{\lambda}$, from the PH model are not directly comparable to the estimates from the other models, because they are on a different scale.

Table 1:
Comparison of regression coefficients between the JM and two-step models fitted to uncensored subjects from Protocol 002.

	JM Model	GC Model	
α_1 (std err)	3.9 (0.058)	3.9 (0.058)	
α_2 (std err)	0.50 (0.056)	0.48 (0.056)	
α_3 (std err)	-0.042 (0.0018)	-0.037 (0.0018)	
		OLS Model	PH Model
λ_0 (std err)	78.2 (1.7)	78.2 (1.7)	
λ_1 (p-value)	-6.9 (0.4)	-3.3 (0.4)	-0.027 (0.7)
λ_2 (p-value)	73.4 (0.002)	51.4 (0.01)	-0.81 (0.02)
λ_3 (p-value)	2903.9 (0.0001)	2050.6 (0.003)	-26.8 (0.006)

The results of fitting the JM and the two-step model to data which included the censored observations are displayed in Table 2. The parameter estimates from model (15) were similar for the two models, except that, once again, the slope was steeper for the JM model. The significance levels for the estimated $\boldsymbol{\lambda}$ based on the JM model are greater than those for the two-step model using proportional hazards. The association of rise and slope with survival was the same as in Table 1.

Table 2:
Comparison of regression coefficients between the JM and two-step models fitted to censored as well as uncensored subjects from Protocol 002.

	JM Model	GC Model
α_1 (std err)	3.9 (0.052)	3.9 (0.052)
α_2 (std err)	0.48 (0.048)	0.45 (0.048)
α_3 (std err)	-0.038 (0.0014)	-0.033 (0.0014)
		PH Model
λ_0 (std err)	90.6 (2.0)	
λ_1 (p-value)	-0.33 (0.4)	-0.02 (0.7)
λ_2 (p-value)	42.2 (0.001)	-0.75 (0.03)
λ_3 (p-value)	2459.4 (0.0001)	-45.6 (0.0001)

Table 3 displays the estimates of the variance parameters for the JM model and two-step models for both data sets. The estimate of s^2 for the two-step model is based on the following relation:

$$E\left[\sum(x_i - \mathbf{w}_i^\top \boldsymbol{\zeta} - \boldsymbol{\lambda}^\top \widehat{\mathbf{b}}_i)^2 | (\mathbf{y}_i)_{1\le i\le n}\right]$$

$$= E\left\{\sum[x_i - E(x_i|(\mathbf{y}_i)_{1\le i\le n})]^2|(\mathbf{y}_i)_{1\le i\le n}\right\} \qquad (16)$$
$$= ns^2 + \sum\left[\boldsymbol{\lambda}^\top\mathbf{D}\boldsymbol{\lambda} - \boldsymbol{\lambda}^\top\mathbf{D}\mathbf{Z}_i^\top(\sigma^2\mathbf{I}_i + \mathbf{Z}_i\mathbf{D}\mathbf{Z}_i^\top)^{-1}\mathbf{Z}_i\mathbf{D}\boldsymbol{\lambda}\right].$$

Table 3:
Comparison of estimates between the JM and two-step models fitted to Protocol data. [a] refers to the $(j,j)^{th}$ element of $\mathbf{D}$, [b] refers to the correlations and [c] is obtained from OLS and corrected by formula (22).

Uncensored		
	JM (No Censoring)	GC (No Censoring)
σ^2	0.59	0.59
d_{11} [a]	0.85	0.85
d_{22}	0.28	0.28
d_{33}	0.00030	0.00029
r_{12} [b]	-0.27	-0.27
r_{13}	0.41	0.41
r_{23}	-0.80	-0.81
s^2	359.63	411.61[c]

Censored		
	JM (Censoring)	GC (Censoring)
σ^2	0.56	0.56
d_{11} [a]	0.84	0.84
d_{22}	0.19	0.18
d_{33}	0.00020	0.00019
r_{12} [b]	-0.25	-0.26
r_{13}	0.33	0.30
r_{23}	-0.50	-0.46
s^2	1108.38	

We obtain our estimate by solving for s^2 in the expression above, and making the following substitutions: the sum of squared residuals for its expectation, ML estimates from the first step for σ^2 and $\mathbf{D}$, and the regression parameter estimate from the second step for $\boldsymbol{\lambda}$. Although this estimate of s^2 is unbiased, it is not necessarily positive. Table 3 shows that all of the estimates of σ^2 were fairly similar, but the estimate of s^2 is greater when the censored observations are included. Conversely, the estimates of d_{22} are greater in the uncensored case.

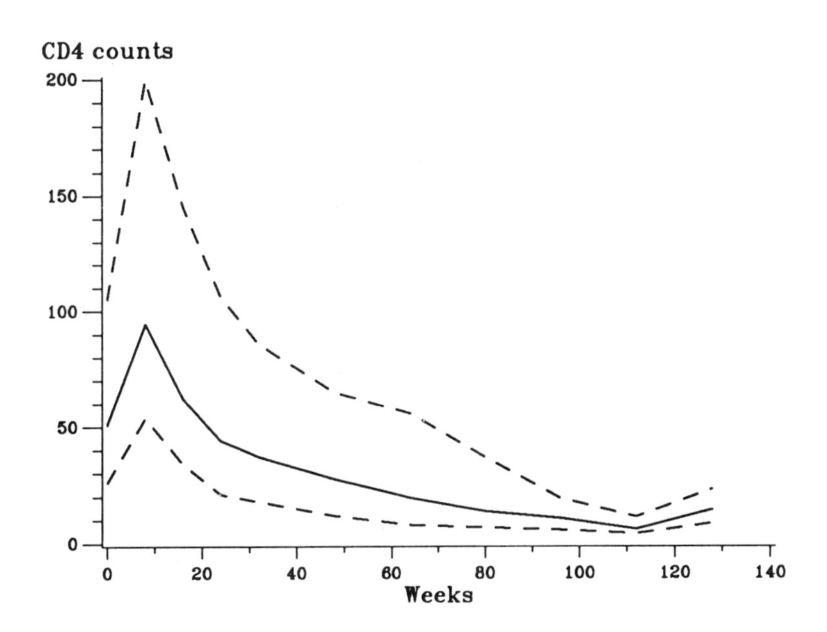

Figure 2: Observed CD4 lymphocyte counts for patients in ACTG 002.
(a) 75th percentile (upper curve).
(b) median (middle curve).
(c) 25th percentile (lower curve).

One useful aspect of our modeling approach is that it permits calculation of the distributions of expected CD4 count among surviving patients and the expected survival curves that correspond to a given CD4 trajectory. Figure 2 displays the median and the upper and lower quartile of observed CD4 lymphocyte counts among patients in ACTG 002. The number of patients who have counts drops from 511 at baseline to 423 at week 8,

361 at week 16, 252 at week 32, 106 at week 64 and 37 at week 96. Because mortality was only about 10% at week 32 and 50% by week 90, much of the reduction in the number of patients with CD4 lymphocyte counts results from missed visits rather than attrition due to death.

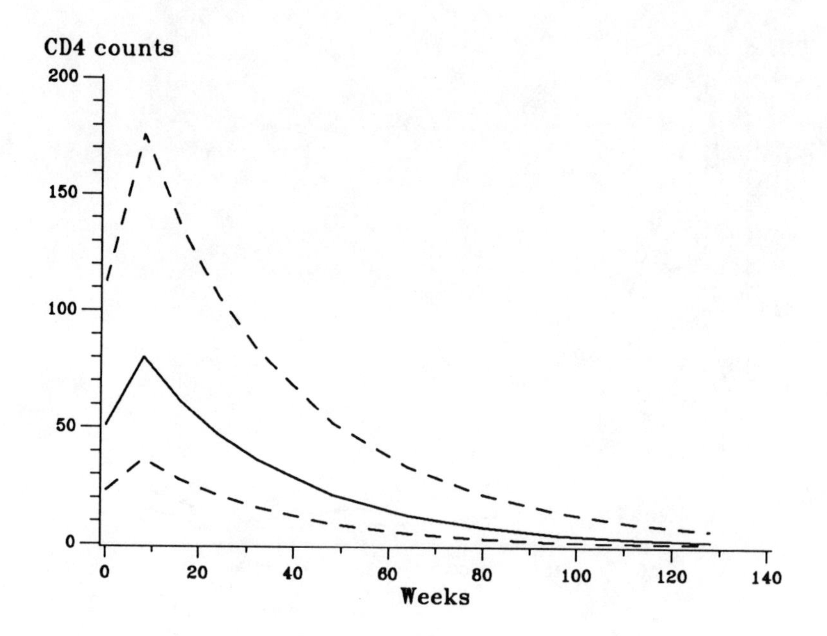

Figure 3: Model-based estimates of CD4 lymphocyte counts among surviving patients (linear model).
(a) 75th percentile (upper curve).
(b) median (middle curve).
(c) 25th percentile (lower curve).

Figure 3 displays the model-based predicted CD4 counts for surviving patients. The upper quartile declines more rapidly than in Figure 2 perhaps reflecting the observation bias. Figure 4 presents the same three curves that would apply to a population with the same CD4 process but no attrition due to death. The major difference between Figure 3 and Figure 4 occurs after week 60. Figure 5 shows the median and quartiles of the empirical Bayes' estimates of the true CD4 counts surviving patients. These estimates correct for the effect of measurement error on the CD4 distribution. Note that the median is similar to Figure 3, but the quartiles have been "shrunken" toward the mean.

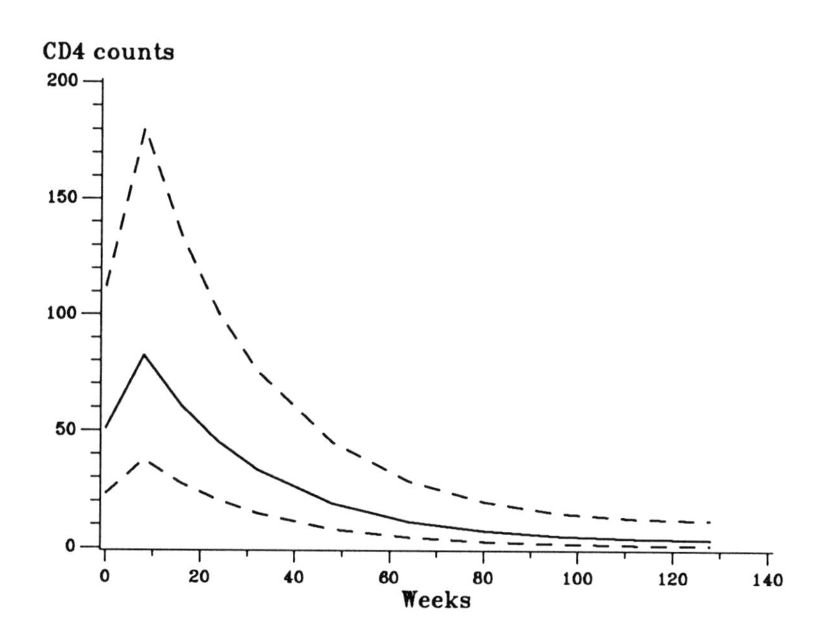

Figure 4: Model-based estimates of CD4 lymphocyte counts for a population with no attrition due to death (linear model).
(a) 75th percentile (upper curve).
(b) median (middle curve).
(c) 25th percentile (lower curve).

Figures 6–8 display the same curves as figures 3–5 assuming a quadratic model for the CD4 progression. This model was similar to model (15) except that a quadratic fixed effect, $\alpha_4(t-8)^2 I_{(t_{ij}\geq 8)}$, was included in the model. No quadratic random effect was included because of collinearity The quadratic term does not greatly affect these estimates, although the peak at 8 weeks is a little higher when this term is included. Figure 9 displays the expected survival distributions for patients with

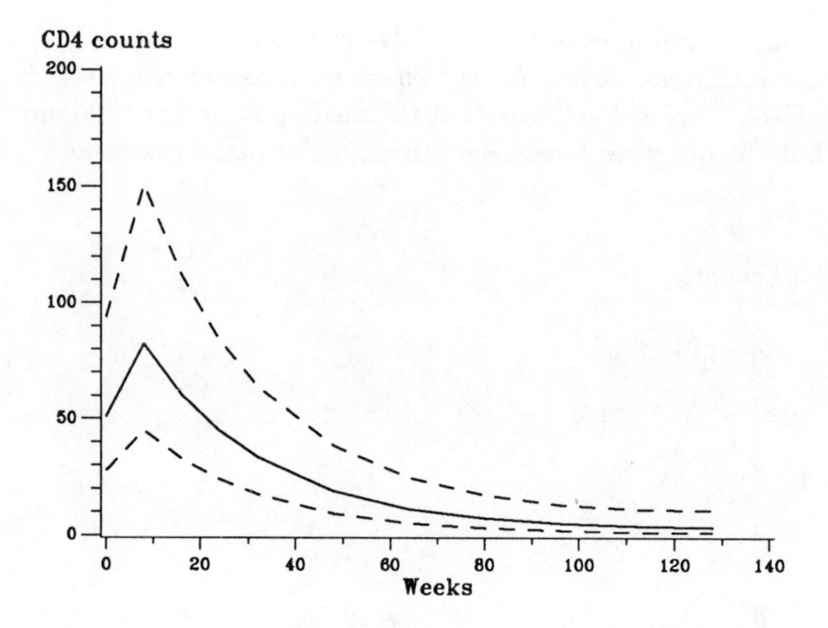

Figure 5: Empirical Bayes estimates of the CD4 lymphocyte counts among surviving patients (linear model).
(a) 75th percentile (upper curve).
(b) median (middle curve).
(c) 25th percentile (lower curve).

three different CD4 trajectories. The three trajectories are those displayed in Figure 5. It is apparent that even major differences in CD4 progression lead to only fairly modest differences in survival distribution.

5 Discussion

In this report, we consider methods for analyzing longitudinal data which include series of repeated measures that cease after removal of a subject resulting from death (which may induce informative censoring) or some other non-informative censoring process. There are a number of advantages in using the

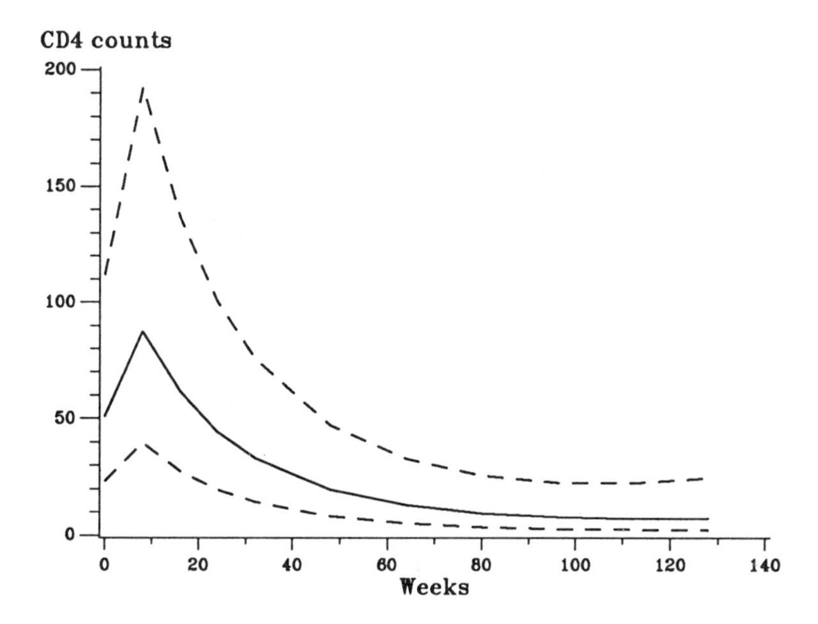

Figure 6: Model based estimates of the CD4 lymphocyte counts among surviving patients (quadratic model).
(a) 75th percentile (upper curve).
(b) median (middle curve).
(c) 25th percentile (lower curve).

JM method compared to the two-step method for analyzing such data. One advantage is a gain in efficiency as illustrated in the simulation. The improvement arises from the fact that survival times contain information about progression that is used in the JM approach. In addition, the likelihood ratio tests for the parameters that link the progression to survival are correct for the model we propose. All of the parameters are estimated by maximum likelihood in the JM approach.

The JM approach also permits fairly easily calculation of the distribution of CD4 counts adjusted for the attrition due to death. Figures 3 and 4 show how the progression of observed counts differs the progression that might be expected if

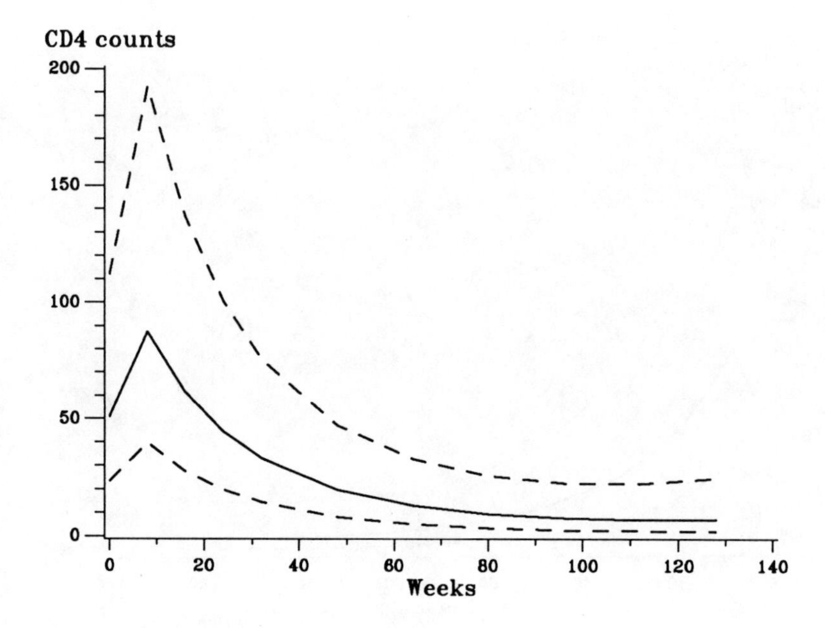

Figure 7: Model-based estimates of CD4 lymphocyte counts for a population with no attrition due to death (quadratic model).
(a) 75th percentile (upper curve).
(b) median (middle curve).
(c) 25th percentile (lower curve).

the same CD4 process applied but there was no attrition due to death. This allows us to look at the treatment effect on CD4 counts adjusting both for the missed observations among the living and the attrition due to death. These results show that the substantial differences in the CD4 trajectories do not seem to translate into large differences in survival.

Under the normality assumption for both the progression of the marker and survival time (or a one-to-one transformation of the survival time), estimation using an EM algorithm is fairly straightforward. The assumption of normality for modeling the survival time may not be met in some applications. In a similar formulation, Wu and Carroll (1988) considered the

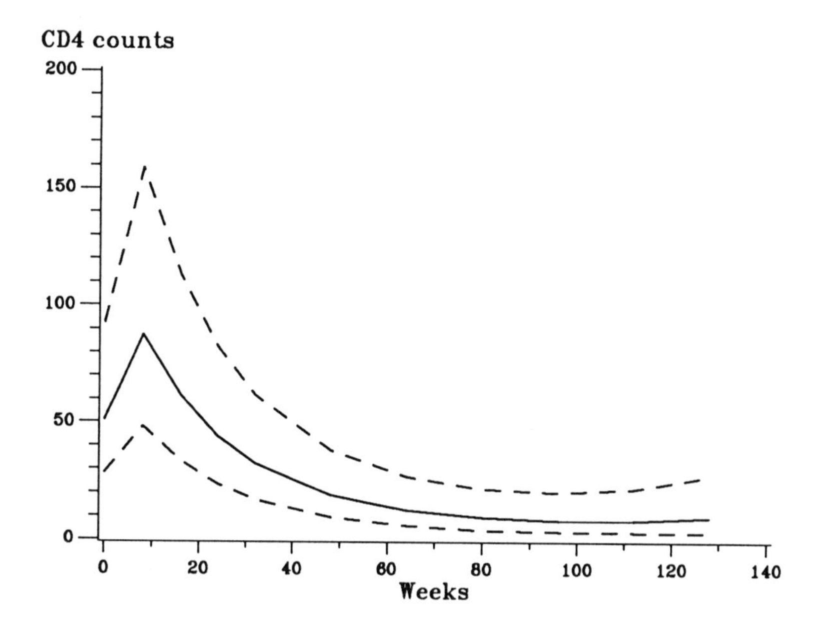

Figure 8: Empirical Bayes estimates of the CD4 lymphocyte counts among surviving patients (quadratic model).
(a) 75th percentile (upper curve).
(b) median (middle curve).
(c) 25th percentile (lower curve).

use of a probit model and obtained estimates using a pseudo-maximum likelihood approach. To relax normality assumptions and use more general models for the survival time, other data-augmentation techniques such as multiple imputation (Rubin 1987a) may prove feasible for estimation. For example, if we can sample from the posterior distribution $\phi(\mathbf{b}_i|Y_{obs})$ to augment the observed data set Y_{obs}, parameter estimates can then be obtained by multiple imputation. The sampling process requires Monte Carlo-based techniques (Rubin, 1987b; Tanner and Wong, 1987; Geman and Geman, 1984; Gelfand and Smith, 1990). Further work is required to explore the potential of these approaches.

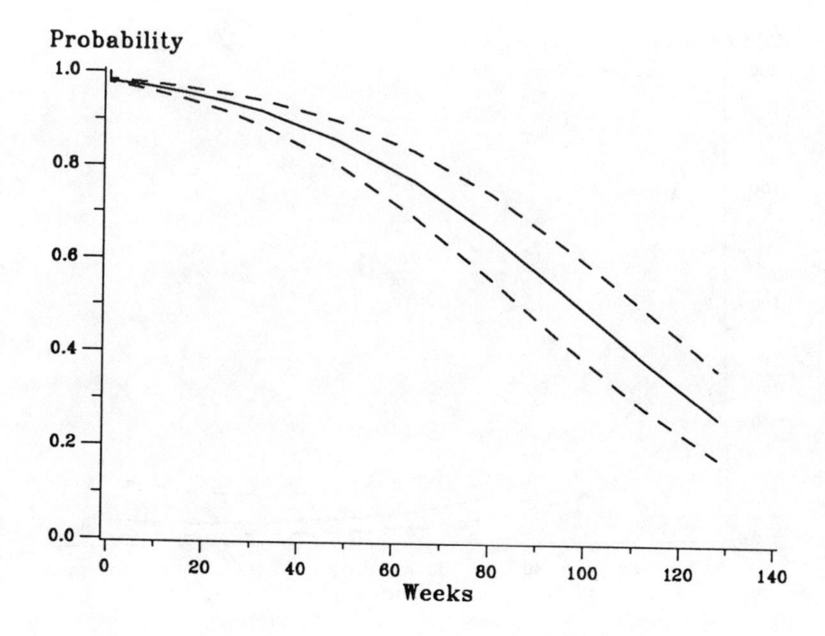

Figure 9: Predicted survival distributions for patients with CD4 trajectories as displayed in Figure 4. Survival curves correspond to:
(a) Upper quartile CD4 trajectory (upper curve).
(b) median CD4 trajectory (middle curve).
(c) Lower quartile CD4 trajectory (lower curve).

Acknowledgements

The authors would like to thank Drs X. Meng at University of Chicago, M. Pagano, A. Tsiatis and S. Choi at Harvard School of Public Health for fruitful discussions. Research supported in part by grants from the National Institutes of Health NIAID 1-R29-AI28905 and NO1-AI-95030.

Bibliography

DeGruttola, V., Wulfsohn, M. and Tsiatis, A. (1990) "Modeling the relationship between survival after AIDS diagnosis and progression of markers of HIV disease," Technical Report, Harvard School of Public Health.

Dempster, A.P., Rubin, D.B. and Laird, N.M. (1977) "Maximum likelihood with incomplete data via the E-M algorithm," *Journal of the Royal Statistical Society, Series B* **39**, 1-38.

Dempster, A.P., Rubin, D.B. and Tsutakawa, R.K. (1981) "Estimation in covariance component models," *Journal of the American Statistical Association*, **76**, 341-353.

Fischl, M., Parker, C., Pettinelli, C., Wulfsohn, M., Hirsch, M., Collier, AC., *et al.* (1990) "A randomized controlled trial of a reduced daily dose of zidovudine in patients with the Acquired Immunodeficiency Syndrome," *New England Journal of Medicine*, **323**, 107-114.

Gelfand, A.E. and Smith, A.F.M. (1990), "Sampling-based approaches to calculating marginal densities," *Journal of the American Statistical Association*, **85**, 398-409.

Geman, S. and Geman, D. (1984), "Stochastic relaxation, Gibbs distributions and the Bayesian restoration of images," *IEEE Transactions on Pattern Analysis and Machine Intelligence*, **6**, 721-741.

Harville, D.A. (1977), "Maximum likelihood approaches to variance component estimation and to related problems," *Journal of the American Statistical Association*, **72**, 320-340.

Laird, N.M. and Ware, J.H. (1982), "Random-effects models for longitudinal data" *Biometrics*, **38**, 963-974.

Meng and Rubin (1990) "Using EM to obtain asymptotic variance-covariance matrices: the SEM algorithm," *Journal of the American Statistical Association*, to appear.

Rubin, D.B. (1976) "Inference and missing data," *Biometrika*, **63**, 57-67.

Rubin, D.B. (1987a) Multiple Imputation for nonresponse in surveys. John Wiley and Sons, New York.

Rubin, D.B. (1987b), Comment on "The calculation of posterior distributions by data augmentation," by M.A. Tanner and W.H. Wong, *Journal of the American Statistical Association*, **82**, 543-546.

Tanner, M. and Wong, W. (1987), "The calculation of posterior distributions by data augmentation," *Journal of the American Statistical Association*, **82**, 528-550.

Turnbull (1976), "The empirical distribution function with arbitrarily grouped, censored, and truncated data," *journal of the Royal Statistical Society, Series B*, **38**, 290-295.

Wu, M.C. and Carroll R.J. (1988), "Estimation and comparison of changes in the presence of Informative right censoring by modeling the censoring process," *Biometrics*, **44**, 175-188.

Department of Biostatistics
Harvard School of Public Health
677 Huntington Avenue
Boston, Massachusetts 02115
U.S.A.

RECOVERY OF INFORMATION AND ADJUSTMENT FOR DEPENDENT CENSORING USING SURROGATE MARKERS

James M. Robins and Andrea Rotnitzky

Abstract: A class of tests and estimators for the parameters of the Cox proportional hazards model, the accelerated failure time model, and a model for the effect of treatment on the mean of a response variable of interest are proposed that use surrogate marker data to recover information lost due to independent censoring and to adjust for bias due to dependent censoring in randomized clinical trials. We construct an adaptive test that (i) is asymptotically distribution free under the null hypothesis of no treatment effect on survival, (ii) incorporates surrogate marker data, and (iii) is guaranteed to be locally more powerful than the ordinary log-rank test against proportional hazards alternatives when the baseline failure time distribution is Weibull. The proposed test is shown to outperform the log-rank test in a series of simulation experiments. We also prove the optimal estimator within our class is semiparametric efficient by first showing that our estimation problem is a special case of the general problem of parameter estimation in an arbitrary semiparametric model with data missing at random, and then deriving a representation for the efficient score in this more general problem.

1. Introduction

Randomized clinical trials of the effect of a new treatment on mortality from a chronic fatal disease such as AIDS must be conducted over prolonged periods of time. It is important to be able to stop such trials the moment that it be determined that the new treatment prolongs survival. To this end, interim analyses comparing the survival experience in the two treatment arms are typically conducted at 6 monthly or yearly intervals. Although subject-specific data on the evolution of time-dependent covariates that predict subsequent survival (such as CD4-count and serum HIV-antigen levels) will often be available at the time of an interim analysis, typically treatment arm specific survival curves are compared using a log-rank or weighted log-rank test that ignores the surrogate marker data. In this paper, we refer to any post treatment variable that, conditional on treatment arm, predicts subsequent survival as a surrogate marker. One major goal of this paper is to develop statistical methods that increase the power to detect a treatment effect by incorporating information on surrogate markers and yet do not compromise the validity of the usual intention to treat analysis of the null hypothesis of no-treatment effect. Specifically, we shall propose a class of tests that are guaranteed to reject, in large samples, at their nominal rate under the null hypothesis of no effect of treatment on survival, but may be much more powerful than any weighted log-rank test when a treatment effect exists. In this paper, we restrict attention to tests conducted at a single point in time. Group sequential procedures, applicable to repeated interim analyses, will be the subject of a separate report.

The second major goal of this paper is to develop statistical methods that can be used to adjust for non-random non-compliance and dependent censoring in randomized clinical trials. In an AIDS randomized trial comparing a treatment A, say high-dose AZT, with a treatment B, say low-dose AZT, it is common for subjects to fail to comply with the assigned treatment protocol and to initiate treatment with a new but unproven therapy C, say, aerosolized pentamidine prophylaxis for pneumocystis carinii pneumonia (PCP). In this setting, in order to obtain some useful information regarding the benefits of high- vs low-dose AZT, suppose it is agreed to regard subjects as censored at the time they initiate treatment with aerosolized pentamidine. Unfortunately, as discussed by Lagakos et al. (1991), the actual level of the associated censored data log-rank intention to treat test may differ from its nominal level if (a) subjects in the low-dose AZT arm are more likely than subjects in the high-dose arm to initiate therapy with aerosolized pentamidine, and (b), within each arm, censoring is not independent of failure (i.e., death) because subjects at high risk of failure (that is, subjects with recurrent episodes of PCP) are more likely to be censored (i.e., to initiate therapy with aerosolized pentamidine). Together (a) and (b) imply that censoring and failure are dependent. Suppose, in this setting, based on substantive considerations, the investigators conducting the trial are willing to assume that, among a subset of subjects in a given treatment arm with identical PCP histories up to time t, the decision to initiate prophylaxis therapy with aerosolized pentamidine at t is unrelated to prognosis. Then, the methods proposed in this paper can be used to construct an asymptotically α-level test of the null hypothesis that the distribution of failure times in the high- and low-dose AZT arms would have been the same had no subject abandoned protocol and initiated therapy with aerosolized pentamidine.

The paper is organized as follows. In Section (2), we (a) specify 3 models whose parameters we shall estimate - the proportional hazards (PH) model, the accelerated failure (AF) time model, and a model for the mean of a random variable measured near the end of follow-up, and (b) formally define dependent and independent censoring mechanisms. The combination of one of these models and a censoring mechanism constitute a semiparametric model for the observed data (Begun et al., 1983).

In Section (3) we show that, under an independent censoring mechanism, (a) the non-centrality parameter of the locally most powerful asymptotically distribution free (ADF) test of the null hypothesis of no treatment effect on survival against PH (or AF) alternatives equals the semiparametric information bound (SIB) for estimating the PH (or AF) model parameter β_0 at $\beta_0=0$ and (b) the SIB is greater when surrogate marker data is available than when it is not.

In Sections (3a)-(3b), we propose a class of tests that (a) incorporate surrogate marker data, (b) are ADF under the null hypothesis of no treatment effect on survival, and (c) contain tests whose non-centrality parameters converge to the SIB. Further, in Sections (3b)-(3c), we explicitly construct an ADF adaptive test that (a) incorporates surrogate marker data, (b) is guaranteed to be locally more powerful than the ordinary log-rank test against PH or AF alternatives when the baseline failure time distribution is Weibull, and (c), as predicted by theory, outperforms the log-rank test in a series of simulation experiments. In Section (3d) we show that our methods allow one to improve upon the Kaplan-

Meier estimate of the baseline survival curve by incorporating surrogate marker data.

In Section (3e), we propose a class of unbiased estimating equations for our 3 models whose solutions are consistent, asymptotically normal even in the presence of dependent censoring. Our class of estimators are based on recent work by Robins (1991) and Robins, Rotnitzky, and Zhao (1992), and can be viewed as a generalization of the Koul et al. (1981) censored linear regression estimator that uses surrogate marker data to recover information and adjust for dependent censoring.

In Section (4), we calculate the semiparametric variance bound for our semiparametric models and show that the asymptotic variance of the optimal estimator in our proposed class attains the bound. We calculate the semiparametric variance bound by showing that the semiparametric problem we are considering is actually a special case of the general problem of estimating the parameters of an arbitrary semiparametric model in the presence of data missing at random [Rubin (1976)]. In Theorems (4.1)-(4.3) we provide a representation for both (a) the efficient score and (b) the influence function of any regular, asymptotically linear estimator in this general estimation problem [provided that, for each subject, the probability of observing complete (i.e., full) data is bounded away from zero]. These representation theorems were derived by Robins, Zhao, Rotnitzky, and Lipsitz (1991). We show that the efficient score is a solution to an operator (i.e., integral) equation which does not in general have a closed form solution. However, we show that, in the special case of our mean model, a closed form solution exists. Although, for the PH and AF model, the efficient score does not exist in closed form, we describe how one can obtain a semiparametric efficient estimator by using linear combinations of estimating equations in our class (Newey, 1992b).

In Section (4e), we show that, in the absence of surrogate marker data, a slightly modified version of the original Koul et al., (1981) estimator is semiparametric efficient in the AF model under an independent censoring mechanism. In addition, as a by product of our investigation of dependent censoring, we construct, in Section (3h) and Appendix 4, a new estimator for the parameters of an AF model when censoring is due solely to a known end-of-follow-up date.

The paper is organized such that a reader who is more interested in the abstract theory of estimation in semiparametric models with data missing at random (rather than in particular applications of this theory) can proceed directly to the general representation theorems (4.1)- (4.3) of Section 4. With the notable exception of the proof of the general representation Theorem (4.1) provided in Appendix 2, the proofs of most theorems are only sketched and regularity conditions largely ignored.

2. A Formalization of the Problem

To be concrete, consider a two-arm double-blind trial comparing the effect of high versus low dose AZT treatment on the survival of AIDS patients in which dependent censoring due to initiation of prophylaxis therapy with aerosolized pentamidine may occur.

Suppose patient enrollment began on August 1, 1989 and continued until follow-up was artificially terminated on July 31, 1990 for the purposes of conducting an interim analysis. The maximum potential follow-up time c_{max} is one year. Many subjects will have been under follow-up for less than a year.

With time measured as time since randomization, define for subject i, $i=1,\cdots,n$,

Q_{1i} - censoring time due to end of follow-up. Thus, $Q_{1i} \le c_{max}=1$.

Q_{2i} - time to initiation of prophlyaxis therapy for PCP

$Q_i = \min(Q_{1i},Q_{2i})$-censoring time

T_i - failure time in the absence of prophylaxis for PCP

$Z_i = (Z_{1i},\cdots,Z_{pi})'$. Z_{1i} is a dichotomous treatment arm indicator. $(Z_{2i},\cdots,Z_{pi})'$ is a vector of pretreatment variables such as age and gender.

$L_i(t)$ and $\bar{L}_i(t) = \{L_i(u)\,;\,0 \le u \le t\}$ are respectively the recorded value at t and the recorded history up to t of a vector of time-dependent covariates such as CD4-count and HIV-antigen level.

For reasons that will become clear below, we may need to consider artificially ending follow-up at a time c^*, $c^* \le c_{max}$. Let $\Delta_i = I(T_i < c^*)$. If we disregard all events occurring subsequent to $\min(c^*,Q_i,T_i)$, the observable random vectors are

$$\{c^*,Z_i,X_i = \min(Q_i,T_i,c^*),\bar{L}_i(X_i),\tau_i = I[X_i \ne Q_i],\Delta_i\tau_i\},i=1,\cdots,n \tag{2.1}$$

which we assume are independent and identically distributed. We call (2.1) the c^*-observed data. Note Δ_i is observed only if $\tau_i=1$. If we do not artificially end follow-up prior to c_{max}, we would have $c^* = c_{max}$, $X_i = \min(Q_i,T_i)$, and $\Delta_i\tau_i = \tau_i$. We shall consider three models for the treatment effect. The PH model

$$pr[T>t \mid Z] = \{\bar{F}_0(t)\}^{\exp(\beta_0' Z)} \tag{2.2a}$$

The AF model

$$pr[T>t \mid Z] = \bar{F}_0(e^{\beta_0' Z}t) \tag{2.2b}$$

and a model for the conditional mean of Δ

$$E[\Delta \mid Z] = g(Z,\beta_0) \tag{2.2c}$$

where $g(\cdot,\cdot)$ is a known function, $\bar{F}_0(t)$ is an unspecified survival curve, and we have suppressed the i subscript. Gray and Tsiatis (1989) discuss the potential usefulness of model (2.2c) in studies of a potentially curative therapy. An investigator may be interested in the mean at time c^* of random variables other than Δ - e.g. the random variable recording HIV-antigen level. The results we obtain for model (2.2c) extend straightforwardly to models for the mean at c^* of any random variable.

If Z_i is the dichotomous treatment arm indicator then the null hypothesis $\beta_0=0$ is equivalent to the usual "intention to treat null hypothesis"

$$\text{pr}[T>t \mid Z] = \bar{F}_0(t) \tag{2.3}$$

of equality of treatment arm specific survival curves under both models (2.2a) and (2.2b). We shall assume the censoring mechanism satisfies

$$\lambda_Q(u \mid \bar{L}(u),Z,T) = \lambda_Q(u \mid \bar{L}(u),Z) \tag{2.4a}$$

where $\lambda_Q(u \mid \cdot) = \lim_{h\to 0} h^{-1}\text{pr}[u\leq X<u+h, \tau=0 \mid X\geq u,\cdot]$. (2.4a) would generally hold under the assumptions concerning initiation of prophylaxis therapy given in the introduction, if data on PCP history was recorded in $\bar{L}(u)$, and if there were no secular trends among patients entering the trial over the year of enrollment. Indeed (2.4a) would hold even if Q_1 and T are dependent given Z due to secular changes in the prognosis of patients at entry over the calendar year of enrollment (e.g., due to improvements in the standard care of AIDS patients), provided these changes could be explained by secular changes in the covariates in $\bar{L}(u)$. [In certain settings, an investigator might believe that there had been important changes in the prognosis of patients at entry over the year of enrollment that could not be explained by secular changes in the variables recorded in $\bar{L}(u)$. In Appendix 4, we show how the methods developed below can be extended to estimate the treatment effect in such settings.] We shall at times consider the implications of assuming the following in addition to (2.4a):

$$\lambda_Q[u \mid Z,T] = \lambda_Q[u \mid Z] \tag{2.4b}$$

$$\lambda_Q[u \mid Z,\bar{L}(T),T] = \lambda_Q[u \mid Z] \tag{2.4c}$$

$$\lambda_Q[u \mid \bar{L}(u),Z,T,\bar{L}(T)] = \lambda_Q[u \mid \bar{L}(u),Z] \tag{2.4d}$$

When (2.4a) holds, but (2.4b) is false, we say we have independent censoring given $\bar{L}(u)$ and Z, but dependent censoring given Z. (2.4c) would hold if no one took PCP prophylaxis (i.e., $Q_i = Q_{1i}$), and (conditional on Z) there exists no secular trends among patients entering the trial over the year of enrollment. (2.4c) implies (2.4a), (2.4b), and (2.4d). Finally, (2.4d) implies (2.4a) and is equivalent to the definition of missing at random (MAR) given by Rubin (1976).

3. Estimation and Testing:

3a. Introduction

Under each of the three models (2.2a)-(2.2c), our estimate $\hat{\beta}$ will be a solution to $S\{\hat{D}(\beta)\} = 0$ with

$$S\{\hat{D}(\beta)\} = \Sigma_i \tau_i \hat{D}_i(\beta)/\hat{K}_i \ ; \tag{3.1}$$

and our tests of the hypothesis that a given value of β equals the true β_0 will be based on $S\{\hat{D}(\beta)\}$ divided by the estimate of its asymptotic standard error given in Section (3j.2), where (i) $\hat{D}_i(\beta)$ depends on the model (2.2a) - (2.2c) and will be defined below, and (ii) $\hat{K}_i \equiv \hat{K}_i(X_i)$ is an estimate of $K_i(X_i)$ with $K(t) \equiv \exp\{-\int_0^t \lambda_Q[u \mid \bar{L}(u),Z]du\}$ and is computed as follows. We suppose we have a correctly specified stratified time-dependent Cox model

$$\lambda_Q[u \mid \bar{L}_i(u),Z_i] = \lambda_{S_i^*}(u)\exp[\alpha_0' W_i(u)] \tag{3.2}$$

where α_0 is a parameter vector, $W_i(u)$ is a vector of functions $w(\bar{L}_i(u),Z_i)$ of $\bar{L}_i(u)$ and Z_i, S_i^* is a discrete stratification variable that is a function of Z_i, and $\lambda_{S_i^*}(u)$ are unspecified stratum specific baseline hazard functions. As an example, $W_i(u)$ might include a subject's most recent CD4-count prior to u, the number of PCP bouts up to u, and their interactions with treatment arm. Let $\hat{\alpha}$ be the Cox maximum partial likelihood estimator of α_0. To obtain $\hat{\alpha}$ one can use standard time-dependent Cox proportional hazards model software by regarding the subjects with $X_i = Q_i$ as the "failures." Let

$$\hat{\lambda}_{S_j^*}(X_j) = (1-\tau_j)\left[\sum_{i=1}^{n} e^{\hat{\alpha}' \cdot W_i(X_j)} Y_i(X_j) I[S_i^* = S_j^*]\right]^{-1} \tag{3.3a}$$

where $Y_i(u) = I[X_i \geq u]$ records "at-risk" status at u. $\hat{\lambda}_{S_j^*}(X_j)$ is the Cox baseline hazard estimator for censoring at X_j in stratum S_j^*. Finally,

$$\hat{K}_i(u) \equiv \prod_{\{j;X_j \leq u, \tau_j = 0\}} I[S_i^* = S_j^*]\left[1 - \hat{\lambda}_{S_j^*}(X_j) e^{\hat{\alpha}' \cdot W_i(X_j)}\right]. \tag{3.3b}$$

We will occasionally write $\hat{K}_i \equiv \hat{K}_i(X_i)$ as $\hat{K}_i^W$ to stress its dependence on $W_i(u)$. $\hat{K}_i$ is an $n^{1/2}$-consistent estimator of $K_i(X_i)$ (Anderson and Gill, 1982).

$\hat{D}_i(\beta)$ is either exactly equal to or is an estimate of a random variable $\tilde{D}_i(\beta)$, where $0 = S^{(F)}\{\tilde{D}(\beta)\} \equiv \Sigma_i \tilde{D}_i(\beta)$ would be an unbiased estimating equation for β with solution $\tilde{\beta}$ if, contrary to fact, there were no Q-censoring and we had thus observed

$$\{c^*, X_i^* \equiv \min(T_i,c^*), \bar{L}_i(X_i^*), Z_i, \Delta_i\}, \; i=1,\cdots,n \tag{3.4}$$

which we shall call the c*-full data. That is, $E[\tilde{D}_i(\beta_0)] = 0$, and further, $\tilde{D}_i(\beta)$ and $\tilde{\beta}$ are functions of the c*-full data. In contrast, $\tau_i \hat{D}_i(\beta)$ and, thus, $S\{\hat{D}(\beta)\}$ and $\hat{\beta}$ will depend only on the c*-observed data. Before providing definitions for $\hat{D}_i(\beta)$ and $\tilde{D}_i(\beta)$ in the general case, we shall consider in Sections (3b)-(3d) tests of the null hypotheses (2.3) (i.e., tests of $\beta_0=0$ in models (2.2a) and (2.2b)) and estimation of the mean model (2.2c) under the assumptions that Z_i and S_i^* are both the (0,1) treatment arm indicator.

3b. <u>Tests of the Null Hypothesis (2.3)</u>

We define $\hat{D}_i(0) \equiv \tilde{D}_i(0) = R_i(Z_i - n^{-1}\Sigma_i Z_i)$ where $R \equiv r(\Delta, \ell n(X^*)) \equiv \Delta r_1\{\ell n(T)\} + (1-\Delta) r_2\{\ell n(c^*)\}$ with $r_1(\cdot)$ and $r_2(\cdot)$ scoring functions chosen by the analyst. Clearly

$E[\tilde{D}_i(0)] = 0$ under (2.3), since (2.3) implies T is independent of Z, and R is random only through its dependence on T. We can construct an ADF test of (2.3) based on $S\{\hat{D}(0)\}$ since the following fundamental lemma, proved in Section (3h), implies that $n^{-1/2}S\{\hat{D}(0)\}$ has asymptotic mean 0 under (2.3) and (2.4a).

Fundamental Lemma: If $K_i(X_i)>\sigma>0$ with probability one (w.p.1) for some $\sigma>0$ and (2.4a) and (2.3) hold, then $E[\tau_i\hat{D}_i(0)/K_i(X_i)] = 0$.

To help understand the lemma, note that when the stronger condition (2.4d) is true, $K_i(X_i)$ is the probability that subject i survived to X_i without being censored. Hence, if subject i is observed to fail at X_i and $K_i(X_i) = .1$, then subject i would need to count for $1/K_i(X_i) = 10$ subjects (himself and 9 others who were censored prior to X_i). Although, under the weaker assumption (2.4a), $K_i(X_i)$ is not the probability of surviving to X_i without being censored, nevertheless the lemma remains true.

To see why the Lemma may not hold if $K_i(X_i)$ is not bounded away from zero, suppose (1) data on $\bar{L}_i(u)$ was not collected or needed; (2) T_i was uniformly distributed on (0,.8) independent of Z_i so (2.3) was true; (3) $Q_i \coprod T_i \mid Z_i$ so (2.4d) was true with (3a) $Q_{1i} = c_{max}=1$ w.p.1, and (3b) Q_{2i} uniformly distributed on (0,.4) given $Z_i = 0$, and $Q_{2i}>1$ w.p.1 given $Z_i = 1$, so that all subjects with $Z_i = 0$ will initiate prophylaxis by time .4 if alive; (4) $c^* \equiv 1.0$; and (5) 50% of subjects were assigned to each treatment arm.

Then $K_i(X_i)>0$ w.p.1, but $K_i(X_i)\to 0$ as $X_i\to .4$ for subjects with $Z_i=0$ and $E[\tau_i\hat{D}_i(0)/K_i(X_i)] = (.25)(.5)$ if $r_1(\ell nT)=0$ if $T\leq .4$, and $r_1(\ell nT)=1$ for $T>.4$ [The 25% of subjects observed to fail between .4 and .8 without having initiated prophylaxis are all in the Z=1 arm with $K_i(X_i)=1$. Hence, for this group $\tau_i\hat{D}_i(0)/K_i(X_i) = \hat{D}_i(0)$ has mean $(1-1/2)E[R_i \mid T_i>.4] = .5$]. Artificially ending follow-up at a time c^* such that $K_i(c^*)>\sigma>0$ w.p.1 will insure that $K_i(X_i)>\sigma>0$ w.p.1, and thus, by the fundamental lemma, that $E[\tau_i\hat{D}_i(0)/K_i(X_i)] = 0$. For example, we can choose $c^* = .4-\epsilon, \epsilon>0$ to ensure that $K_i(c^*)>\sigma>0$ w.p.1 for some σ.

In the remainder of this subsection, we shall suppose that no subject initiates PCP prophylaxis so that $Q_i=Q_{1i}$, and that there are no secular trends so that censoring mechanism (2.4c) holds. Eq. (2.4c) implies the Cox model (3.2) is guaranteed to be correctly specified with $\alpha_0=0$. Nonetheless, as we shall see, the estimation of the coefficients α_0 that are known to be zero is the key to recovery of information from the surrogate markers $L_i(u)$.

Write $S\{\hat{D}(0)\}$ divided by the standard error estimate of Section 3j.2 as $\psi(r,w,c^*)$ to emphasize its dependence on r, w, and c^*. $\psi(r,w,c^*)$ is asymptotically distribution free under (2.3) and (2.4c). Specifically, a corollary of Theorem 3.4 of Section (3j.2) is

Theorem 3.1: If $K(X)>\sigma>0$ with probability one, then $\psi(r,w,c^*)$ is asymptotically N(0,1) under (2.3) and (2.4c). Further, under local AF or PH alternatives with $\beta_0=n^{-1/2}$, $\psi(r,w,c^*)$ is asymptotically normal with variance 1 and mean $[NC(r,w,c^*)]^{1/2}$, say.

Notational Convention: The value of the non-centrality parameter NC(r,w,c*) in Theorem (3.1) depends on whether we are considering AF or PH model alternatives. When a quantity such as NC(r,w,c*) depends on the model, we shall write it as $NC^{PH}(r,w,c^*)$ or $NC^{AF}(r,w,c^*)$, as appropriate, whenever it is important to indicate the model. However, when, as in Theorem (3.1), we leave off the model-identifying superscript, a quantity such as NC(r,w,c*) will be used to generically refer to either model.

We briefly discuss how to choose c* to ensure that $K(X)>\sigma>0$ with probability one. If, as we shall allow, the distribution of Q has a point mass at c_{max} (as would be the case if an initial group of subjects were enrolled simultaneously), then K(X)=0 with positive probability if $c^* = c_{max}$, but $K(X)>\sigma>0$ if $c^*=c_{max}^-$. If Q is absolutely continuous with respect to Lebesgue measure with support on (0,1) then (a) $K(X)\geq K(c^*)>\sigma>0$ for all $c^*<c_{max}$ where σ may depend on c*, and (b) K(X)>0 if $c^* = c_{max}$ but will not be bounded away from zero which can create problems (even asymptotically) due to division by $\hat{K}_i(X_i)$. As discussed in Section 3c, the problems associated with setting $c^* = c_{max}$ might be solved practically (and presumably theoretically) by treating the last observation in each stratum S* as a failure when computing $\hat{K}_i(X_i)$ and/or by choosing R such that $R/K(X)$ is bounded as $X\to c_{max}$.

Let $\hat{K}_i^0$ be $\hat{K}_i$ with $\hat{\alpha} \equiv 0$ in (3.3a) and (3.3b) and let $\psi(r,0,c^*)$ be the associated test statistic. $\hat{K}_i^0$ is the treatment-arm-specific Kaplan-Meier estimator of K(u) evaluated at $u = X_i$ and does not depend on surrogate marker data L(u). Let α_j and $W_j(u)$, j=1,···,J, represent the parameter and covariate vector in the jth of J nested Cox models (3.2) ordered by increasing dimension of $W_j(u)$. For a given choice of $R = r[\Delta,\ell n(X^*)]$, the optimal covariate is $W_{op}^r(u) \equiv \{Z-E(Z)\}\{K(u)\}^{-1}E[R \mid \bar{L}(u),Z,Y(u)=1] =$ $\{Z-E(Z)\}E[\tau R/K(X) \mid \bar{L}(u),Z,Y(u)=1]$ where the equality is by (3.10f) below. In Section (4c), we prove

Lemma 3.1: (a) Under censoring mechanism (2.4c), if $j^*>j$ $NC(r,0,c^*)\leq NC(r,w_j,c^*)\leq NC(r,w_{j^*},c^*)\leq NC(r,w_{op}^r,c^*)$ where the last inequality is strict unless there exists a constant matrix b such that $W_{op}^r(u) = b\, W_{j^*}(u)$ with probability one. (b) For

$$W(u) = (W^*(u)',ZW^*(u)')' \tag{3.5a}$$

with $W^*(u) = w^*\{\bar{L}(u)\}$, NC(r,0,c*) is strictly less than NC(r,w,c*) if, for a component $W_m^*(u)$ of W*(u),

$$E[\{Z-E(Z)\}^2 \int_0^\infty dN_Q(u)Cov\{R,W_m^*(u) \mid Z,T\geq u\}] \neq 0 \tag{3.5b}$$

with $N_Q(u) = I[X\leq u, \tau=0]$.

Inequality (3.5b) will generally hold if $W_m^*(u)$ and R are dependent given Z. [To obtain a test that is strictly more powerful than $\psi(r,0,c^*)$, it is often important to use covariates of the form (3.5a)]. Lemma (3.1a) implies that increasing the number of covariates in the Cox model (3.2) usually leads to improvements in power. We can obtain an asymptotically distribution-free test of (2.3) with non-centrality parameter approximating that of $NC(r,w^r_{op},c^*)$ either by (i) specifying a richly parameterized Cox model (3.2); or, possibly, by (ii) extending (3.2) by adding, as a covariate, an estimate of $W^r_{op}(u)$ given by $(Z-n^{-1}\Sigma_i Z_i)$ times $\hat{pr}[\tau=1 \mid \bar{L}(u),Z,Y(u)=1]$ multiplied by the predicted value from the least squares fit of a linear regression of $R/\hat{K}(X)$ on functions of $\bar{L}(u)$ and Z among those subjects with $Y(u)=1$ and $\tau=1$. Here $\hat{pr}[\tau=1 \mid \bar{L}(u),Z,Y(u)=1]$ is the predicted value from the fit of a logistic model for the probability that $\tau=1$ on functions of $\bar{L}(u)$ and Z among subjects with $Y(u)=1$. Separate linear and logistic models may be fit at each u in the set of observed Q-censoring times. The resulting test, $\psi(r,\hat{w}^r_{op}, c^*)$, (a) will have the same limiting distribution and thus non-centrality parameter as $\psi(r,w^r_{op},c^*)$ if each of the linear and logistic regression models are correctly specified, and (b) will still be asymptotically N(0,1) under (2.3) and (2.4c) if the models are misspecified or even incompatible with any joint distribution for the data (see Appendix 3). This robustness to model misspecification is convenient since $\bar{L}(u)$ is the entire history of a complex process up to u, and, thus, estimation of $E[\tau R/K(X) \mid \bar{L}(u),Z,Y(u)=1]$ by non-parametric regression is not practical due to the curse of dimensionality.

Since (2.4c) implies independent censoring given Z, ADF competitors to $\psi(r,w,c^*)$ will be the standard intention-to-treat weighted log rank tests $\psi_{LR} \equiv \psi_{LR}(c^*)$ with $c^* = c_{max}$, where $\psi_{LR}(c^*) \equiv \Sigma_i\Delta_i\tau_i\omega_i(Z_i-E_i)/[\Sigma_i\Delta_i\tau_i\omega_i^2E_i(1-E_i)]^{1/2}$, ω_i is a weight function, $E_i = \Sigma_jY_j(T_i)Z_j/\Sigma_jY_j(T_i)$. $\psi_{LR}(c^*)$ and $\psi(r,0,c^*)$, in contrast to $\psi(r,w,c^*)$, do not depend on the surrogates $\bar{L}(u)$, but only on

$$\{c^*, \tau_i, \Delta_i\tau_i, X_i, Z_i\},\ i=1,\cdots,n\ ,$$

which we call the <u>c*-$\overline{\text{sur}}$-data</u>.

<u>Remark</u>: Another test that incorporates surrogate marker data could be based on modifying the generalized "Buckley-James" estimating function considered by Ritov (1990) to $\sum_{i=1}^{n}(Z_i-n^{-1}\Sigma_jZ_j)\{\tau_iR_i+(1-\tau_i)\tilde{E}[R_i \mid \bar{L}_i(u),Y_i(u)=1,Z_i]\}$ evaluated at $u=X_i$ divided by its estimated asymptotic standard error. However, this test is guaranteed to be asymptotically N(0,1) under (2.3) and (2.4c) only if the estimate of the conditional expectation $E[R \mid \bar{L}(u),Z,Y(u)=1] = E[\tau K(u)R/K(X) \mid \bar{L}(u),Z,Y(u)=1]$ is based on a non-parametric regression of $\tau K(u)R/K(X)$ on $\bar{L}(u)$ and Z given $Y(u)=1$, which, as discussed above, is usually not practical due to the curse of dimensionality. Further, it follows from Theorem (3.2f) below that, if $\bar{L}(u)$ was a sufficiently simple process so that the non-parametric regression was practical and, thus, the modified "Buckley-James" test was asymptotically N(0,1), then the test would be asymptotically equivalent to and would have the same non-centrality parameter as some test $\psi(r^{(1)},w,c^*)$, where, in general $R_i \neq R_i^{(1)} \equiv r^{(1)}(\Delta_i,\ell nX_i^*)$.

Write ψ_{LR}^{PH} and ψ_{LR}^{AF} respectively for the tests that have $\omega_i=1$ and $\omega_i = \partial \ell n\lambda_{\ell nT}(u)/\partial u\,|_{u=\ell nT_i}$ where $\lambda_{\ell nT}(u)$ is the hazard of ℓnT. $\psi_{LR}^{PH}(c^*)$ and $\psi_{LR}^{AF}(c^*)$ are locally optimal in the class of weighted log-rank tests against their respective alternatives and are equal when $\bar{F}_0(t)$ is Weibull (Gill, 1980). In fact, results due to Begun et al. (1983) and Ritov and Wellner (1988) imply that, under (2.4c), they are locally optimal in the much larger class of regular, asymptotically linear (RAL) tests of (2.3) that use only the c^*-$\overline{sur}$-data. Informally, RAL tests are ones which are asymptotically N(0,1) under (2.3) and (2.4c), are asymptotically equivalent to a sample average, and whose convergence is uniform under Pitman sequences of distributions all satisfying the null hypothesis (2.3). See Section (4a) for a formal definition.

In Appendix 1, we show that the non-centrality parameter of the locally most powerful RAL test of (2.3) against PH (or AF) alternatives with $\beta_0=n^{-1/2}$ is the semiparametric information bound (SIB) for the estimation of $\beta_0=0$ in the PH (AF) model under censoring mechanism (2.4c). The SIB is defined in Section (4a) below and in Begun et al. (1983). The SIB depends on the available data. Write $NC_s^{c^*}$ and $NC_{\bar{s}}^{c^*}$ for the SIB at $\beta_0=0$ based on the c^*-observed data and the c^*-$\overline{sur}$-data respectively [where, in accord with the convention described previously, $NC_s^{c^*}$ refers to $NC_s^{c^*,PH}$ if we are considering the PH model and to $NC_s^{c^*,AF}$ if we are considering the AF model.] $NC_s^{c^*} \rightarrow NC_s^{c_{max}} \equiv NC_s$ and $NC_{\bar{s}}^{c^*} \rightarrow NC_{\bar{s}}^{c_{max}} \equiv NC_{\bar{s}}$ as $c^* \rightarrow c_{max}$. In Theorem (3.2), we shall show $NC_{\bar{s}} \leq NC_s \leq NC_{full}$ where NC_{full} is the SIB at $\beta_0=0$ based on the c^*-full-data (3.4) with $c^*=c_{max}$; and, further, in the absence of staggered entry (i.e., $Q_i = c_{max}$ for all i), $NC_{\bar{s}} = NC_s = NC_{full}$ and no information is gained from surrogate marker data. Thus we can view $(NC_{full} - NC_{\bar{s}})$ as the amount of information lost due to staggered entry in the absence of surrogate data and $(NC_s - NC_{\bar{s}})/(NC_{full} - NC_{\bar{s}})$ as the fraction of the lost information that can be recovered by optimally utilizing surrogate data. Begun et al. (1983) and Ritov and Wellner (1988) prove that the non-centrality parameter of ψ_{LR}^{PH} and ψ_{LR}^{AF} equal $NC_{\bar{s}}^{PH}$ and $NC_{\bar{s}}^{AF}$ respectively. We prove in Section (4e)

<u>Theorem 3.2</u>: Under (2.4c) and with Z dichotomous, (a) $NC_{\bar{s}} \leq NC_s$. Sufficient (and nearly necessary) conditions for equality are that either (i) $Q_i = c_{max}$ for all i or (ii), for all u, $\bar{L}(u)$ and T are conditionally independent given $(Z,X>u,T<c_{max})$. (b) $NC_s \leq NC_{full}$. Sufficient (and nearly necessary) conditions for equality are that either (i) $Q_i = c_{max}$ for all i, or (ii), for all u, $Var[T\,|\,Z,\bar{L}(u),X>u,T<c_{max}]=0$ in which case we call L(u) a perfect surrogate. (c) There exists $r_s \equiv r_s[\Delta,\ell n(X^*)]$ such that $NC(r_s, w_{op}^{r_s}, c^*) = NC_s^{c^*}$. In general, r_s is a solution to an integral equation which has a closed form solution only in special cases. (d) In particular, if L(u) is a perfect surrogate, $r_s = r_{pf} \equiv r_{pf}[\Delta,\ell n(X^*)] = \Delta r_{pf,1}(\ell nT) + (1-\Delta)r_{pf,2}(\ell nc^*)$. r_{pf} depends on the alternative. Specifically $r_{pf,1}^{AF}(u) = \partial \ell nf_{\ell nT}(u)/\partial u$, $r_{pf,1}^{PH}(u) = 1 - \int_{-\infty}^{u} \lambda_{\ell nT}(u)du$, $r_{pf,2}(u) = E[r_{pf,1}(\ell nT)\,|\,\ell nT>u]$, so $r_{pf,2}^{AF}(u) =$

$-\lambda_{\ell nT}(u)$ and $r^{PH}_{pf,2}(u) = -\int_{-\infty}^{u} \lambda_{\ell nT}(u)du$. r^{AF}_{pf} is proportional to r^{PH}_{pf} if $\bar{F}_0(u)$ is Weibull. (e) There exists $r_{\bar{s}} \equiv r_{\bar{s}}[\Delta, \ell n(X^*)]$ such that $NC(r_{\bar{s}},0,c^*)$ equals $NC_{\bar{s}}^{c^*}$. In particular, if $\lambda_Q(u \mid Z) = \lambda_Q(u)$, then for m = 1,2,

$$r_{\bar{s},m}(u) = r_{pf,m}(u)K(e^u) + \int_0^{e^u} r_{pf,2}\{\ell nx\}\lambda_Q(x)K(x)dx.$$

(f) Any RAL modified Buckley-James test of (2.3) is asymptotically equivalent to [i.e. has the same influence function as] some test $\psi(r,w^r_{op},c^*)$.

Since r_s does not exist in closed form, it is rather difficult to construct an adaptive test with non-centrality parameter $NC_s^{c^*}$. However, because $r_{\bar{s}}$ exists in closed form, we can use Lemma (3.1) to construct a simple adaptive ADF test $\psi(\hat{r}_{\bar{s}},w,c^*)$ of (2.3) that incorporates surrogate marker data and is guaranteed to be more powerful than the log-rank test against AF (or PH) alternatives if $\bar{F}_0(u)$ is in a specified parametric family $\bar{F}(u;\theta)$, such as the Weibull family. [Note, if $\bar{F}_0(u)$ is Weibull with $\lambda_0(u) = au^b$, then, under (2.3), $r^{AF}_{pf,2}(u) = -\lambda_{\ell nT}(u) = -ae^{u(b+1)}$ and $r^{AF}_{pf,1}(u) = (b+1) - \lambda_{\ell nT}(u)$ for Weibull parameters $\theta=(a,b)$.] We construct $\hat{r}_{\bar{s}}$ as follows.

Obtain "maximum likelihood" estimates of θ [and, thus, of $r_{pf,m}(u)$, for m = 1,2] based on the data (X_i, τ_i),i=1,⋯,n, with $c^* \equiv c_{max}$ under the assumption of independent censoring. Let $\hat{K}^{\dagger}(u)$ be the Kaplan-Meier estimate of K(u) and $\hat{\lambda}^{\dagger}_Q(u)$ be the Nelson-estimator of $\lambda_Q(u)$ based on all the data, i.e., based on (X_i, τ_i),i=1,⋯,n, with $c^* = c_{max}$. Let $\hat{r}_{\bar{s},1}(u)$ and $\hat{r}_{\bar{s},2}(u)$ be as in Theorem 3.2e except K(u), $\lambda_Q(u)$, and $r_{pf,m}(u)$ are replaced by these estimates. Then, as is argued in Appendix 3,

Lemma 3.2: $\psi(\hat{r}_{\bar{s}},w,c^*)$ will be asymptotically N(0,1) under (2.3) and (2.4c) even if the model for $\bar{F}_0(u)$ is misspecified. Further, if the parametric model for $\bar{F}_0(u)$ is correctly specified, $\lambda_Q(u) = \lambda_Q(u \mid Z)$ and Eqs. (3.5a)-(3.5b) hold with $R = R_{\bar{s}}$, then, $NC(\hat{r}_{\bar{s}},w,c^*) = NC(r_{\bar{s}},w,c^*) > NC(r_{\bar{s}},0,c^*) = NC_{\bar{s}}^{c^*}$. Thus, as $c^* \rightarrow c_{max}$, the non-centrality parameter of our adaptive test will eventually exceed that of the optimal log-rank test based on all the data. By Lemma 3.1, a high-dimensional w in (3.2) would lead to further gains in power.

3c. Simulation Experiment

The use of marker data can lead to particularly large increases of power in trials in which (1) new subjects are still being enrolled at the time of the first interim analysis, (2) the observed failures are concentrated amongst subjects who enrolled early in the study and (3) there exists a marker whose values soon after enrollment are good predictors of subsequent failure-time. Excellent candidates for trials in which the proposed methods can lead to substantial increases in power are the ACTG pediatric AIDS protocols, such as protocol 152 and 154. In these protocols, an infant's "failure time" is defined to be the time at which the infant's development falls below a prespecified level. For example, an infant is considered to have "failed" when the infant's head circumference first falls below the second percentile for age. Because of strong tracking in the rate of head growth, estimated rates of growth based on measurements made in the first several months after enrollment should be highly predictive of subsequent "failure." Thus, we assumed there was an interim analysis conducted exactly one year after initial enrollment into the trial began and patient accrual was uniform over the year, so that the censoring variable was uniformly distributed on (0,1). We assumed that no subject failed in the first six months after his/her enrollment. After six months, in our simulations under the null hypothesis (2.3), failure time in both arms was exponentially distributed with a hazard of 3.22. We used a PH model with β_0=-.35 under the alternative. To keep the analysis simple, we chose, as a surrogate, a single time-independent marker measured immediately after initiation of treatment. In the first set of trials, we unrealistically assumed that the surrogate was perfectly correlated with (and in fact equal to) subsequent failure time. In a second set of trials we made the more realistic assumption that the value of the surrogate for subject i was obtained by multiplying his/her failure time by an independent uniform random variable on (.75, 1.33). The results reported in each row of Table 1 are based on

TABLE 1. Results of a Simulation Experiment

Row	Surrogate Strength	Scoring Function r	Artificial End of F/U c* in yrs	W(u) Cox Model Covariates	Tail Method	Actual Rejection Rate under Null in %	Asymptotic Relative Efficiency
1	Perf	$r_{\bar{s}}$	.9	W_{op}^{r}	3	4.0	236
2	Perf	$r_{\bar{s}}$	1.0	W_{op}^{r}	3	4.0	237
3	Perf	$r_{\bar{s}}$	.9	Ind	3	3.5	148
4	Perf	$r_{\bar{s}}$	1.0	Ind	3	3.5	165
5	Mod or Perf	$r_{\bar{s}}$	.9	0	3	5.0	94
6	Mod or Perf	$r_{\bar{s}}$	1.0	0	3	7.0	100
7	Mod	$r_{\bar{s}}$	.9	W_{op}^{r}	3	6.0	158
8	Mod	$r_{\bar{s}}$	1.0	W_{op}^{r}	3	6.0	163
9	Mod	$r_{\bar{s}}$	.9	Ind	3	5.5	135
10	Mod	$r_{\bar{s}}$	1.0	Ind	3	5.0	141
11	Mod	$\hat{r}_{\bar{s}}$	1.0	0	3, 4	7.0	102
12	Mod	$\hat{r}_{\bar{s}}$	1.0	Ind	2, 3, 4	5.0	141
13	Mod	$\hat{r}_{\bar{s}}$	1.0	0	1	14.0	-
14	Mod	$\hat{r}_{\bar{s}}$	1.0	Ind	1	17.5	-
15	Mod	$\hat{r}_{\bar{s}}$	1.0	0	2	11.5	-

200 realizations. Each realization represented a trial with 300 subjects in each treatment arm. The column labeled "rejection rate" is the actual rejection rates of the nominal 5% tests $|\psi(r,w,c^*)| > 1.96$ based on simulations conducted under the null hypothesis. Column 7 gives the estimated asymptotic relative efficiency (ARE) of our tests compared to the standard log-rank test based on the ratios of the square of the average Z-values (under the alternative), where ARE $\equiv NC(r,w,c^*)/NC_{LR}$. The log-rank test is based on follow-up through $c_{max} = 1$ year.

Column 2 characterizes the surrogate strength as perfect or moderate [uniform (.75, 1.33) noise]. Columns 3, 4, and 5 describe r,w, and c* for our tests $\psi(r,w,c^*)$. w^r_{op} is the optimal covariate [depending on r and c*] defined in Section 3b. The covariate "Ind" is given by (3.5a) with W*(u) a time-independent dichotomous covariate recording whether a subject's surrogate is above the population median, and thus is not optimal. "None" implies that no covariates were used in model (3.2) to estimate K(u) and thus refers to the test $\psi(r,0,c^*)$.

The numbers in column 5 refer to modifications to $\psi(r,0,c^*)$ to prevent large values of $R_i/\hat{K}_i(X_i)$as $X_i \rightarrow 1$ when $c^*=c_{max}=1$. The number "1" represents the unmodified $\psi(r,0,c^*)$. Modification 2 replaces $R_i \equiv r(\Delta_i,X_i^*)$ by R_i-$r(\Delta_i,1)$. In modification 3, if the last subject, say j, at risk in a given treatment arm is Q-censored (i.e., $Q_j=X_j$), subject j is treated as a failure at X_j in the analysis. In modification 4, c* is replaced by the minimum of c* and the earliest time t at which in either treatment arm only one subject remains at risk.

In rows 1 and 2 we obtain striking ARE's of 236 and 237 while preserving the nominal α-level under the null hypothesis (2.3). The relative efficiencies of 148 and 165 in rows 3 and 4 demonstrate the loss of efficiency from using a non-optimal w. Rows 5-6 demonstrate the further loss of efficiency when we fail to use the surrogate data. As predicted by our theoretical calculations, the ARE is equal to that of the log-rank test when c*=1.0, although, even using modification 3, the rejection rate (RR) of 7% slightly exceeds the nominal. Rows 7-15 present the results of more realistic simulation experiments that use a surrogate with a moderate correlation with failure time. The ARE's of our tests in rows 7-10 are considerably less than when we had a perfect surrogate, although the ARE of 163 in row 8 is certainly great enough to be important.

In rows (11)-(12), we observe, that, as predicted by theory, $\psi(\hat{r}_{\bar{s}},w,c^*)$ performs similarly to $\psi(r_{\bar{s}},w,c^*)$. [In computing $\hat{r}_{\bar{s}}$, we took the guarantee period of .5 years as known, but estimated the Weibull parameters a=3.22 and b=1.] Again at c*=1.0, the actual 7% RR of $\psi(\hat{r}_{\bar{s}},0,c^*)$ under tail methods (3) and (4) slightly exceeds the nominal. In contrast, the RR with c*=1.0 is equal to the nominal for $\psi(\hat{r}_{\bar{s}},w,c^*)$ with w the indicator covariate, provided we use a tail modification. The slight elevation of the RR in row 11 is attibutable to the standard error estimator of $S\{\hat{D}(0)\}$ underestimating the actual standard error (data not shown). In contrast, the RR of 14% and 17.5% in rows (13) and (14) of the unmodified $S\{\hat{D}(0)\}$ reflects the fact that the unmodified $S\{\hat{D}(0)\}$ is not centered and clearly demonstrates the need for modification. On the other hand, the elevation of the

RR in row (15) is solely due to bias in the standard error estimate when using method (2). [Choosing c^* to be .9 (or less) guarantees the actual α-level equals the nominal (whether or not a modification is used), although some efficiency is thereby lost.] Finally, we note that if one uses modification (3) or (4), it is an algebraic fact that the value of $\psi(r,0,c^*)$ does not further depend on whether modification (2) is also used.

3d. Estimation of the Mean Model

For dichotomous Z, we consider a saturated model (2.2c) for the mean of Δ. Specifically, $g(Z,\beta_0) = \beta_{0,0}+\beta_{0,1}Z$, with $\beta_0=(\beta_{0,0},\beta_{0,1})'$. Define $\hat{D}(\beta) = (\Delta-g(Z,\beta),Z\{\Delta-g(Z,\beta)\})'$, and $W^{\Delta}_{op}(u) = \{Z-E(Z)\}E[\Delta \mid \bar{L}(u),Z,Y(u)=1]$. Let $\hat{\beta}^0$ and $\hat{\beta}^w$ be the estimators based on $\hat{K}^0_i$ and $\hat{K}^w_i$. In Section (4c), we prove

Lemma 3.3: Under (2.4c), (a) $\hat{\beta}^{w^{\Delta}_{op}}$ and $\hat{\beta}^0$ are semiparametric efficient based on the c^*-observed and c^*-$\overline{sur}$ data respectively; (b) $\hat{\beta}^0$ is never more and is usually less efficient than $\hat{\beta}^w$; and (c) as an estimator of $\beta_{0,0} = pr[T<c^* \mid Z=0]$, $\hat{\beta}^0_0$ is asymptotically equivalent to the usual Kaplan-Meier estimator $1-\Pi\{1-[\Sigma_j I(Z_j=0)Y_j(X_i)]^{-1}\}$, with the product over the set $\{i;\ \tau_i=1,Z_i=0,\Delta_i=1\}$ of observed failures in treatment arm Z=0, so $\hat{\beta}^w_0$ usually improves upon the Kaplan-Meier estimator by using surrogate marker data.

3e. Definition of $S\{\hat{D}(\beta)\}$ and $S^{(F)}\{\tilde{D}(\beta)\}$

With one exception, the estimating functions $S^{(F)}\{\tilde{D}(\beta)\}=\Sigma_i\tilde{D}_i(\beta)$ are not new. We review their definitions here both (a) to fix notation and (b) because the $S\{\hat{D}(\beta)\}$ are closely related to the $S^{(F)}\{\tilde{D}(\beta)\}$.

Let h(Z), h(u,Z), and θ(u,Z) be fixed functions taking values in R^p. For any V(u) define $\tilde{E}[V(u)] \equiv n^{-1}\Sigma_i V_i(u)$ and $\hat{E}\{V(u)\} \equiv n^{-1}\Sigma_i(\tau_i/\hat{K}_i)V_i(u)$.

For model (2.2c), $\tilde{D}^{MN}(\beta) \equiv \hat{D}^{MN}(\beta) \equiv \tilde{D}^{MN}(\beta,h) \equiv h(Z)\{\Delta-g(Z,\beta)\}$.

For model (2.2a), $\tilde{D}^{PH}(\beta) \equiv \tilde{D}^{PH}(\beta,h) \equiv \int_0^{\infty} dN_T(u)\{h(u,Z) - \tilde{\mathscr{L}}^{PH}(u,\beta,h)\}$, where $N_T(u) = I[X^*\le u,\Delta=1]$, $X^*=\min(T,c^*)$, $\tilde{\mathscr{L}}^{PH}(u,\beta,h) = \tilde{E}[e^{\beta' Z}I\{X^*>u\}h(u,Z)]/\tilde{E}[I\{X^*>u\}e^{\beta' Z}]$. Ritov and Wellner (1988) discuss the estimating functions $S^{(F)}\{\tilde{D}^{PH}(\beta)\}$. $\hat{D}^{PH}(\beta)$ replaces $\tilde{\mathscr{L}}$ by $\hat{\mathscr{L}}$ in the definition of $\tilde{D}^{PH}(\beta)$, where $\hat{\mathscr{L}}$ is defined like $\tilde{\mathscr{L}}$ but with $\hat{E}$ replacing $\tilde{E}$. Note $\tau\hat{D}^{PH}(\beta)$, in contrast to $\tau\tilde{D}^{PH}(\beta)$, can be computed from the c^*-observables (2.1).

For model (2.2b) we consider two choices of $\tilde{D}(\beta)$, namely, $\tilde{D}^{AF1}(\beta)$ and $\tilde{D}^{AF2}(\beta)$. $\tilde{D}^{AF1}(\beta) \equiv \tilde{D}^{AF1}(\beta,h) \equiv \int_{-\infty}^{\infty} dN_{\epsilon(\beta)}(u)\{h(u,Z) - \tilde{\mathscr{L}}^{AF1}(u,\beta,h)\}$ where $N_{\epsilon(\beta)}(u) = I[\nu(\beta) \le u,\Delta=1]$, $\nu(\beta) = \min\{\epsilon(\beta),\mu(\beta)\}$, $\mu(\beta) = \ell n c^* + \beta' Z$, $\epsilon(\beta) = \ell n T+\beta' Z$, and $\tilde{\mathscr{L}}^{AF1}(u,\beta,h) = \tilde{E}[I\{\nu(\beta)>u\}h(u,Z)]/\tilde{E}[I\{\nu(\beta)>u\}]$. Tsiatis (1990), Ritov (1990), Wei, Ying, and Lin (1990), and Kalbfleisch and Prentice (1980) discuss the estimating function $S^{(F)}\{\tilde{D}^{AF1}(\beta)\}$. $\hat{D}^{AF1}(\beta)$ replaces $\tilde{\mathscr{L}}$ by $\hat{\mathscr{L}}$ in the definition of $\tilde{D}^{AF1}(\beta)$.

We define $\tilde{D}^{AF2}(\beta) \equiv \hat{D}^{AF2}(\beta) \equiv \tilde{D}^{AF2}(\beta,h,\theta) \equiv [\int_{-\infty}^{\infty} dN_{\epsilon(\beta)}(u)\{h(u,Z) - \tilde{\mathscr{L}}^{AF2}(u,\beta,h)\}] -$

$\int_{-\infty}^{\infty} du I\{\nu(\beta)\geq u\}\{\theta(u,Z) - \tilde{\mathscr{L}}^{AF2}(u,\beta,\theta)\}$, where $\tilde{\mathscr{L}}^{AF2}(u,\beta,h) = \tilde{E}[I\{\mu(\beta)>u\}h(u,Z)]/\tilde{E}[I\{\mu(\beta)>u\}]$. $S^{(F)}\{\tilde{D}^{AF2}(\beta)\}$ is a new estimating function for β_0 in the AF model with a fixed known potential censoring time c^*. In practice, one would select $\theta(u,Z)$ to be a step function so the integral could be easily evaluated. Note $\tau_i\tilde{D}_i^{AF2}(\beta)$, in contrast to $\tau_i\tilde{D}_i^{AF1}(\beta)$, can be computed from the c^*-observables (2.1) since $\mu(\beta)$, in contrast to $\nu(\beta)$, is always observed.

$\tilde{D}^{AF2}(\beta,h,\theta)$ has a particularly simple form when Z is a dichotomous (0,1) variable. Using the fact that, for dichotomous Z, we can uniquely represent any function g(u,Z) as $g_1(u)Z+g_0(u)$, define $r_2(u) = -\int_{-\infty}^{u}\theta_1(x)dx$, and $r_1(u) = h_1(u) + r_2(u)$. Then $\tilde{D}^{AF2}(\beta,h,\theta) = \tilde{D}^{AF2}(\beta,r) \equiv R(\beta)[Z-\tilde{E}(Z)]$ where $R(0)=\{\Delta r_1(\ell nT)+(1-\Delta)r_2\{\ell n(c^*)\}$ as in Section 3b; and, more generally, $R(\beta) \equiv r\{\Delta(\beta),X^*(\beta)\} \equiv \Delta(\beta)r_1[\epsilon(\beta)] + \{1-\Delta(\beta)\}\{r_2[c^*(\beta)]\}$, where $c^*(\beta) \equiv \min(\ell nc^*, \ell nc^*+\beta)$, $X^*(\beta) \equiv \min[\epsilon(\beta),c^*(\beta)]$ and $\Delta(\beta) = I[\epsilon(\beta)<c^*(\beta)]$. We call $\Delta(\beta)$ an artificial (full-data) censoring indicator since if either (a) $\beta<0$ and Z=1 or (b) $\beta>0$ and Z=0, $\Delta(\beta)$ need not equal Δ. Note $\Delta(\beta)$ is discontinuous in β and $\Delta(0)=\Delta$.

3f. Asymptotic Distribution Theory for $\tilde{\beta}$ and $S^{(F)}\{\tilde{D}(\beta_0)\}$

$S\{\hat{D}(\beta)\}$ and $S^{(F)}\{\tilde{D}(\beta)\}$ are discontinuous in β under model the AF model (2.2b). In this instance, we define $\hat{\beta}$ and $\tilde{\beta}$ to be solutions to $n^{-1/2} S\{\hat{D}(\beta)\} = o_p(1)$ and $n^{-1/2}S^{(F)}\{\tilde{D}(\beta)\} = o_p(1)$, and one would compute $\hat{\beta}$ and $\tilde{\beta}$ respectively by minimizing $S\{\hat{D}(\beta)\}'S\{\hat{D}(\beta)\}$ and $S^{(F)}\{\tilde{D}(\beta)\}'S^{(F)}\{\tilde{D}(\beta)\}$ in a neighborhood of β_0. It will be useful to discuss the asymptotic distribution of $\tilde{\beta}$ based on the c^*-full data (3.4) before that of $\hat{\beta}$ based on c^*-observed data (2.1). Except for $\tilde{\beta}^{AF2}$, the following results are not new. Let $\mathscr{L}$ be defined like $\tilde{\mathscr{L}}$ but with a true expectation replacing $\tilde{E}$. Let $D(\beta)$ be defined like $\tilde{D}(\beta)$ except with $\mathscr{L}$ replacing $\tilde{\mathscr{L}}$.

Theorem 3.3: Under regularity conditions, for $|\beta-\beta_0|$ of $O(n^{-1/2})$, under the models (2.2), $n^{-1/2}S^{(F)}\{\tilde{D}(\beta_0)\} = n^{-1/2}\Sigma_i U_f + o_p(1)$,

$$n^{-1/2}S^{(F)}\{\tilde{D}(\beta)\} = n^{-1/2}S^{(F)}\{\tilde{D}(\beta_0)\} - \kappa(\beta-\beta_0) + o_p(1) \quad , \tag{3.6}$$

$n^{-1/2}S^{(F)}\{\tilde{D}(\beta_0)\}$ and $n^{1/2}(\tilde{\beta}-\beta_0)$ are asymptotically normal with mean 0 and asymptotic variance $Var(U_f)$ and $\kappa^{-1}Var(U_f)\kappa^{-1\prime}$ respectively .

Under model (2.2c), $U_f^{MN} \equiv U_f^{MN}(h) = D^{MN}(\beta_0,h) = \tilde{D}^{MN}(\beta_0,h)$, $\kappa^{MN} = E[U_f^{MN}(h)U_f^{MN}(h_{op}^{MN})'] = E[h(Z)\partial g(Z,\beta_0)/\partial\beta']$, $h_{op}^{MN}(Z) = [\partial g(Z,\beta_0)/\partial\beta]\{Var[\varsigma \mid Z]\}^{-1}$, $\varsigma \equiv \Delta-g(Z,\beta_0)$.

Under (2.2a), $U_f^{PH} \equiv U_f^{PH}(h) = \int_0^{\infty} dM_T(u)\{h(u,Z) - \mathscr{L}^{PH}(u,\beta_0,h)\}$, where $dM_T(u) = dN_T(u) - \lambda_0(u)I\{X^*\geq u\}du$, and $\lambda_0(u) = -\partial\ell n\bar{F}_0(u)/\partial u$. Set $h_{op}^{PH}(u,Z) = Z$. $\kappa^{PH} \equiv \kappa^{PH}(h) = E[U_f^{PH}(h)U_f^{PH}(h_{op}^{PH})'] = E[\int_0^{\infty}\lambda_0(u)I(X^*\geq u)\Phi^{PH}(h)\Phi^{PH}(h_{op}^{PH})'du] = E[\int_0^{\infty} dN_T(u)\{\mathscr{L}^{PH}(u,\beta_0,hh_{op}^{PH\prime}) - \mathscr{L}^{PH}(u,\beta_0,h)\mathscr{L}^{PH}(u,\beta_0,h_{op}^{PH})'\}]$, where

$\Phi(h) \equiv h(u,Z) - \mathscr{L}(u,\beta_0,h)$ and $\mathscr{L}(u,\beta_0,h_1h_2')$ is a pxp matrix.

Under (2.2b), $U_f^{AF1} \equiv U_f^{AF1}(h) = \int_{-\infty}^{\infty} dM_\epsilon(u)\{h(u,Z) - \mathscr{L}^{AF1}(u,\beta_0,h)\}$, $\kappa^{AF1} \equiv \kappa^{AF1}(h) =$

$E[U_f^{AF1}(h)U_f^{AF1}(h_{op}^{AF})'] = E[\int_{-\infty}^{\infty} dN_\epsilon(u)\{\mathscr{L}^{AF1}(u,\beta_0,hh_{op}^{AF}{}') - \mathscr{L}^{AF1}(u,\beta_0,h)\mathscr{L}^{AF1}(u,\beta_0,h_{op}^{AF})'\}]$,

$\epsilon \equiv \epsilon(\beta_0)$, $\nu \equiv \nu(\beta_0)$, $dM_\epsilon(u) = dN_\epsilon(u) - I\{\nu \geq u\}\lambda_\epsilon(u)du$, $\lambda_\epsilon(u)$ is the hazard function of ϵ, and $h_{op}^{AF}(u,Z) = Z\partial \ell n\lambda_\epsilon(u)/\partial u$.

Further, $U_f^{AF2} \equiv U_f^{AF2}(h,\theta) = D^{AF2}(\beta_0) - E[D^{AF2}(\beta_0) \mid Z]$, $\kappa^{AF2} \equiv \kappa^{AF2}(h,\theta) =$ $E[U_f^{AF2}(h,\theta)U_f^{AF2}(h_{op}^{AF},\theta_{op}^{AF})']$ where $\theta_{op}^{AF}(u,Z) = Z\partial\lambda_\epsilon(u)/\partial u$. If $Z \in \{0,1\}$, $U_f^{AF2} \equiv U_f^{AF2}(r) =$ $\{R(\beta_0)-E[R(\beta_0)]\}\{Z-E[Z]\}$.

Remarks: For $\tilde{\beta}^{AF1}$ and $\tilde{\beta}^{PH}$, Theorem 3.3 is a direct consequence of Anderson and Gill (1982), Ritov and Wellner (1988), Tsiatis (1990), and Ritov (1990), among others. For $\tilde{\beta}^{MN}$, Theorem 3.3 is standard. The key step in the proof for $\tilde{\beta}^{AF2}$ is given in Theorem A.2 of Appendix 3. A key identity is based on the following lemma which can be proved by integration by parts.

Lemma 3.4: Any $U_f^{AF1}(h)$ can be written as $U_f^{AF2}(h,\theta)$ with $\theta(u,Z) \equiv \lambda_\epsilon(u)\, h(u,Z)$. Conversely any $U_f^{AF2}(h,\theta)$ can be written as $U_f^{AF1}(g)$ for g=h+h** with $h^{**}(u,Z) \equiv$ $\int_u^\mu \{h^*(x,Z) - \mathscr{L}^{AF2}(u,\beta_0,h^*)\}\bar{F}_\epsilon(x)dx/\bar{F}_\epsilon(u)$, $\mu = \ell nc^* + \beta_0'Z$, $\bar{F}_\epsilon(u) \equiv pr(\epsilon > u)$, and $h^*(u,Z) \equiv$ $\lambda_\epsilon(u)h(u,Z) - \theta(u,Z)$. In particular $U_f^{AF2}(h_{op}^{AF},\theta_{op}^{AF}) = U_f^{AF1}(h_{op}^{AF})$.

3.g. Asymptotic Distribution Theory for $\hat{\beta}$ and $S\{\hat{D}(\beta_0)\}$

The next theorem states that the asymptotic distribution of $\hat{\beta}$ and $S\{\hat{D}(\beta_0)\}$ differ from that of $\tilde{\beta}$ and $S^{(F)}\{\tilde{D}(\beta_0)\}$ only in that the asymptotic variance of $n^{-1/2}S\{\hat{D}(\beta_0)\}$ exceeds that of $n^{-1/2}S^{(F)}\{\tilde{D}(\beta_0)\}$ by the non-negative quantity $Var(U_{mis}) - Var(U_{rec})$, where (a) $Var(U_{mis})$ represents additional uncertainty attributable to observing the c*-observed data rather than the c*-full data, if, when computing $\hat{K}_i(X_i)$, we had used the true value α_0 rather than $\hat{\alpha}$ in formulas (3.3a) and (3.3b), and (b) $Var(U_{rec})$ represents the part of the additional uncertainty that can be recovered by estimating α_0 by $\hat{\alpha}$, even were α_0 known. Define $N_Q(x) = I[X \leq x, \tau = 0]$, $Y(u) = I[X \geq u]$, $M_Q(x) \equiv N_Q(x) - \int_0^x \lambda_Q[u \mid \bar{L}(u),Z]Y(u)du$. $M_Q(x)$ is, by (2.4a), a subject-specific martingale with respect to the filtration $\mathbf{F}(u)$ that records $[c^*,T,Z,\bar{L}\{\min(T,u)\}, \{N_Q(x), 0 \leq x \leq u\}]$. For a random H(u), define $\Phi^Q(H,u,s) \equiv H(u) -$ $\mathscr{L}^Q(H,u,s)$ with $\mathscr{L}^Q(H,u,s) \equiv E\{H(u)Y(u)e^{\alpha_0'W(u)}I[S^*=s]\}/E\{Y(u)e^{\alpha_0'W(u)}I[S^*=s]\}$. Set $\Gamma(H)$ $\equiv \int_0^\infty dM_Q(u)\Phi^Q(H,u,S^*)$.

Theorem 3.4: Under regularity conditions, for $|\beta - \beta_0|$ of $O(n^{-1/2})$, under models (2.2), (3.2), and (2.4a), if $K(X) > \sigma > 0$ for some σ w.p.1

$$n^{-1/2}S\{\hat{D}(\beta_0)\} = n^{-1/2}\Sigma_i U_i + o_p(1)\ , \qquad (3.7)$$

$$n^{-1/2}S\{\hat{D}(\beta)\} = n^{-1/2}S\{\hat{D}(\beta_0)\} - \kappa(\beta-\beta_0) + o_p(1)\ , \qquad (3.8)$$

$$n^{1/2}(\hat{\beta}-\beta_0) = n^{-1/2}\Sigma_i \kappa^{-1} U_i + o_p(1) \quad , \tag{3.9}$$

$n^{-1/2}S\{\hat{D}(\beta_0)\}$ and $n^{1/2}(\hat{\beta}-\beta_0)$ are asymptotically normal with mean 0 and asymptotic variances $Var(U) = Var(U_f) + Var(U_{mis}) - Var(U_{rec})$ and $\kappa^{-1}Var(U)\kappa^{-1\prime}$; $U = U_f - U_{mis} + U_{rec}$; $U_{mis} = \Gamma(H_{mis})$, with $H_{mis}(u) = U_f/K(u)$ except that $H^{AF2}_{mis}(u) = D^{AF2}(\beta_0)/K(u)$; and $U_{rec} = \rho(U_{mis}, U_w) \equiv E[U_{mis}U_w{}']\{E[U_w U_w{}']\}^{-1}U_w$, where $U_w = \Gamma(W)$ with W the function W(u). [$\rho(A,B)$ is, by definition, the predicted value from the population least squares regression of A on B.] Further $Var[U_{rec}] = E[U_{mis}U_w{}']\{E[U_w U_w{}']\}^{-1}E[U_w U_{mis}{}']$ and $E[U_{mis}U_{rec}{}'] = E[U_{rec}U_{rec}{}']$ where $E[\Gamma(H_1)\Gamma(H_2)'] = E[\int_0^\infty dN_Q(u)\{\mathscr{L}^Q(H_1 H_2{}', u, S^*) - \mathscr{L}^Q(H_1,u,S^*)\mathscr{L}^Q(H_2,u,S^*)'\}]$ when $H_1(u)$, $H_2(u)$ are $\mathbf{F}(u)$ predictable. Note $E[U_f U_{mis}{}'] = E[U_f U_{rec}{}'] = 0$ since U_f is $\mathbf{F}(0)$-predictable. $NC\{\hat{D}(\beta)\}$, the non-centrality parameter of the test based on $S\{\hat{D}(\beta)\}$, is $\{\kappa^{-1}Var(U)\kappa^{-1\prime}\}^{-1}$.

A sketch of the proof of Theorem 3.4 is given in Section (3i). Consistent estimators for the asymptotic variance of $\hat{\beta}$ and $S\{\hat{D}(\beta_0)\}$ are given in Section 3j.2.

3h. Fundamental Identities:

The following identities are fundamental to our results. In particular, as described below, they motivated the estimating function $S\{\hat{D}(\beta)\}$.

$$1/K(t) = 1/K(u) + \int_u^t dx \lambda_Q(x)/K(x) \tag{3.10a}$$

$$\tau/K(t) = 1/K(u) - (1-\tau)/K(t) + \int_u^t dx \lambda_Q(x)/K(x) \tag{3.10b}$$

$$Y(u)\tau/K(X) = Y(u)/K(u) - \int_u^\infty dM_Q(x)/K(x) \tag{3.10c}$$

$$\tau/K(X) = 1 - \int_0^\infty dM_Q(x)/K(x) \tag{3.10d}$$

If $K(X)>\sigma>0$ w.p.1, and (2.4a) holds,

$$E[\tau h(T,Z)/K(X)] = E[h(T,Z)] \quad , \tag{3.10e}$$

and

$$E[h(T,Z,\bar{L}(u))/K(u) \mid \bar{L}(u),Z,Y(u)=1] = E[\tau h(T,Z,\bar{L}(u))/K(X) \mid \bar{L}(u),Z,Y(u)=1] \,. \tag{3.10f}$$

(3.10a) is proved by integration from which (3.10b) follows. (3.10c) and (3.10d) follow immediately from (3.10b). (3.10e) follows by multiplying both sides of (3.10d) by h(T,Z) taking expectations, and noting that $\int_0^t h(T,Z)M_Q(x)/K(x)$ is a mean zero $\mathbf{F}(t)$-adapted martingale since $h(T,Z)/K(x)$ is $\mathbf{F}(x)$-predictable and $K(x)$ is bounded away from zero. (3.10f) follows similarly from (3.10c) except we take conditional expectations.

Since $E[D(\beta_0)]=0$ and $D(\beta_0)$ is a function of T,Z and c* only, it follows from (3.10e) that $E[\tau D(\beta_0)/K(X)]=0$, proving the fundamental lemma of Section (3b). Thus we would expect, under suitable regularity conditions, that $\hat{\beta}$ solving $0 = S\{\hat{D}(\beta)\}$ will be an asymptotically normal and unbiased estimator of β_0 since $\hat{D}(\beta)$ is an $n^{1/2}$-consistent estimator of $D(\beta)$ and $\hat{K}_i(X_i)$ is an $n^{1/2}$-consistent estimator $K_i(X_i)$. In this paper, we do not specify these regularity conditions in detail.

3.i Sketch of the Derivation of Asymptotic Distribution Theory for $\hat{\beta}$ and $S\{\hat{D}(\beta_0)\}$

Our derivation of Theorem 3.4 is based on the following algebraic identity which is a sample analogue of (3.10d). For any B_i, $\Sigma_i \tau_i B_i/\hat{K}_i = \Sigma_i B_i - \Sigma_i \Psi_i(\hat{H}_i)$ with $\hat{H}_i(u) \equiv B_i/\hat{K}_i(u)$, $\Psi(H) \equiv \int_0^\infty dN_Q(u)\{H(u) - \tilde{\mathscr{L}}^Q(H,u,S^*)\}$ and $\tilde{\mathscr{L}}^Q(H,u,s) \equiv$ $\tilde{E}[H(u)Y(u)e^{\hat{\alpha}' W(u)} I(S^*=s)]/\tilde{E}[Y(u)e^{\hat{\alpha}' W(u)} I(S^*=s)]$. But Robins (1991) shows by expanding around α_0, that, if $B=b(T,Z,c^*)$ and $K(X)>\sigma>0$, $n^{-1/2}\Sigma_i\Psi_i(\hat{H}_i) = n^{-1/2}\Sigma_i\Psi_i(H_i) + o_p(1)$ for $H_i(u) = B_i/K_i(u)$. But, under (2.4a), $n^{-1/2}\Sigma_i\Psi_i(H_i)$ is exactly the Cox partial likelihood score test of the true hypothesis $\theta_0=0$ in the correctly specified PH model for Q that adds $\theta_0'H(u)$ to $\alpha_0'W(u)$ in (3.2). But, Anderson and Gill (1982), Ritov and Wellner (1988), and Begun et al., (1983) show $n^{-1/2}\Sigma_i\Psi_i(H_i) = n^{-1/2}\Sigma_i U_{\theta|\alpha,i} + o_p(1)$ where $U_{\theta|\alpha} \equiv \Gamma(H) - \rho(\Gamma(H),\Gamma(W))$ is the Cox efficient score for θ. Hence, we have proved

Lemma 3.5: If (3.2) holds, $K(X)>\sigma>0$ w.p.1, and $B=b(T,Z,c^*)$, $n^{-1/2}\Sigma_i \tau_i B_i/\hat{K}_i \equiv n^{1/2}\hat{E}[B] = n^{-1/2}\Sigma_i[B_i - U_{\theta|\alpha,i}] + o_p(1)$. Further B_i is uncorrelated with $U_{\theta|\alpha,i}$ since B_i is $\mathbf{F}(0)$-predictable.

We establish (3.7) for the mean model (2.2c) by applying Lemma (3.5) to $n^{-1/2}S\{\hat{D}(\beta_0)\} \equiv n^{1/2}\hat{E}[D(\beta_0)]$. The key to establishing (3.7) for the PH model (2.2a) is the identity $n^{-1/2}S\{\hat{D}^{PH}(\beta_0)\} = n^{1/2}\hat{E}[\int_0^\infty dM_T(u)\{h(u,Z)-\hat{\mathscr{L}}^{PH}(u,\beta_0,h)\}]$. Using this identity one can show that, under regularity conditions, $n^{-1/2}S\{\hat{D}^{PH}(\beta_0)\} = n^{1/2}\hat{E}\{U_f^{PH}\}+o_p(1)$, although, the proof of this result is non-standard in that $\hat{\mathscr{L}}^{PH}(u,\beta_0,h)$ depends on the data obtained at times past u. Lemma (3.5) is then applied to $n^{1/2}\hat{E}\{U_f^{PH}\}$. A similar argument establishes (3.7) for $n^{-1/2}S\{\hat{D}^{AF1}(\beta_0)\}$.

We establish (3.7) for $n^{-1/2}S\{\hat{D}^{AF2}(\beta_0,r)\}$ with Z dichotomous from the identity $n^{-1/2}S\{\hat{D}^{AF2}(\beta_0,r)\} = n^{1/2}\hat{E}[D^{AF2}(\beta_0,r)] + \hat{E}\{R(\beta_0)\}n^{1/2}\tilde{E}[Z-E(Z)]$. We then apply Lemma (3.5) to $n^{1/2}\hat{E}[D^{AF2}(\beta_0,r)]$ and note $\hat{E}\{R(\beta_0)\} \xrightarrow{P} E[R(\beta_0)]$. Establishing Eq. (3.7) for $n^{-1/2}S\{\hat{D}^{AF2}(\beta_0)\}$ with Z non-dichotomous is discussed in Appendix (3).

Having established (3.7), we can establish (3.8) and (3.9) for the PH model and the mean model by a Taylor series expansion around β_0. Since, for the AF model, $S\{\hat{D}(\beta)\}$ is non-differentiable, one would establish (3.8) and (3.9) using the approach of Pakes and Pollard (1989) and Huber (1981) for non-differentiable m-estimators. κ is shown to be as stated in Theorems 3.3 and 3.4 in Section (4b).

3j. Variance Estimation

3j.1 c*-full data

To fix notation, we review previously derived estimators $\tilde{V}ar\{U_f(\tilde{\beta})\}$ and $\tilde{\kappa}(\tilde{\beta})$ of $Var(U_f)$ and κ when c*-full data is available. $\tilde{V}ar\{U_f(\beta)\} \equiv \tilde{E}[\tilde{\Omega}(\beta)]$, with $\tilde{\Omega}^{PH}(\beta,h) = \int_0^{\infty} dN_T(u)\tilde{J}^{PH}(u,\beta,h,h)$ and $\tilde{J}(u,\beta,h_1,h_2) \equiv \tilde{\mathscr{L}}(u,\beta,h_1h_2{}') - \tilde{\mathscr{L}}(u,\beta,h_1)\tilde{\mathscr{L}}(u,\beta,h_2)'$ (Kalbfleisch and Prentice, 1980); $\tilde{\Omega}^{AF1}(\beta,h) = \int_{-\infty}^{\infty} dN_{\epsilon(\beta)}(u)\tilde{J}^{AF1}(u,\beta,h,h)$; $\tilde{\Omega}^{MN}(\beta) = \tilde{D}^{MN}(\beta)\tilde{D}^{MN}(\beta)'$; and $\tilde{\Omega}^{AF2}(\beta) = \tilde{U}_f^{AF2}(\beta)\tilde{U}_f^{AF2}(\beta)'$, where $\tilde{U}_{f,i}^{AF2}(\beta) \equiv \tilde{U}_{f,i}^{AF2}(\beta,h,\theta) = \tilde{D}_i^{AF2}(\beta,h,\theta) - \sum_{j=1}^{n} n^{-1}P_{ji}(\beta,h,\theta)$ and $P_{ji}(\beta) \equiv P_{ji}(\beta,h,\theta) = [\int_{-\infty}^{\infty} dN_{\epsilon_j(\beta)}(u)\{h(u,Z_i) - \tilde{\mathscr{L}}^{AF2}(u,\beta,h)\}] - \int_{-\infty}^{\infty} duI\{\epsilon_j(\beta)>u\}I\{\mu_i(\beta)>u\}[\theta(u,Z_i) - \tilde{\mathscr{L}}^{AF2}(u,\beta,\theta)]$ since, by the independence of ϵ and Z, $n^{-1}\sum_{j=1}^{n} P_{ji}(\beta_0)$ is consistent for $E[D^{AF2}(\beta_0) \mid Z_i]$. $\tilde{V}ar\{U_f^{AF2}(\beta)\}$ is a new estimator.

If Z is dichotomous (0,1), we use $\tilde{V}ar(U_f^{AF2}(\beta)) \equiv \tilde{V}ar\{U_f^{AF2}(\beta,r)\} = \tilde{E}[\{R(\beta) - \tilde{E}[R(\beta)]\}^2]\tilde{E}[\{Z-\tilde{E}(Z)\}^2]$.

Next define $\tilde{\kappa}^{PH}(\beta,h) = \tilde{E}[\int_0^{\infty} dN_T(u)\tilde{J}^{PH}(u,\beta,h,h_{op}^{PH})]$ and $\tilde{\kappa}^{MN}(\beta,h) = \tilde{E}[h(Z)\partial g(Z,\beta)/\partial\beta']$. Since h_{op}^{AF} and θ_{op}^{AF} depend on the derivative of the unknown density $\lambda_\epsilon(u)$ which we may wish to avoid estimating, we set $\tilde{\kappa}^{AF1}(\beta)$ and $\tilde{\kappa}^{AF2}(\beta)$ to be the matrix of symmetric partial numerical derivatives of the corresponding $n^{-1}S^{(F)}\{\tilde{D}(\beta)\}$ with respect to β' based on a step size of $O(n^{-1/2})$ (Pakes and Pollard, 1989; Robins and Tsiatis, 1991). Eq. (3.6) implies $\tilde{\kappa}(\tilde{\beta})$ is consistent for κ.

3j.2 c*-Observed Data

We shall provide consistent estimators $\hat{V}ar\{U(\hat{\beta})\}$ and $\hat{\kappa}(\hat{\beta})$ of $Var(U)$ and κ depending on $\hat{\beta}$. In particular, the estimate $[\hat{V}ar\{U^{AF2}(0)\}]^{1/2}$, for dichotomous Z and a given $r \equiv r(\Delta(0),X^*(0)) \equiv r[\Delta,\ell n(X^*)]$, is the denominator of the test statistic $\psi(r,w,c^*)$ of Section (3b) used in the simulations in Section (3c).

It follows from the decomposition of Var(U) in Section 3g that $\hat{V}ar\{U(\hat{\beta})\}$ can be based on consistent estimators of $Var(U_f)$ and $E[\Gamma(H_1)\Gamma(H_2)']$ for $H_1(u),H_2(u)\in\{H_{mis}(u),W(u)\}$.

A consistent estimator $\hat{V}ar\{U_f(\hat{\beta})\}$ of $Var(U_f)$ is $\hat{V}ar[U_f(\hat{\beta})] \equiv \hat{E}\{\hat{\Omega}(\hat{\beta})\}$ where $\hat{\Omega}(\beta)$ is defined like $\tilde{\Omega}(\beta)$ except $\hat{J}$ replaces $\tilde{J}$ (by replacing $\tilde{\mathscr{L}}$ with $\hat{\mathscr{L}}$), n^{-1} is replaced by $n^{-1}\tau_j/\hat{K}_j$ in the definition of $\tilde{U}_{f,i}^{AF2}(\beta)$, $P_{ji}(\beta)$ is unchanged and, for dichotomous Z, $\hat{V}ar[U_f^{AF2}(\beta,r)] = \hat{E}[\{R(\beta)-\hat{E}[R(\beta)]\}^2]\ \tilde{E}[\{Z-\tilde{E}(Z)\}^2]$. $\hat{\kappa}^{PH}(\beta)$ and $\hat{\kappa}^{MN}(\beta)$ are defined as above with $\hat{E}$ and $\hat{J}$ replacing $\tilde{E}$ and $\tilde{J}$. Finally $\hat{\kappa}^{AF1}(\beta)$ and $\hat{\kappa}^{AF2}(\beta)$ are numerical partial derivative matrices of the corresponding $n^{-1}S\{\hat{D}(\beta)\}$.

$E[\Gamma(H_1)\Gamma(H_2)']$ can be consistently estimated by $\tilde{E}[\int_0^{\infty} dN_Q(u)\ \{\hat{\mathscr{L}}^Q(\hat{H}_1\hat{H}_2{}',u,S^*) - \hat{\mathscr{L}}^Q(\hat{H}_1,u,S^*)\hat{\mathscr{L}}^Q(\hat{H}_2,u,S^*)'\}$ where $\hat{H}_1(u)$ and $\hat{H}_2(u)$ are consistent for $H_1(u)$ and $H_2(u)$; $\hat{\mathscr{L}}^Q(H,u,s) = B(H,u,s)/B(\mathbf{1},u,s)$ with $\mathbf{1}(u)=1$, and $B(H,u,s) =$

$\sum_{i=1}^{n}\{\tau_i\hat{K}_i(u)/\hat{K}_i(X_i)\}Y_i(u)H_i(u)e^{\hat{\alpha}'W_i(u)}I[S_i^*=s]$. Note $\hat{\mathcal{L}}^Q(H,u,s)$ is consistent for $\mathcal{L}^Q(H,u,s)$ by Eq. (3.10f) and the weak law of large numbers.

Thus, it only remains to provide consistent estimators $\hat{H}_{mis}(u,\hat{\beta})$ for the $H_{mis}(u)$ as follows. $\hat{H}^{AF2}_{mis}(u,\hat{\beta}) = \hat{D}^{AF2}(\hat{\beta})/\hat{K}(u)$. $H^{MN}_{mis}(u,\hat{\beta}) = \hat{D}^{MN}(\hat{\beta})/\hat{K}(u)$. $\hat{H}^{PH}_{mis}(u,\hat{\beta}) \equiv \{\hat{K}(u)\}^{-1}\hat{U}^{PH}_f(\hat{\beta})$ where $\hat{U}^{PH}_f(\beta) \equiv \hat{U}^{PH}_f(\beta,h) = \int_0^\infty[dN_T(u) - I(X^*\geq u)e^{\beta'Z}\hat{\lambda}_0(u)du]\{h(u,Z) - \hat{\mathcal{L}}^{PH}(u,\beta,h)\}$ and $\hat{\lambda}_0(u) \equiv \hat{\lambda}_0(u,\beta) \equiv \hat{E}[dN_T(u)]/\hat{E}[e^{\beta'Z}I\{X^*\geq u\}]$. $\hat{H}^{AF1}_{mis}(u,\hat{\beta}) = \{\hat{K}(u)\}^{-1}\,\hat{U}^{AF1}_f(\hat{\beta})$, where $\hat{U}^{AF1}_f(\beta) = \int_{-\infty}^{\infty}[dN_{\epsilon(\beta)}(u) - I[\nu(\beta)\geq u]\hat{\lambda}_{\epsilon(\beta)}(u)du]\{h(u,Z) - \hat{\mathcal{L}}^{AF1}(u,\beta,h)\}$ with $\hat{\lambda}_{\epsilon(\beta)}(u) = \hat{E}[dN_{\epsilon(\beta)}(u)]/\hat{E}[I\{\nu(\beta)\geq u\}]$.

3k. Efficiency of $\hat{\beta}$

Write $\hat{\beta}^* \equiv \hat{\beta}^*(h)$ for an estimator $\hat{\beta}(h)$ solving $S\{\hat{D}(\beta,h)\}=0$ in which the components of $W^{mis}(u) \equiv E[H_{mis}(u) \mid \bar{L}(u),Z,Y(u)=1]$ are included as additional covariates in a correctly specified model (3.2). $\hat{\beta}^*$ is not a feasible estimator since it depends on unknown population quantities. Hence, given preliminary consistent estimates $\hat{\beta}$, $\hat{K}(u)$, $\hat{H}_{mis}(u,\hat{\beta})$, define for each u separately, $\hat{W}^{mis}(u)$ to be a subject's predicted value from a non-parametric (e.g., kernel) regression of $[\hat{K}(u)\,\tau\,\hat{H}_{mis}(u,\hat{\beta})/\hat{K}(X)]$ on $\bar{L}(u)$ and Z given $Y(u)=1$. Eq. (3.10f) implies $\hat{W}^{mis}(u)$ is consistent for $W^{mis}(u)$ under appropriate smoothness and regularity conditions guaranteeing the consistency of kernel regression estimators. Let $\hat{\hat{\beta}}^*(h)$ be a feasible second stage estimate in which the components of $\hat{W}^{mis}(u)$ are included as additional covariates in a correctly specified model (3.2). In Section (4c), we prove

Theorem 3.5: Subject to regularity conditions, under the semiparametric model defined by a model (2.2), (2.4a) and a particular model (3.2), the limiting distributions of $\hat{\beta}^*(h)$ and $\hat{\hat{\beta}}^*(h)$ are identical with asymptotic variance less than or equal to that of $\hat{\beta}(h)$ with $\hat{K}_i$ used in calculating $\hat{\beta}(h)$ based on any correctly specified model (3.2). Further, there exists h_{eff} such that the asymptotic variance of $\hat{\beta}^*(h_{eff})$ equals the semiparametric variance bound based on the c*-observed data (2.1). Theorem (3.5) also holds for the estimators $\hat{\beta}^{AF2}$ with (h,θ) replacing h and (h_{eff},θ_{eff}) replacing h_{eff}. [Also, if, in computing $\hat{\beta}(h)$, we replaced $\hat{K}_i$ by an appropriate completely non-parametric estimate, then, even without imposing (3.2), any $\hat{\beta}(h)$ would be asymptotically equivalent to $\hat{\beta}^*(h)$.]

Remark: Since $\bar{L}(u)$ is the history of a complex process up to u, the "feasible estimators" $\hat{\hat{\beta}}^*(h)$ are largely of theoretical interest, since, non-parametric estimation of $W^{mis}(u)$ is not practical due to the "curse of dimensionality." Thus, in practice, $\hat{W}_{mis}(u)$ would be replaced by the predicted value from the fit of a regression model.

4. Semiparametric Efficiency and Estimation in Missing Data Models

4a. Main Theorems

In Theorem 4.1, we provide representations for (a) the efficient score and (b) the influence function of a regular, asymptotically linear estimator in an arbitrary (discrete time) semiparametric model with the data missing at random. We specialize to the case of monotone missingness in Theorem (4.2) and extend our results to continuous time censoring processes in Theorem (4.3). Finally, in Theorems (4.4)-(4.6), we specialize Theorem (4.3) to the models (2.2a)-(2.2c). We start with a review of the theory of semiparametric efficiency bounds that borrows heavily from the survey paper of Newey (1990) and the monograph of Bickel, Klassen, Ritov, and Wellner (BKRW, 1991).

Suppose the data consists of n independent copies of an observed random variable V. Let $Lik(\beta,\theta; V)$ be the likelihood for a single subject in a semiparametric model indexed by a parameter $\beta \epsilon R^p$ of interest and a nuisance parameter θ taking values in some infinite dimensional set. Let (β_0,θ_0) index the distribution generating V. Define a regular parametric submodel to be a regular (fully) parametric model with parameters (β,η) and likelihood $Lik(\beta,\eta ; V)$ with true values β_0,η_0, where the "sub" prefix refers to the fact that for each η the distribution $Lik(\beta,\eta ; V)$ equals a distribution $Lik(\beta,\theta; V)$ allowed by the semiparametric model. Define the nuisance tangent space Λ to be the mean square closure of the set of all random vectors bS_η, where S_η is the score for η in some regular parametric submodel (usually, $S_\eta = \partial \ell n L(\beta_0,\eta_0 ; V)/\partial\eta$) and b is a conformable constant matrix with p rows; i.e. $\Lambda = \{A \epsilon R^p : E[\| A \|^2]<\infty$, and there exists $b_j S_{\eta,j}$ with $\lim_{j\to\infty} E[\| A-b_jS_{\eta,j} \|^2] = 0\}$, where each b_j is a matrix of constants and $\| A \| = A'A$. We shall consider Λ as a subset of the Hilbert space of px1 random vectors H with inner product $E[H'H]$. In our examples, Λ is a linear subspace. The projection of any vector H on a closed linear space, such as Λ, exists and is the unique vector $\Pi(H \mid \Lambda)$ in Λ satisfying $E[\{H-\Pi(H \mid \Lambda)\}'A] = 0$ for all $A \epsilon \Lambda$. Π is the projection operator. Henceforth we restrict attention to random vectors H for which $E[H'H]<\infty$. The semiparametric variance bound for regular estimators of β_0 is, by definition, the supremum of the Cramer-Rao bounds for β_0 over all regular parametric submodels and equals the inverse of the variance of $S_{eff} \equiv S_\beta-\Pi[S_\beta \mid \Lambda]$ where S_β is the score for β (usually, $S_\beta = \partial \ell n L(\beta_0,\theta_0 ; V)/\partial\beta$). S_{eff} is called the efficient score (Begun et al. 1983) and $Var[S_{eff}]$ is called the SIB.

We shall need the following definitions.

<u>Def</u>: (a) A test statistic $n^{-1/2}S(\beta)$ or (b) an estimator $\hat{\beta}$ is asymptotically linear at β_0 in a semiparametric model $Lik(\beta,\theta; V)$ with influence function $D=d(V)$ if (a) $n^{-1/2}S(\beta_0) = n^{-1/2}\Sigma_i D_i + o_p(1)$ or (b) $n^{1/2}(\hat{\beta}-\beta_0) = n^{-1/2}\Sigma_i D_i + o_p(1)$, where $E(D_i) = 0$ and $E(D_i'D_i) < \infty$ whatever be θ_0. D_i may depend on (β_0,θ_0). We shall impose the additional condition that $E_{\beta,\eta}[D_i]$ is continuous at (β_0,η_0) for each regular parametric submodel.

<u>Def</u>: A local data generating process (LDGP) at (β_0,θ_0) in a regular parametric submodel is one in which the data is generated according to $Lik(\beta_n,\eta_n ; V)$ with $n^{1/2}(\beta_n-\beta_0)$ and $n^{1/2}(\eta_n-\eta_0)$ bounded.

<u>Def</u>: (a) A test statistic $n^{-1/2}S(\beta_0)$ or (b) an estimator is regular at β_0 if (a) the limiting distribution of $n^{-1/2}S(\beta_0)$ is the same for all LDGP $Lik(\beta_0,\eta_n ; V)$ in all regular parametric

submodels or (b) the distribution of $n^{1/2}(\hat{\beta}-\beta_0)$ is the same for all LDGP Lik$(\beta_n,\eta_n;V)$ in all regular parametric submodels. The limiting distribution may depend on (β_0,θ_0).

Def: For any set $\mathcal{F}$ of random variables, let $\mathcal{F}_0$ be the subset with mean 0.

Lemma 4.1: In any semiparametric model, the influence function of any regular asymptotic linear (RAL) test of the true hypothesis $\beta=\beta_0$ is in $\Lambda_0^\perp \equiv (\Lambda^\perp)_0$, where "$\perp$" denotes an orthogonal complement. The influence function of any RAL estimator of β_0 is in $\Lambda_{0*}^\perp \equiv \{A\in\Lambda_0^\perp; E[AS_\beta'] = I_{p\times p}\}$. Theorem (2.2) in Newey (1990a) implies Lemma 4.2 for RAL estimators. Theorem A.1 in Appendix 1 implies the lemma for RAL tests.

We now specialize the above general results to "full" and "missing data" models. Henceforth let $V = (V^{(1)},\cdots,V^{(K)})'$ be a multivariate random variable with each $V^{(k)}$ univariate and

$$L^{(F)}(\beta,\theta;V) \tag{4.1}$$

be the likelihood for a single subject when V is fully observed in a semiparametric model indexed by $\beta\in R^p$ and an infinite dimensional nuisance parameter θ and let $S_\beta^{(F)}$, $\Lambda^{(F)}$, and $S_{eff}^{(F)}$ be the score for β, the nuisance tangent space, and the efficient score in the full data model. Suppose now V may not be fully observed and let $R = (R^{(1)},\cdots,R^{(K)})$ be a random variable such that $R^{(k)}=1$ if $V^{(k)}$ is observed and $R^{(k)}=0$ otherwise. R has 2^K possible realizations (r). Let $V_{(r)}$ be the vector of observed components of V when R=(r) so that the observable random variables are $(R,V_{(R)})$. Suppose the data is missing at random (Rubin, 1976) i.e.,

$$pr[R=r \mid V] = pr[R=r \mid V_{(r)}] \equiv \pi(r,V_{(r)}) \equiv \pi(r) \tag{4.2}$$

and that

$$\pi(\mathbf{1}) > \sigma > 0 \text{ with probability one} \tag{4.3}$$

where $\mathbf{1}$ is the K-vector of 1's. Often it is assumed

$$\pi(r,V_{(r)})\in\{\pi(r,V_{(r)};\gamma) : \gamma\in \boldsymbol{\Upsilon}\} \tag{4.4}$$

where, for each γ, $\Pi(r,V_{(r)};\gamma)$ is a density for $pr[R=r \mid V]$ satisfying (4.2) and $\boldsymbol{\Upsilon}$ may be infinite dimensional. Henceforth let S_β,Λ, and S_{eff} be the score for β, the nuisance tangent space, and the efficient score in the missing data model defined by (4.1)-(4.4) based on the data $(R,V_{(R)})$.

Define the tangent space for model (4.4) to be $\Lambda^{(3)} = \{A^{(3)}\in R^p$; there exists $b_j\ S_{\psi,j}$ with $\lim_{j\to\infty} E[\| A^{(3)}-b_jS_{\psi,j} \|^2] = 0\}$ where S_ψ is the score at the truth for a regular parametric submodel $\pi(r,V_{(r)},\psi)$ of the model $\pi(r,V_{(r)},\gamma)$ satisfying $\pi(r,V_{(r)},\psi_0) = \pi(r,V_{(r)})$ for some ψ_0 and the b_j are constant matrices. Define $\Lambda^{(2)} \equiv \{A^{(2)} = a^{(2)}(R,V_{(R)})\in R^P$; $E[A^{(2)} \mid V] = 0\}$.

In Appendix 2, we prove

Lemma 4.2: (a) $\Lambda^{(3)} \subseteq \Lambda^{(2)}$. (b) If the model (4.4) is completely non-parametric in the sense that it is unrestricted except for the condition $\Sigma_r \pi(r, V_{(r)}; \gamma) = 1$, then $\Lambda^{(2)} = \Lambda^{(3)}$.

Let $H = h(V)$ and $D = d(V)$ be generic functions of V. Define the operators $\mathbf{g}(H)$, $\mathbf{m}(H)$, and $\mathbf{u}(H)$ by $\mathbf{g}(H) = \Sigma_r I(R=r)E[H \mid V_{(r)}]$, $\mathbf{m}(H) = \Sigma_r \pi(r)E[H \mid V_{(r)}]$, $\mathbf{u}(H) = \pi(\mathbf{1})^{-1}I(R=\mathbf{1})H$ where the sums are over the 2^K possible value of r. Here and throughout bold lower case letters represent operators. Define $\Lambda^{(1)} = \{\mathbf{g}(A^{(F)}) : A^{(F)} \in \Lambda^{(F)}\}$.
In Appendix 2, we prove

Theorem (4.1): In the missing data model defined by (4.1)-(4.4), (a) $S_\beta = \mathbf{g}(S_\beta^{(F)})$ is the score for β, (b) $\Lambda^{(1)}$ and $\Lambda^{(3)}$ are mutually orthogonal closed linear spaces; (c) $\Lambda = \Lambda^{(1)} \oplus \Lambda^{(3)}$ is the nuisance tangent space where $\oplus$ denotes the direct sum of two spaces, (d) $\Lambda_0^\perp = \{A_0^\perp \equiv A_0^\perp(D, A^{(2)}) \equiv \mathbf{u}(D) + A^{(2)} - \Pi[\mathbf{u}(D) + A^{(2)} \mid \Lambda^{(3)}]; D \in \Lambda_0^{(F),\perp}, A^{(2)} \in \Lambda^{(2)}\}$ where $\Lambda_0^{(F),\perp} \equiv (\Lambda^{(F),\perp})_0$. (e) $E[A_0^\perp(D, A^{(2)}) S_\beta{}'] = E[D S_\beta^{(F)\prime}] = E[D S_{eff}^{(F)\prime}]$ for $D \in \Lambda_0^{(F),\perp}$. Further $\Lambda_{0*}^\perp \equiv \{A \in \Lambda_0^\perp; E[A S_\beta{}'] = I_{p \times p}\}$ is the set $\{\mathbf{u}(D) + A^{(2)} - \Pi[\mathbf{u}(D) + A^{(2)} \mid \Lambda^{(3)}]; D \in \Lambda_{0*}^{(F),\perp}, A^{(2)} \in \Lambda^{(2)}\}$, where $\Lambda_{0*}^{(F),\perp} \equiv \{D \in \Lambda_0^{(F),\perp}; E[D S_\beta^{(F)\prime}] = I_{p \times p}\}$. (f) The efficient score $S_{eff} \equiv S_\beta - \Pi[S_\beta \mid \Lambda]$ is given by $\mathbf{u}(D_{eff}) - \Pi[\mathbf{u}(D_{eff}) \mid \Lambda^{(2)}]$ with D_{eff} the unique D in $\Lambda^{(F),\perp}$ solving $\Pi[\mathbf{m}^{-1}(D) \mid \Lambda^{(F),\perp}] = S_{eff}^{(F)}$, where $\mathbf{m}^{-1}(D)$ is the unique H solving $\mathbf{m}(H) = D$. (g) $\Pi[\mathbf{u}(D) \mid \Lambda^{(2)}] = \mathbf{u}(D) - \mathbf{g}[\mathbf{m}^{-1}(D)]$, and thus $S_{eff} = \mathbf{g}[\mathbf{m}^{-1}(D_{eff})]$. We now indicate the importance of this rather abstract theorem.

By Lemma (4.1), it follows that part e (d) of Theorem (4.1) says that the influence function of any RAL estimator (test) in the missing data model (4.1)-(4.4) is obtained by first applying the operator $\mathbf{u}$ to the influence function of an RAL estimator (test) in the full data model $L^{(F)}(\beta, \theta; V)$, adding an arbitrary element of $\Lambda^{(2)}$, and finally subtracting off the projection on the tangent space $\Lambda^{(3)}$ of the model (4.4) for the missingness process. Part f of the Theorem says that the efficient score for β_0 does not depend on $\Lambda^{(3)}$ and thus on the model (4.4) for the missingness process.

In a general missing data model, the characterization of S_{eff} given in part f of the theorem may be of little practical help since, for a given H, $\mathbf{m}^{-1}(H)$ and $\Pi[\mathbf{u}(H) \mid \Lambda^{(2)}]$ may not exist in closed form. However, $\Pi[\mathbf{u}(H) \mid \Lambda^{(2)}]$ and $\mathbf{m}^{-1}(H)$ exist in closed form when there is a monotone missing data pattern, where a monotone missing data pattern is defined as follows. Suppose we have a sequence of sets $S_0, S_1, \cdots, S_M$ satisfying $\phi = S_0 \subsetneq S_1 \subsetneq S_2 \cdots \subsetneq S_M \equiv \{1, \cdots, K\}$. For $1 \le m \le M+1$, let $\bar{V}_m$ be the vector comprised of the components $V^{(k)}$ of V for $k \in S_{m-1}$. For $0<m<M+1$, let $R_m = 1$ if $\bar{V}_{m+1}$ is fully observed and $R_m=0$ otherwise. Let $R_0=1$. Note $R_m=1$ if $R_{m+1}=1$. We say that the missing data pattern is monotone if whenever $R_{m+1}=0$ and $R_m=1$, $\bar{V}_{m+1}$ constitutes all the observed elements of V. Let $\pi_0=1$ and, for $m>1$, $\pi_m = P[R_m=1 \mid R_{m-1}=1, \bar{V}_m]$. Set $\bar{\pi}_m = \prod_{j=1}^{m} \pi_m$ and $\bar{\pi}_0=1$.

Theorem 4.2: If missingness is monotone in the missing data semiparametric model (4.1)-(4.4),

$E[D \mid \bar{V}_m] = E[D \mid \bar{V}_m, R_{m-1}=1]$; $\mathbf{g}(D) = R_M D + \sum_{m=1}^{M} (R_{m-1}-R_m)E[D \mid \bar{V}_m]$;

$\mathbf{m}(D) = \bar{\pi}_m D + \sum_{m=1}^{M} (1-\pi_m)\bar{\pi}_{m-1}E[D \mid \bar{V}_m]$; $\mathbf{u}(D) = D + \sum_{m=1}^{M} (R_m - \pi_m R_{m-1})\bar{\pi}_m^{-1} D$;

$\mathbf{m}^{-1}(D) = D + \mathbf{v}(D)$, where $\mathbf{v}(D) = \sum_{m=1}^{M} (1-\pi_m)\bar{\pi}_m^{-1}\{D - E[D \mid \bar{V}_m]\}$;

$\Lambda^{(2)} = \{A^{(2)} = \sum_{m=1}^{M} (R_m - \pi_m R_{m-1}) a(\bar{V}_m)$ for some $a(\bar{V}_m) \in R^P\}$;

$\Pi[\mathbf{u}(D) \mid \Lambda^{(2)}] = \sum_{m=1}^{M} (R_m - \pi_m R_{m-1})\bar{\pi}_m^{-1} E[D \mid \bar{V}_m]$; and D_{eff} is the unique $D \in \Lambda^{(F),\perp}$ solving

$$S_{eff}^{(F)} = D + \Pi[\mathbf{v}(D) \mid \Lambda^{(F),\perp}] \tag{4.5}$$

Continuous Time Models:

An example of monotone missingness occurs when missingness is solely due to right censoring by a random variable Q^* where Q^* has a discrete sample space $\{t_1, t_2, \cdots, t_M, t_{M+1}\}$ with $\bar{V}_{M+1} \equiv V$ being the full-data and $\bar{V}_m$ the observed data for a subject with $Q^* = t_m$. Suppose now $V \equiv \bar{V}(C) = \{V(t) ; 0 \le t \le C\}$ is a continuous time process, Q^* is a continuous censoring variable, and C may be random. We obtain a continuous time version of Theorem (4.2) by taking limits as $\Delta t \equiv t_{m+1} - t_m \to 0$. Specifically we assume a full data model (4.1) for $V \equiv \bar{V}(C)$ but we only observe for each subject

$$C, \min(Q^*, C), \tau = I(C \le Q^*), \bar{V}\{\min(Q^*, C)\} \ . \tag{4.6}$$

We assume

$$\lambda_{Q^*}[u \mid \bar{V}(C)] = \lambda_{Q^*}[u \mid \bar{V}(u)\} \ , \tag{4.2$'$}$$

$$K^*(C) > \sigma > 0 \text{ with probability one } , \tag{4.3$'$}$$

and

$$\lambda_{Q^*}[u \mid \bar{V}(u)] \in \{\lambda_{Q^*}[u \mid \bar{V}(u) ; \gamma] ; \gamma \in \boldsymbol{\Upsilon}\} \ . \tag{4.4$'$}$$

Here $K^*(t) = \exp\{-\int_0^t \lambda_{Q^*}[u \mid \bar{V}(u)]du\}$. A continuous time version of Theorem (4.2) follows by making the formal identifications; $(1-\pi_m) = \lambda_{Q^*}(t_m \mid \bar{V}(t_m))\ \Delta t + o(\Delta t)$; $\bar{\pi}_m = K^*(t_m)$, $R_m = 1 - N_{Q^*}(t_m)$, where $N_{Q^*}(t) = I[Q^* \le t]$. Specifically, define $M_{Q^*}(u) = N_{Q^*}(u) - \int_0^u \lambda_{Q^*}[t \mid \bar{V}(t)] Y^*(t) dt$, with $Y^*(t) = I[Q^* \ge t]$. Then we have

Theorem 4.3: In the semiparametric model defined by (4.1), (4.2$'$)-(4.4$'$), Theorem (4.1) and Eq. (4.5) continue to hold with $D = d\{\bar{V}(C)\}$, $E[D \mid \bar{V}(u), Y^*(u)=1] = E[D \mid \bar{V}(u)]$,

$\mathbf{g}(D) = \tau D + (1-\tau) E[D \mid \bar{V}(Q^*)]$;

$\mathbf{m}(D) = K^*(C) D + \int_0^C du\ E[D \mid \bar{V}(u)]\{K^*(u)\}\lambda_{Q^*}[u \mid \bar{V}(u)]$

$\mathbf{v}(D) = \int_0^C du \lambda_{Q^*}[u \mid \bar{V}(u)]\{K^*(u)\}^{-1}\{D - E[D \mid \bar{V}(u)]\}$

$\mathbf{m}^{-1}(D) = D+\mathbf{v}(D)$, $\mathbf{u}(D) \equiv \tau D/K^*(C) = D - \int_0^C dM_{Q^*}(u)\{K^*(u)\}^{-1}D$

$\Lambda^{(2)} = \{A^{(2)} \equiv \int_0^C dM_{Q^*}(u)a\{\bar{V}(u)\}\ ;\ a\{\bar{V}(u)\}\in R^p\}$

$\Pi[\mathbf{u}(D) \mid \Lambda^{(2)}] = -\int_0^C dM_{Q^*}(u)\{K^*(u)\}^{-1}E[D \mid \bar{V}(u)]$;

$\Lambda^{(3)}$ is the closed linear span of the set $\{A^{(3)} \equiv bS_\psi\}$ where S_ψ is the score for a regular parametric submodel $\lambda_{Q^*}[u \mid \bar{V}(u);\psi]$ for model (4.4′) and b is a conformable matrix with p rows. Typically $S_\psi = \frac{\partial \ell n}{\partial \psi}\Big[\{\lambda_{Q^*}[Q^* \mid \bar{V}(Q^*),\psi]\}^{1-\tau}\exp\Big\{-\int_0^{\min(Q^*,C)}\lambda_{Q^*}[t \mid \bar{V}(t),\psi]\Big\}\Big]_{\psi=\psi_0}$.

We have as yet specified neither the full data $V=\bar{V}(C)$ or the semiparametric model (4.1). Let $C=c^*$ and, for $u\le c^*$, $\bar{V}(u) = \{c^*,Z,\bar{L}(\min\{T,u\}), TI\{T<u\}, I(T<u)\}$ so that $V = \bar{V}(c^*)$ is the c^*-full data (3.4). Now define $Q^* = Q$ if $Q<X^*$, where $X^* \equiv \min(T,c^*)$, and $Q^* = \infty$ otherwise, so once a subject has failed un-Q-censored (i.e., $T<Q$), he cannot be Q^* censored (since $Q^* = \infty$). Then $\lambda_{Q^*}[u \mid \bar{V}(u)] = \lambda_Q[u \mid \bar{L}(u), Z]$ and $K^*(u) = K(u)$ for $u\le X^*$; $\lambda_{Q^*}[u \mid \bar{V}(u)]=0$ and $K^*(u) = K(X^*)$ for $X^*\le u<c^*$; and the observed data (4.6) is the c^*-observed data (2.1). Further censoring mechanism (A.2′) is equivalent to the censoring mechanism (2.4d) rather than (2.4a). Hence, we can restate Theorem (4.3) as follows

Theorem (4.4): With V and $\bar{V}(u)$ as just defined, if (4.1), (2.4d), (4.3′) and model (3.2) for censoring by Q hold, then Theorem (4.1) and Eq. (4.5) remain true with

$E[D \mid \bar{L}(u),Z,Y(u)=1] = E[D \mid \bar{L}(u),Z,X^*>u]$

$\mathbf{g}(D) = \tau D + (1-\tau)E[D \mid \bar{L}(Q),Z,X^*>Q]$,

$\mathbf{m}(D) = K(X^*)D + \int_0^{X^*} du\lambda_Q[u \mid \bar{L}(u),Z]K(u)E[D \mid \bar{L}(u),Z,Y(u)=1]$, $\mathbf{m}^{-1}(D) = D + \mathbf{v}(D)$,

$\mathbf{v}(D) = \int_0^{X^*} du\lambda_Q[u \mid \bar{L}(u),Z]\{K(u)\}^{-1}\{D-E[D \mid \bar{L}(u),Z,Y(u)=1]\}$,

$\Lambda^{(2)} = \{A^{(2)} \equiv \int_0^\infty dM_Q(u)a(\bar{L}(u),Z)\}$,

$\Pi[\mathbf{u}(D) \mid \Lambda^{(2)}] = -\int_0^\infty dM_Q(u)\{K(u)\}^{-1}E[D \mid \bar{L}(u),Z,Y(u)=1]$,

$\mathbf{u}(D) = D - \int_0^\infty dM_Q(u)\{K(u)\}^{-1}D$, and

$\Lambda^{(3)} = \{A^{(3)} = b_1\Gamma(W) + b_2\int_0^\infty dM_Q(u)r(u,S^*)\}$ where $r(u,S^*)$ is any vector-valued function and b_1 and b_2 are constant conformable matrices with p rows. This characterization of $\Lambda^{(3)}$ follows from the results of Ritov and Wellner (1988) on the PH model.

4b. Semiparametric Models (2.2a)-(2.2c)

We now consider the semiparametric models for $V = \bar{V}(c^*)$ induced by (2.2a)-(2.2c). The semiparametric missing data model for the c^*-observed data (2.1) defined by a model (2.2a)-(2.2c) and censoring mechanism (2.4d) can be shown to be identical to that defined by the corresponding model (2.2a)-(2.2c) and (2.4a) in the sense that, for each β, the allowable distributions for the c^*-observables (2.1) are the same. Hence, assuming (2.4d) rather than (2.4a) can make no inferential difference. In particular, S_{eff} will be the same function of the c^*-observables and their joint distribution. Hence, one can calculate S_{eff}

under (2.4d) and then re-express S_{eff} in terms of the c*-observables and their distribution to obtain S_{eff} under (2.4a). The following Theorem can be proved using results in Chamberlain (1987), Ritov and Wellner (1988), and Robins and Rotnitzky (1992).

Theorem 4.5: In the "full-data" semiparametric model for the c*-full data V induced by (2.2a)-(2.2c), (a) $\Lambda^{(F)} = \Lambda_1^{(F)} \oplus \Lambda_2^{(F)} \oplus \Lambda_3^{(F)}$; (b) $\Lambda_1^{(F)}, \Lambda_2^{(F)}$, and $\Lambda_3^{(F)}$ are mutually orthogonal closed subspaces; (c) $\Lambda_1^{(F)} = \{A_1 = a_1(Z); E[A_1]=0\}$; (d) $\Lambda_3^{(F)} = \{A_3 = a_3(V); E[A_3 \mid Z, X^*, \Delta]=0\}$ except $\Lambda_3^{(F),MN} = \{A_3 = a_3(V); E[A_3 \mid Z, \Delta]=0\}$; (e) $\Lambda_2^{(F),MN} = \{A_2^{(F)} = r\{\varsigma, Z\}; E[A_2^{(F)} \mid Z]=0$, $E[\varsigma A_2^{(F)\prime} \mid Z]=0\}$; $\Lambda_2^{(F),AF} = \{ \int_{-\infty}^{\infty} r(u) dM_\epsilon(u)\}$; and $\Lambda_2^{(F),PH} = \{ \int_0^{\infty} r(u) dM_T(u)\}$; (f) $\Lambda_0^{(F),\perp} = \{U_f\}$ with $U_f^{AF} \equiv U_f^{AF1}$. [Note, however, $\{U_f^{AF1}\} = \{U_f^{AF2}\}$ by Lemma 3.4.]; (g) $S_{eff}^{(F)} = U_f(h_{op})$.

To use Eq. (4.5) to find D_{eff}, we need to be able to compute $\Pi(D \mid \Lambda_0^{(F),\perp})$ for D=d(V). One can prove the following using the definition of a projection.

Theorem 4.6: $\Pi(D \mid \Lambda_0^{(F),\perp,AF)}) = U_f^{AF1}(h)$ with $h(u,Z) = \mathbf{r}\{d^{*,AF}(u,Z)\}$ with $d^{*,AF}(u,z) = E[D \mid \Delta=1, \epsilon=u, Z]$ if $u<\mu$ and $d^{*,AF}(u,Z) = E[D \mid \Delta=0, \epsilon>u, Z]$ if $u \geq \mu$, where $\mathbf{r}^{AF}\{g(u,Z)\} \equiv g(u,Z) - E[g(\epsilon,Z) \mid Z, \epsilon>u]$ as in Ritov and Wellner (1988).

$\Pi[D \mid \Lambda_0^{(F),\perp,PH}] = U_f^{PH}(h)$ with $h(u,Z) = \mathbf{r}^{PH}\{d^{*,PH}(u,Z)\}$, with $d^{*,PH}(u,Z) = E[D \mid \Delta=1, T=u, Z]$ if $u<c^*$ and $d^{*,PH}(u,Z) = E[D \mid \Delta=0, T>c^*, Z]$ if $u \geq c^*$, where $\mathbf{r}^{PH}\{g(u,Z)\} = g(u,Z) - E[g(T,Z) \mid Z, T>u]$.

$\Pi[D \mid \Lambda_0^{(F),\perp,MN}] = U_f^{MN}(h)$, with $h(Z) = E[D\varsigma \mid Z]\{E[\varsigma^2 \mid Z]\}^{-1}$.

We next demonstrate that the influence function U of $n^{-1/2}S\{\hat{D}(\beta_0)\}$ and the influence function $-\kappa^{-1}U$ of $\hat{\beta}$ given in Theorem (3.4) satisfy, as they must, (d) and (e) of Theorem (4.1). Using the projection arguments for the Cox model in Ritov and Wellner (1988), for any D=d(V), $\mathbf{u}(D) - \Pi[\mathbf{u}(D) \mid \Lambda^{(3)}] = D - \Gamma(D/K) + \rho[\Gamma(D/K), \Gamma(W)]$ where D/K is the function D/K(u). For any $A^{(2)} \equiv \int_0^{\infty} dM_Q(u) H^{(2)}(u)$ with $H^{(2)}(u)$ being $\mathbf{F}(u)$-predictable, $A^{(2)} - \Pi[A^{(2)} \mid \Lambda^{(3)}] = \Gamma(H^{(2)}) - \rho[\Gamma(H^{(2)}), \Gamma(W)]$. Thus, from their definitions, $U \equiv U_f - U_{mis} + U_{rec} = \mathbf{u}(U_f) + A_{mis}^{(2)} - \Pi[\mathbf{u}(U_f) + A_{mis}^{(2)} \mid \Lambda^{(3)}]$ where $A_{mis}^{(2)} = 0$ except that $A_{mis}^{(2),AF2} = -\int_0^{\infty} dM_Q(u) E[D^{AF2}(\beta_0) \mid Z]/K(u) \in \Lambda^{(2)}$ and $U_f \in \Lambda_0^{(F),\perp}$ as required by part d of Theorem 4.1. Similar arguments show $\kappa^{-1}U$ satisfies part (e) of Theorem (4.1). Since, under regularity conditions, $\hat{\beta}$ will be RAL, Lemma (4.2) and Theorem (4.1) imply that the value of κ in Theorem (3.4) must be $E[U_f\, S_{eff}^{(F)\prime}]$.

4c. Proof of Lemmas 3.1 and 3.3 and Theorem 3.5

Consider any two correctly specified models (a) and (b) for the censoring process satisfying (3.2) with the first model nested within the second, so that $\Lambda^{3,(a)} \subseteq \Lambda^{3,(b)} \subseteq \Lambda^{(2)}$ in obvious notation. Then we have

Theorem (4.7): For a given $\hat{D}(\beta)$, $\kappa^{-1}Var(U^{(a)})\kappa^{-1\prime} \geq \kappa^{-1}Var(U^{(b)})\kappa^{-1\prime} \geq \kappa^{-1}Var\{\mathbf{u}(U_f) - \Pi[\mathbf{u}(U_f) \mid \Lambda^{(2)}]\}\kappa^{-1\prime} = Var^A\{n^{1/2}(\hat{\beta}^* - \beta_0)\}$. The last inequality is strict unless $\Pi[\mathbf{u}(U_f) +$

$A^{(2)}_{mis} \mid \Lambda^{(3),b}] = \Pi[\mathbf{u}(U_f) + A^{(2)}_{mis} \mid \Lambda^{(2)}]$ with probability one which will occur if $W^{mis}_{(u)}$ is included in (3.2) for model b.

Proof: For any A and closed subspace Ω, it is straightforward to show $Var[A-\Pi(A \mid \Omega)] = Var(A) - Var\{\Pi(A \mid \Omega)\}$. Further $Var\{\Pi[A \mid \Omega^{(1)}]\} \le Var\{\Pi[A \mid \Omega^{(2)}]\}$, in the positive definite sense, if $\Omega^{(1)} \subseteq \Omega^{(2)}$ with strict inequality unless the projections are equal with probability one. The theorem follows by setting $A = \mathbf{u}(U_f) + A^{(2)}_{mis}$, noting $\hat{D}(\beta)$ determines A, and calculating the projections using the formulae given in Theorem (4.4) and in the last subsection.

Except for the asymptotic equivalence of $\hat{\beta}^*$ and $\hat{\hat{\beta}}^*$ discussed in Appendix 3, Theorem (3.5) now follows from Theorems (4.1f), (4.5), and (4.7) with h_{eff} defined by $D_{eff} = U_f(h_{eff})$. Part (a) of Lemma (3.1) follows from Theorem (4.7). Part (b) follows by noting, by Theorem 3.4, $Var(U_{rec}) \neq 0 \Leftrightarrow E[\Gamma(H_{mis})\Gamma(W)']\neq 0$ and then evaluating this expectation under (2.4c). Part (a) of Lemma (3.3) follows from Theorem (4.7) and part (e) of Theorem (4.1), upon noting that $\Lambda^{(F),\perp,MN}_{0^*}$ has a single member when Z is dichotomous (since all functions h(Z) lead to the same estimate $\tilde{\beta}^{MN}$). Part (b) is a corollary of Theorem (4.7). Finally part (c) follows from the fact that the usual KM-estimator is known to be the non-parametric MLE based on the c^*-$\overline{sur}$-data.

4d. Semiparametric Efficient Estimation

For the models (2.2a)-(2.2c), the solution $D_{eff} \equiv U_f(h_{eff})$ to Eq. (4.5) does not generally exist in closed form except for the mean model (2.2c).

Specifically, since, by Theorem (4.5f), $\Lambda^{(F),\perp,MN}_0 = \{h(Z)\varsigma\}$, we can write $D_{eff} \equiv h_{eff}(Z)\varsigma$. Theorems (4.5g) and (4.6) and Eq. (4.5) imply $S^{(F)}_{eff} = [\partial g(Z,\beta_0)/\partial\beta]\{E[\varsigma^2 \mid Z]\}^{-1}\varsigma = h_{eff}(Z)\varsigma + E[\mathbf{v}(D_{eff})\varsigma \mid Z]\{E[\varsigma^2 \mid Z]\}^{-1}\varsigma$. But, by Theorem (4.4), $E[\mathbf{v}(D_{eff})\varsigma \mid Z] = h_{eff}(Z)P^{MN}(Z)$ where $P^{MN}(Z) = E\{\int_0^{X^*} du\lambda_Q[u \mid \bar{L}(u),Z]\{K(u)\}^{-1}Var[\varsigma \mid \bar{L}(u),Z,Y(u)=1] \mid Z\}$. Hence $h^{MN}_{eff}(Z) = [\partial g(Z,\beta_0)/\partial\beta]\{E[\varsigma^2 \mid Z] + P^{MN}(Z)\}^{-1}$. Thus, as argued in Appendix 3, $\hat{\hat{\beta}}^*(\hat{h}_{eff})$ is a semiparametric efficient adaptive estimator where $\hat{h}_{eff}(Z)$ is estimated by applying (nested) non-parametric regression estimates to each conditional expectation in the RHS of the identities $E[\varsigma^2 \mid Z] = E[\tau\varsigma^2/K(X) \mid Z]$ and $P^{MN}(Z) =$

$E[\int_0^\infty dN_Q(u)\{E[\tau\varsigma^2/K(X) \mid \bar{L}(u),Z,Y(u)=1] - [K(u)]E^2[\tau\varsigma/K(X) \mid \bar{L}(u),Z,Y(u)=1]\} \mid Z]$ with K(X) and ς replaced by preliminary estimates with $E^2(A) = [E(A)]^2$.

When, as in the PH or AF model, Eq. (4.5) does not admit a closed form solution but $\Lambda^{(F),\perp}_0$ can be explicitly exhibited as $\{U_f(h)\}$, one can obtain semiparametric efficient estimators via "linear combinations of estimating functions" as in Newey (1992). Specifically, let $g_1(u,Z),g_2(u,Z),\cdots$ be an infinite complete basis sequence of real-valued functions in the sense that if $\iint_{u\in[0,c_{max}]} h^2(u,z)dudF(z)<\infty$, then there exists constants c_j such that $\lim_{k\to\infty} \iint_{u\in[0,c_{max}]}[h(u,z) - \sum_{j=1}^{k} c_jg_j(u,z)]^2dudF(z)$ is zero. Sequences of polynomials (i.e., power series) in (u,Z) are known to be complete. Let $g^{[k]}(u,Z)$ be the K-vector $(g_1,\cdots,g_k)', k>p, \beta_0 \in R^p$. Following Newey (1992b), $\hat{h}^{[k]}(u,Z) = \hat{b}^{[k]} g^{[k]}(u,Z)$ is the estimated optimal linear combination of the $g^{[k]}$ in the sense that $Var^A\{n^{1/2}[\hat{\hat{\beta}}^*(\hat{h}^{[k]})-\beta_0]\} \leq Var^A\{n^{1/2}[\hat{\hat{\beta}}^*(bg^{[k]})-\beta_0]\}$ for any pxk matrix b. Here $\hat{b}^{[k]}$ is the pxk matrix $\hat{\kappa}(\hat{\beta},g^{[k]})'\{\hat{Var}[U(\hat{\beta},g^{[k]})]\}^{-1}$, $\hat{\beta}$ is a preliminary estimate, and e.g., $\hat{\kappa}(\hat{\beta},g^{[k]})$ is $\hat{\kappa}(\hat{\beta},h)$ with $g^{[k]}$ replacing h, and, finally, the covariates W(u) used in computing $\hat{Var}[U(\hat{\beta},g^{[k]})]$ include $\hat{W}^{mis}(u)$ as defined in Section 3k except based on $\hat{H}_{mis}(u,\hat{\beta},g^{[k]})$ rather than $\hat{H}_{mis}(u,\beta) \equiv \hat{H}_{mis}(u,\beta,h)$. It follows from the completeness of $g_1,g_2,\cdots$ and the optimality (for fixed k) of $\hat{\hat{\beta}}^*(\hat{h}^{[k]})$ that the asymptotic variance of $\hat{\hat{\beta}}^*(\hat{h}^{[k]})$ can be made arbitrarily close to that of $\hat{\beta}^*(h_{eff})$ (and thus to the semiparametric variance bound) for k sufficiently large, provided the linear operator mapping h to U(h) is mean-square continuous. In fact, Newey (1992b) shows that, under regularity conditions, if we let the dimension $k \equiv k(n)$ increase with sample size n at an appropriate rate $\hat{\hat{\beta}}^*(\hat{h}^{[k(n)]})$ is a feasible semiparametric efficient estimator. The results obtained in this subsection will be largely of theoretical rather than practical interest due to the "curse of dimensionality."

4e. Proof of Theorem 3.2 and an Efficient Koul et al. Estimator

We first prove part e of Theorem 3.2. Ritov and Wellner (1988) proved that, for the AF model, the efficient score $S_{eff,\bar{s}}$ based on the c*-$\overline{sur}$-data, under the independent censoring mechanism (2.4b), is

$$\int_{-\infty}^{\infty} \{dN_\epsilon^*(u) - \lambda_\epsilon(u)\, I(\omega>u)du\} b^{AF}(u,Z) \tag{4.8}$$

with $N_\epsilon^*(u) = I\{\omega \leq u, \Delta\tau=1\}$ and $b^{AF}(u,Z) = \{d\ell n\lambda_\epsilon(u)/du\}\{Z-E[Z \mid \omega>u]\}$, and $\omega = \ell nX+\beta_0 Z$ where $\bar{s}$ in $S_{eff,\bar{s}}$ specifies the c*-$\overline{sur}$-data. Suppose we could find a function $\rho(\Delta,\nu,Z)$ of the c*-full data (3.4) (i.e., of V) such that $S_{eff,\bar{s}} = \mathbf{g}[\rho(\Delta,\nu,Z)]$ with $\mathbf{g}(\cdot)$ as in Theorem 4.4. Then since, by Theorem (4.1g), $S_{eff,\bar{s}} = \mathbf{g}\{\mathbf{m}^{-1}(D_{eff,\bar{s}})\}$, we would obtain $D_{eff,\bar{s}} = \mathbf{m}\{\rho(\Delta,\nu,Z)\}$ without solving (4.5). Now, since $D_{eff,\bar{s}} \in \Lambda_0^{(F),\perp}$ and, for dichotomous Z, $\Lambda_0^{(F),\perp} = \{U_f^{AF2}(r)\}$, we can write $D_{eff,\bar{s}} = U_f^{AF2}(r_{\bar{s}}) \equiv D^{AF2}(\beta_0,r_{\bar{s}}) = R_{\bar{s}}(\beta_0)\{Z-E(Z)\}$ with $E[R_{\bar{s}}(\beta_0)] = 0$. Hence $\hat{\beta}_{\bar{s}}$ solving $0 = S\{\hat{D}^{AF2}(\beta,r_{\bar{s}})\} = \Sigma_i \tau_i R_{\bar{s},i}(\beta)\{Z_i-\hat{E}(Z)\}/\hat{K}_i^0$ is semiparametric efficient in the absence of surrogate marker data. We call $\hat{\beta}_{\bar{s}}$ the efficient Koul et al., estimator due to its similarity to the estimator in Koul et al. (1981). (Even if Q is independent of Z, we must divide by the Z-specific KM estimator $\hat{K}_i^0$ rather than the marginal KM estimator for censoring to "fully project on $\Lambda^{(2)}$" and thus to be efficient.) If Z is not dichotomous, $D_{eff,\bar{s}}$ will not be a multiplicatively separable function of (Δ,ν) and Z.

A calculation shows Eq. (4.8) equals $\mathbf{g}\{\rho(\Delta,\nu,Z)\}$ for $\rho(\Delta,\nu,Z) = \Delta \boldsymbol{\ell}\, b^{AF}(\epsilon,Z) + (1-\Delta)b^{*,AF}(\mu,Z)$ where $\boldsymbol{\ell}\, b^{AF}(\epsilon,Z) = b^{AF}(\epsilon,Z) + b^{*,AF}(\epsilon,Z)$, and

$b^{*,AF}(u,Z) = -\int_{-\infty}^{u} \lambda_\epsilon(x) b^{AF}(x,Z)dx = E[\boldsymbol{\ell}\, b^{AF}(\epsilon,Z) \mid Z,\epsilon>u]$ (Ritov and Wellner, 1988). Hence, by Theorem (4.4), $D_{eff,\bar{s}} = \mathbf{m}\{\rho(\Delta,\nu,Z)\} = K(X^*)\rho(\Delta,\nu,Z) + \int_0^{X^*} \lambda_Q[u \mid Z]K(u)b^{*,AF}\{\ell nu+\beta_0 Z,Z\}$. Specializing to dichotomous Z and $\beta_0 = 0$, $\rho(\Delta,\nu,Z) = [\Delta r^{AF}_{pf,1}(\ell nT) + (1-\Delta)\, r^{AF}_{pf,2}(\ell n(c^*))][Z-E(Z)]$ and $b^{*,AF}(u,Z) = r^{AF}_{pf,2}(u)[Z-E(Z)]$. It follows that $r^{AF}_{\bar{s}}(u)$ is as given in part e of Theorem (3.2) if $\lambda_Q[u \mid Z] = \lambda_Q(u)$. To proof part e for the PH model, we note $S^{PH}_{eff,\bar{s}}$ at β_0=0 is given by (4.8) with $\epsilon=\ell nT$ and with $b^{PH}(u,Z) \equiv Z-E[Z \mid \ell nX>u]$ replacing b^{AF} (Ritov and Wellner, 1988).

Theorem (3.2a) follows by noting $NC_s^{c^*} = NC_{\bar{s}}^{c^*}$ if and only if $D_{eff,\bar{s}}$ still solves (4.5) given data on L(u). That is, by Theorem (4.4), if and only if $\int_0^{X^*} du\{E[D_{eff,\bar{s}} \mid \bar{L}(u),Z,Y(u)=1] - E[D_{eff,\bar{s}} \mid Z,Y(u)=1]\} = 0$ w.p.1. Theorem (3.2c) follows from Theorem 4.4 and the relations $NC_s^{c^*} = NC_{full}^{c^*} \Leftrightarrow S_{eff} = S^{(F)}_{eff} \Leftrightarrow S^{(F)}_{eff} = D_{eff} \Leftrightarrow \mathbf{v}(D_{eff}) = 0$ and $\mathbf{u}(D_{eff}) - \Pi[\mathbf{u}(D_{eff}) \mid \Lambda^{(2)}] = D_{eff}$ w.p.1. Theorem (3.2d) then follows from $S^{(F)}_{eff} = D_{eff}$ and the expressions for $S^{(F),PH}_{eff}$ and $S^{(F),AF}_{eff}$ at β_0=0, e.g., as given in Ritov and Wellner (1988).

To prove part (f), note that, by Lemma (4.1) and Theorem (4.1d), the influence function of any RAL modified Buckley-James test of the hypothesis β_0=0 in model (2.2b), under (2.2c), must be of the form $\mathbf{u}(D) - \Pi[\mathbf{u}(D) \mid \Lambda^{(2)}]$ for some $D \in \Lambda_0^{(F),\perp}$ [since the fact that the test does not use the information that $\lambda_Q[u \mid \bar{L}(u),Z] = \lambda_Q(u \mid Z)$ implies that it must be RAL even if only (2.4d) rather than (2.4c) were imposed, and, thus, $\Lambda^{(3)}$ were $\Lambda^{(2)}$]. But, by Theorems (4.5f) and (4.7), this is exactly the influence function of the test $\psi(r,w^r_{op},c^*)$ with $r[\Delta,\ell n(X^*)] = D/\{Z-E(Z)\}$.

Appendix 1

Theorem (A.1): A RAL test statistic $n^{-1/2}S(\beta_0)$ at β_0 with influence function D is asymptotically normal with mean $c_1 E[DS_{eff}']$ and variance $E[DD']$ under a LDGP $Lik(\beta_n,\eta_n;V)$ in any regular parametric submodel such that $n^{1/2}(\beta_n-\beta_0)\rightarrow c_1, n^{1/2}(\eta_n-\eta_0)\rightarrow c_2$. Further, $D \in \Lambda_0^{(F),\perp}$. The NC parameter, $E[D'S_{eff}]\{E(DD')\}^{-1}E[DS_{eff}']$, is less than or equal to $E[S_{eff}S_{eff}']$ with equality if $D = S_{eff}$.

Proof: $n^{-1/2}S(\beta_0) = \Sigma_i D_i + o_p(1)$ under any LDGP by contiguity of a LDGP to the fixed process (β_0,η_0). Hence, $n^{-1/2}S(\beta_0) = n^{-1/2}\Sigma_i[D_i - E_n(D_i)] + n^{1/2}E_n(D_i)$ where E_n is an expectation with respect to the density $Lik(\beta_n,\eta_n,V)$. But, $n^{-1/2}\Sigma_i[D_i-E_n(D_i)] \xrightarrow{d} N\{0,E(DD')\}$ under the LDGP as discussed in the proof of Theorem 2.2 of Newey (1990a). Also, as in Newey (1990a, Theorem 2.2), by regularity of the submodel, $n^{1/2}E_n[D] = E[DS_\beta']c_1 + E[DS_\eta']c_2 + o(1)$. Consider now a LDGP with $\beta_n = \beta_0$, i.e., $c_1 = 0$. Then, by the assumption of regularity of $n^{-1/2}S(\beta_0)$, $E[DS_\eta'] = 0$ for all regular submodels so $D \in \Lambda_0^{(F),\perp}$. Hence $E[DS_\beta'] = E[DS_{eff}']$ and the theorem follows by Slutsky's theorem and the fact that the maximum possible value of the NC parameter is $E[S_{eff}S_{eff}']$ by the Cauchy-Schwartz inequality.

Appendix 2

Proofs of Lemma (4.1a) and Theorems (4.1) and (4.2)

Proof of Lemma (4.1a): $\Lambda^{(3)} \subseteq \Lambda^{(2)}$ since (a) any score S_ψ of (4.4) is in $\Lambda^{(2)}$ by the conditional mean zero property of scores, and (b) $\Lambda^{(2)}$ is closed since it is the inverse image of the closed set of {0} under the continuous mapping $E\{\cdot \mid V\}$. To prove (4.1b), note for any bounded $A^{(2)}$ in $\Lambda^{(2)}$, the submodel $\pi(R,V_{(R)})(1+\psi' A^{(2)})$ defined on a sufficiently small open ball around $\psi_0=0$ is regular with score $A^{(2)}$ by Lemma C.4 of Newey (1990b). But any function in $\Lambda^{(2)}$ can be approximated in mean square by bounded functions.

Proof of Theorem 4.1: Part (a) follows from Lemma A5.5 of BKRW. Proof of (b): Since $\Lambda^{(3)} \subset \Lambda^{(2)}$, in order to prove $\Lambda^{(3)} \perp \Lambda^{(1)}$, it suffices to show that for any H=h(V),

$$E[\mathbf{g}(H)A^{(2)\prime}]=0 \tag{A.1}$$

But $E[\mathbf{g}(H)A^{(2)\prime}] = E\{E[\mathbf{g}(H)A^{(2)\prime} \mid V]\} = E[\Sigma_r \pi(r,V_{(r)})E[H \mid V_{(r)}]a^{(2)}(r,V_{(r)})'] = E\{HE[A^{(2)} \mid V]'\}=0$, where the 2nd identity is by (4.2), and the third by iterated expectations. Now $\Lambda^{(3)}$ is closed by definition. To prove $\Lambda^{(1)}$ is closed, we note that $\Lambda^{(1)}$ is the image of the closed set $\Lambda^{(F)}$ under the linear operator $\mathbf{g}(\cdot)$. Hence it suffices to show $\mathbf{g}(\cdot)$ has a continuous inverse. But $\mathbf{g}(\cdot)$ has a continuous inverse by part a) of proposition A1.5 of BKRW (1991) since $E[\,\|\mathbf{g}(A^{(F)})\|^2] \geq E[I(R=\mathbf{1})A^{(F)\prime}A^{(F)}] = E[\pi(\mathbf{1})A^{(F)\prime}A^{(F)}] \geq \sigma E[\,\|A^{(F)}\|^2]$ where the equality is by (4.2) and the final inequality by (4.3). To prove part (c), it follows from Lemma A5.5 of BKRW and Lemma C.4 of Newey (1990b) that Λ is the closure of $\{\mathbf{g}(A^{(F)}) + A^{(3)}; A^{(3)} \in \Lambda^{(3)}, A^{(F)} \in \Lambda^{(F)}\}$ which is $\Lambda^{(1)} \oplus \Lambda^{(3)}$ by part (b).

To prove (d) and (e), note that if $B \in \Lambda_0^{\perp}$, then for some D^{**}, $B=D^{**}-\Pi[D^{**} \mid \Lambda]$ with $E[D^{**}]=0$. Hence, by $\Lambda^{(1)} \perp \Lambda^{(3)}$, $B = D^*-\Pi[D^* \mid \Lambda^{(3)}]$, where $D^* \equiv D^{**}-\Pi[D^{**} \mid \Lambda^{(1)}] \in \Lambda_0^{(1),\perp}$. Now, for any $H^*=h^*(R,V_{(R)})$, (4.2) implies

$$H^*-\mathbf{u}(H) \in \Lambda^{(2)} \ , \tag{A.2a}$$

with $H \equiv E[H^* \mid V]$. Thus,

$$E[H^*\mathbf{g}(A^{(F)\prime})] = E[\mathbf{u}(H)\mathbf{g}(A^{(F)})'] = E[HA^{(F)\prime}] \tag{A.2b}$$

where the first equality is by (A.2a) and $\Lambda^{(1)} \perp \Lambda^{(2)}$, and the second uses (4.2). Hence,

$$H^* \in \Lambda_0^{(1),\perp} \Rightarrow H \in \Lambda_0^{(F),\perp} \ . \tag{A.3}$$

Now write $D^* = \mathbf{u}(D) + \{D^*-\mathbf{u}(D)\}$, and note $D \equiv E[D^* \mid V] \in \Lambda_0^{(F),\perp}$ and $D^*-\mathbf{u}(D) \in \Lambda^{(2)}$ by (A.2a), proving part (d). Further, part (e) follows from $E[BS_\beta'] = E[B\mathbf{g}(S_\beta^{(F)})'] = E[\mathbf{u}(D)\mathbf{g}(S_\beta^{(F)})'] = E[DS_\beta^{(F)\prime}]$ where the second equality uses (A.2b) and $\Lambda^{(1)} \perp \Lambda^{(3)}$ and the third uses (4.2).

Proof of part (f): $S_{eff} = S_\beta - \Pi[S_\beta \mid \Lambda] = S_\beta - \Pi[S_\beta \mid \Lambda^{(1)}] \in \Lambda_0^{(1),\perp}$ since, by (A.1), $S_\beta \equiv \mathbf{g}(S_\beta^{(F)}) \perp \Lambda^{(3)}$. Since $\Pi[S_\beta \mid \Lambda^{(1)}] = \mathbf{g}(A_\beta^{(F)})$ for some $A_\beta^{(F)} \in \Lambda^{(F)}$ by $\Lambda^{(1)}$ closed, $S_{eff} =$

$\mathbf{g}(A_\beta) = \mathbf{u}\{\mathbf{m}(A_\beta)\} + [\mathbf{g}(A_\beta)-\mathbf{u}\{\mathbf{m}(A_\beta)\}]$, where $A_\beta = S_\beta^{(F)}-A_\beta^{(F)}$. Since for any $H^*\equiv h^*(V)$, $E[\mathbf{g}(H^*) \mid V] = \mathbf{m}(H^*)$ and, so by (A.2a), $\mathbf{g}(H^*)-\mathbf{u}[\mathbf{m}(H^*)]\in\Lambda^{(2)}$, it follows from (A.1), that

$$\mathbf{u}[\mathbf{m}(H^*)]-\mathbf{g}(H^*) = \Pi[\mathbf{u}\{\mathbf{m}(H^*)\} \mid \Lambda^{(2)}] \quad . \tag{A.4}$$

Letting $D_{eff} = \mathbf{m}(A_\beta)$, we have $S_{eff} = \mathbf{u}(D_{eff}) - \Pi[\mathbf{u}(D_{eff}) \mid \Lambda^{(2)}]$, with $D_{eff}\in\Lambda_0^{(F),\perp}$ by (A.3).

To show D_{eff} is the unique $D\in\Lambda_0^{(F),\perp}$ solving

$$\Pi[\mathbf{m}^{-1}(D) \mid \Lambda_0^{(F),\perp}] = S_\beta^{(F)}-\Pi[S_\beta^{(F)} \mid \Lambda_0^{(F),\perp}] \quad , \tag{A.5}$$

we first show $\mathbf{m}^{-1}(D)$ is well-defined, i.e., for any $D=d(V)$, there exists a unique $H=h(V)$ such that $D=\mathbf{m}(H)$. To do so, we note $D=\mathbf{m}(H)$ is equivalent to $\pi(\mathbf{1})^{-1}D=H+\pi(\mathbf{1})^{-1}\Sigma_{r\neq\mathbf{1}}\pi(r)E[H \mid V_{(r)}] \equiv (\mathbf{i}+\mathbf{k})H$, where $\mathbf{i}$ is the identity operator and $\mathbf{k}=\pi(\mathbf{1})^{-1}\Sigma_{r\neq\mathbf{1}}\Pi(r)E[\cdot \mid V_{(r)}]$. Thus, by the Riesz theory for type 2 Fredholm operator equations $D=\mathbf{m}(H)$ will have a unique solution H if the bounded linear operator $\mathbf{k}$ is compact and the null space of $(\mathbf{i}+\mathbf{k})$ is $\{0\}$. [Note $\mathbf{k}$ is bounded since $\pi(\mathbf{1})^{-1}$ is bounded by (4.3)]. But $E(\cdot \mid V_{(r)})$ is Hilbert-Schmidt and, thus compact (BKRW, Section A.4). Since the product of two bounded linear operators is compact if either is compact, $\mathbf{k}$ is compact (Kress, 1990). To show that if $H\neq 0$, $(\mathbf{i}+\mathbf{k})(H)\neq 0$, write $E[\{\pi(\mathbf{1})\}H\}'[\mathbf{i}+\mathbf{k}](H)] = E\{H'[\Sigma_r\pi(r)E(H \mid V_{(r)})]\} \geq E[\pi(\mathbf{1}) \| H \|^2] \geq \sigma E[\| H \|^2]$ where the last inequality uses (4.3). Now, D_{eff} satisfies (A.5) by $\mathbf{m}^{-1}(D_{eff}) = S_\beta^{(F)}-A_\beta^{(F)}, A_\beta^{(F)}\in\Lambda^{(F)}$.

To show uniqueness of D_{eff}, suppose (A.5) holds for $\tilde{D}\in\Lambda_0^{(F),\perp}, \tilde{D} \neq D_{eff}$. Then $\mathbf{m}^{-1}(\tilde{D}) = S_\beta^{(F)} + \tilde{A}^{(F)}$ for $\tilde{A}^{(F)} \neq -A_\beta^{(F)}$, $\tilde{A}^{(F)}\in\Lambda^{(F)}$. Hence, $-\mathbf{g}(\tilde{A}^{(F)}) \neq \Pi[\mathbf{g}(S_\beta^{(F)}) \mid \Lambda^{(1)}]$, so, by definition, $A^{(F)}$ exists such that $0 \neq E[\mathbf{g}(S_\beta^{(F)}+\tilde{A}^{(F)})\mathbf{g}(A^{(F)})']$, i.e., $0 \neq E[\mathbf{u}\{\mathbf{m}(S_\beta^{(F)}+\tilde{A}^{(F)})\}\mathbf{g}(A^{(F)})'] = E[\mathbf{u}(\tilde{D})\mathbf{g}(A^{(F)})'] = E[\tilde{D}A^{(F)'}]$ so $\tilde{D}$ is not in $\Lambda_0^{(F),\perp}$ where we have used (A.2b) and (4.2). Thus we have proved uniqueness by contradiction.

Proof of (g): g is just (A.4) above.

Proof of Theorem 4.2: If missingness is monotone and (4.2) holds, (a)-(d) of Theorem 4.2 follow directly from their definitions. Part (f) follows from the fact that under monotone missingness $f[R \mid V] = \prod_{m=1}^{M} \{f(R_m \mid R_{m-1}=1,\overline{V}_m)\}^{R_{m-1}}$ with parametric submodels $\prod_{m=1}^{M} \{f(R_m \mid R_{m-1}=1,\overline{V}_m;\psi)\}^{R_{m-1}}$. It is straightforward to show (f) implies (g). Part (e) can be shown to hold by induction. Part (h) follows from part (c) of Theorem (4.2) and part (f) of Theorem 4.1.

Appendix 3:

In this Appendix, we further discuss the asymptotic distribution of some of our proposed tests and estimators. Under sufficient regularity and smoothness conditions, the estimators $\hat{\hat{\beta}}^*(h)$ of Section 3k and $\hat{\hat{\beta}}^*(h_{eff}^{MN})$ of Section 4c, the test statistic $\psi(\hat{r}_{\bar{g}},w,c^*)$ of Lemma 3.2, and the adaptive test $\psi(r,\hat{w}_{op}^r,c^*)$ discussed following Lemma 3.1 will be RAL.

If RAL, the equality of the limiting distributions of (a) $\hat{\hat{\beta}}^*(h)$ with that of $\hat{\beta}^*(h)$ and (b) $\hat{\hat{\beta}}^*(\hat{h}_{eff})$ with that of $\hat{\beta}^*(h_{eff})$ are a consequence of Proposition (3) in Newey (1992a) since, in Newey's notation, $E[M(z) \mid v]=0$. Newey's Proposition (3) gives conditions under which substituting estimates for an unknown population quantity has no effect on the limiting distribution of a statistic. Similarly, if RAL, Newey's Proposition (3) implies that (a) the limiting distribution of $\psi(\hat{r}_{\bar{g}},w,c^*)$ is as stated in Lemma (3.2), and (b) that $\psi(r,\hat{w}^r_{op},c^*)$ has the same limiting distribution as $\psi(r,w^*,c^*)$ where w^* is the limit of $\hat{w}^r_{op}$.

We now sketch the derivation of the limiting distribution (3.7) of $n^{-1/2}S\{\hat{D}^{AF2}(\beta_0)\}$. By the identity in the first paragraph of Section (3e), $n^{-1/2}S\{\hat{D}(\beta_0)\} = n^{-1/2}\Sigma_i\tilde{D}_i(\beta_0) - n^{-1/2}\Sigma_i\Psi_i(\hat{H}_{1i})$ with $\hat{H}_{1i}(u) = \tilde{D}_i(\beta_0)/\hat{K}_i(u)$, where we have suppressed the AF2 superscript. Proposition (3) of Newey (1992a) implies that $n^{-1/2}\Sigma_i\Psi_i(\hat{H}_{1i}) = n^{-1/2}\Sigma_i\Psi_i(\hat{H}_{2i}) + o_p(1)$ where $\hat{H}_{2i}(u) = D_i(\beta_0)/\hat{K}_i(u)$. Thus, by Lemma 3.5, (3.7) follows from

Theorem A.2: Under (2.2b) $n^{-1/2}S^{(F)}\{\tilde{D}(\beta_0)\} \equiv n^{-1/2}\Sigma_i\tilde{D}_i(\beta_0) = n^{-1/2}\Sigma_iU_f + o_p(1)$ (A.6) with $U_f = D(\beta_0)-E[D(\beta_0) \mid Z]$.

Sketch of Proof: With $\tilde{D}(\beta_0) = \tilde{D}(\beta_0,h,\theta), n^{-1/2}S^{(F)}\{\tilde{D}(\beta_0)\} = A_1+A_2$, where $A_1 = n^{1/2}\tilde{E}\{\int_{-\infty}^{\infty} dM_\epsilon(u)[h(u,Z)-\tilde{\mathscr{L}}(u,\beta_0,h)]\}$, $A_2 = n^{1/2}\tilde{E}\{\int_{-\infty}^{\infty} duI\{\nu>u\}[h^*(u,Z)-\tilde{\mathscr{L}}(u,\beta_0,h^*)]\}$, with $h^*(u,Z) = \lambda_\epsilon(u)h(u,Z) - \theta(u,Z)$. Now, by a standard argument using Lenglart's inequality, $A_1=A_{11}+o_p(1)$ with $A_{11} = n^{1/2}\tilde{E}[\int_{-\infty}^{\infty} dM_\epsilon(u)[h(u,Z)-\mathscr{L}(u,\beta_0,h)]]$. Further $A_2=A_{21}+A_{22}+A_{23}$, where, with $\mathscr{L}(u) \equiv \mathscr{L}(u,\beta_0,h^*)$, $\tilde{\mathscr{L}}(u) \equiv \tilde{\mathscr{L}}(u,\beta_0,h^*)$, $\bar{F}_\nu(u) = \bar{F}_\mu(u)\bar{F}_\epsilon(u)$ with $\bar{F}_\mu(u) = pr(\mu>u)$, $A_{21} = n^{1/2}\tilde{E}[\int_{-\infty}^{\infty} duI(\nu>u)\{h^*(u,Z)-\mathscr{L}(u)\}]$, $A_{22} = n^{1/2}\int_{-\infty}^{\infty} du\bar{F}_\nu(u)[\mathscr{L}(u)-\tilde{\mathscr{L}}(u)]$, $A_{23} = \int_{-\infty}^{\infty} du\, n^{1/2}\tilde{E}[I\{\nu>u\}-\bar{F}_\nu(u)][\mathscr{L}(u)-\tilde{\mathscr{L}}(u)]$. Now, under regularity conditions, A_{23} is $o_p(1)$ since $\int_{-\infty}^{\infty} n^{1/2}\tilde{E}[I\{\nu>u\}-\bar{F}_\nu(u)]$ is $O_p(1)$ by the CLT, and $\mathscr{L}(u)-\tilde{\mathscr{L}}(u)$ converges to zero uniformly in u. Thus $n^{-1/2}S^{(F)}\{\tilde{D}(\beta_0)\} = n^{-1/2}\Sigma_iD_i(\beta_0)+A_{22}+o_p(1)$ since $A_{11}+A_{21} = n^{-1/2}\Sigma_iD_i(\beta_0)$. Thus, it remains to show $A_{22} = -n^{-1/2}\Sigma_iE[D_i(\beta_0) \mid Z_i] + o_p(1)$.

Since $\tilde{\mathscr{L}}(u) = \tilde{\mathscr{L}}_1(u)/\tilde{\mathscr{L}}_2(u)$ with $\tilde{\mathscr{L}}_1(u) = \tilde{E}[I\{\mu>u\}h^*(u,Z)]$, $\tilde{\mathscr{L}}_2(u) = \tilde{E}[I\{\mu>u\}]$, a Taylor expansion around $\mathscr{L}_1(u)$ and $\mathscr{L}_2(u)$ gives $A_{22} = A_{22}^* + o_p(1)$, where

$$A_{22}^* = n^{1/2}\int_{-\infty}^{\infty} du\bar{F}_\epsilon(u)\bar{F}_\mu(u)\left\{\frac{\tilde{\mathscr{L}}_1(u)-\mathscr{L}_1(u)}{\bar{F}_\mu(u)} + \frac{\mathscr{L}_1(u)[\tilde{\mathscr{L}}_2(u)-\bar{F}_\mu(u)]}{[\bar{F}_\mu(u)]^2}\right\} =$$

$$-n^{1/2}\int_{-\infty}^{\infty} du\bar{F}_\epsilon(u)[\tilde{\mathscr{L}}_1(u) - \tilde{\mathscr{L}}_2(u)\mathscr{L}_1(u)/\bar{F}_\mu(u)] = -n^{-1/2}\Sigma_i\int_{-\infty}^{\infty} du\bar{F}_\epsilon(u)I\{\mu>u\}$$

$$\left\{h^*(u,Z) - \frac{E[h^*(u,Z)I(\mu>u]}{E[I(\mu>u)]}\right\} = -n^{-1/2}\Sigma_iE[D_i(\beta_0) \mid Z_i].$$ A more abstract approach to the proof of Theorem A.2 is to use Theorem 4.3 in Newey (1990a).

Appendix 4

In this Appendix, we assume that (i) time to potential end of follow-up Q_1 and T are dependent due to rapid secular changes in the prognosis of patients at entry into the trial over the calendar year of enrollment; but (ii), in contrast with Section 2, we no longer assume that these changes can be fully explained by secular changes in the covariates recorded in $\bar{L}(u)$. Hence (2.4a) will be false when, as in Section 2, $Q \equiv \min(Q_1,Q_2)$.

Redefine Q to be Q_2, time to initiation of prophylaxis, and, for notational convenience, write time to potential end of follow-up Q_1 as C, and include C in $\bar{L}(u)$ for each $u, u \geq 0$. (Note C is observed even for subjects failing prior to C.) Replace c^* by C wherever c^* occurs in the paper, so, for example, henceforth, $X = \min(T,Q,C)$; $X^* = \min(T,C)$; $\Delta = I(T<C), \tau = I(X \neq Q)$, and the C-observed and C-full data are given by (2.1) and (3.4) with C replacing c^*. With Q,X, and $\bar{L}(u)$ so redefined, (2.4a) will again hold under the assumptions concerning initiation of prophylaxis given in the introduction (provided data on PCP history was recorded in $\bar{L}(u)$). If Z were the treatment indicator, by Z assigned completely at random, we would have

$$C \amalg Z \; . \tag{A.7}$$

Consider the conditional AF models

$$\mathrm{pr}[T>t \mid Z,C] = \bar{F}_0(e^{\beta_0' Z} t \mid C) \; , \tag{A.8}$$

and the more general model

$$\mathrm{pr}[T>t \mid Z,C] = \bar{F}_0[e^{g(Z,C,\beta_0)} t \mid C] \tag{A.9}$$

where $g(Z,C,\beta) = 0$ if $Z = 0$ or $\beta = 0$, $g(\cdot,\cdot,\cdot)$ is a fixed real-valued function, and $\bar{F}_0(t \mid c)$ is, for each c, an unspecified survival function. If $g(Z,C,\beta_0)$ depends on C, we say there is a C-treatment interaction. We will show how to generalize the AF2 method of estimation to consistently estimate the parameters of (A.9) from the C-full data under (A.7) and from the C-observed data under (2.4a) and (A.7) [provided K(X) is bounded away from zero]. Only the (generalized) AF2-method allows one to obtain asymptotically normal and unbiased estimators of β_0 from the C-observed data without having to use non-parametric methods to estimate the conditional law of either $\epsilon = \ell n T + g(Z,C,\beta_0)$ or Z given C. Furthermore, since (A.8) and (A.7) together imply the marginal AF model (2.2b), it follows that the parameters of (2.2b) can still be estimated when (A.8), (A.7), and (2.4a) [as redefined] hold.

Let, h(u,Z,C), and $\theta(u,Z,C)$ be fixed functions taking values in R^p. Redefine $\tilde{D}^{AF2}(\beta) \equiv \hat{D}^{AF2}(\beta) \equiv \tilde{D}^{AF2}(\beta,h,\theta) \equiv [\int_{-\infty}^{\infty} dN_{\epsilon(\beta)}(u)\{h(u,Z,C) - \tilde{\mathscr{L}}^{AF2}(u,\beta,h,C)\}] - \int_{-\infty}^{\infty} du I\{\nu(\beta) \geq u\}\{\theta(u,Z,C) - \tilde{\mathscr{L}}^{AF2}(u,\beta,\theta,C)\}$, where $N_{\epsilon(\beta)}(u) = I[\nu(\beta) \leq u, \Delta=1]$, $\nu(\beta) = \min\{\epsilon(\beta),\mu(\beta)\}$, $\mu(\beta) = \ell n C + g(Z,C,\beta)$, $\epsilon(\beta) = \ell n T + g(Z,C,\beta)$, $\tilde{\mathscr{L}}^{AF2}(u,\beta,h,c) = \tilde{E}[I\{\ell n c + g(Z,c,\beta) > u\} h(u,Z)] / \tilde{E}[I\{\ell n c + g(Z,c,\beta) > u\}]$ and $\tilde{E}[I\{\ell n c + g(Z,c,\beta) > u\}] =$

$n^{-1}\sum_{i=1}^{n} I\{\ell nc+g(Z_i,c,\beta)>u\}$. $\tilde{D}^{AF2}(\beta,h,\theta,C)$ has a particularly simple form when Z is a dichotomous (0,1) variable. Specifically $\tilde{D}^{AF2}(\beta,h,\theta) \equiv \tilde{D}^{AF2}(\beta,r) = R(\beta)[Z-\tilde{E}(Z)]$, where $R(\beta) \equiv r\{\Delta(\beta),X^*(\beta),C\} \equiv \Delta(\beta)r_1[\epsilon(\beta),C] + \{1-\Delta(\beta)\}\{r_2[C(\beta),C]\}$, $C(\beta) \equiv \min(\ell nC, \ell nC+g(1,C,\beta))$, $X^*(\beta) \equiv \min[\epsilon(\beta),C(\beta)]$, $\Delta(\beta) = I[\epsilon(\beta)<C(\beta)]$, $r_2(u,C) = -\int_{-\infty}^{u}\theta_1(x,C)dx$, $r_1(u,C) = h_1(u,C) + r_2(u,C)$, and, e.g., we write $\theta(u,Z,C)$ as $Z\theta_1(u,C) + \theta_0(u,C)$.

Noting (A.7) and (A.9) imply that

$$(\epsilon,C)\coprod Z \tag{A.10}$$

with $\epsilon \equiv \epsilon(\beta_0)$, we see that $\tilde{\mathscr{L}}^{AF2}(u,\beta_0,h,c)$ converges in probability under (A.7) and (A.9), to $\mathscr{L}^{AF2}(u,\beta_0,h,c) \equiv E[h(u,Z,C)\mid \mu>u,C=c] = E[h(u,Z,C)\mid \nu>u,C=c]$ with $\mu=\mu(\beta_0)$ and $\nu=\nu(\beta_0)$.

With the above redefinitions, Theorem (3.3) [under model (A.9) and (A.7)] and Theorem (3.4) [under model (A.9), (A.7), and (2.4a)] remain true for $\tilde{\beta}^{AF2}$ and $\hat{\beta}^{AF2}$, with $U_f^{AF2} \equiv U_f^{AF2}(h,\theta) = D^{AF2}(\beta_0) - E[D^{AF2}(\beta_0)\mid Z]$, $\kappa^{AF2} \equiv \kappa^{AF2}(h,\theta) = E[U_f^{AF2}(h,\theta)U_f^{AF2}(h_{op}^{AF},\theta_{op}^{AF})']$ where $h_{op}^{AF}(u,Z,C) = Z\partial\ell n\lambda_\epsilon(u\mid C)/\partial u$ and $\theta_{op}^{AF}(u,Z,C) = Z\partial\lambda_\epsilon(u\mid C)/\partial u$. If $Z\in\{0,1\}$, $U_f^{AF2} \equiv U_f^{AF2}(r) = \{R(\beta_0)-E[R(\beta_0)]\}\{Z-E[Z]\}$. The formulae for the variance estimates in Section 3j.1 and 3j.2 need to be modified only in that, now, $P_{ji}(\beta) \equiv P_{ji}(\beta,h,\theta) \equiv [\int_{-\infty}^{\infty} dN_{\epsilon_j(\beta)}(u)\{h(u,Z,C_j) - \tilde{\mathscr{L}}^{AF2}(u,\beta,h,C_j)\}] - \int_{-\infty}^{\infty} du I\{\epsilon_j(\beta)>u\}I\{\ell nC_j+g(Z_i,C_j,\beta)>u\}[\theta(u,Z_i,C_j) - \tilde{\mathscr{L}}^{AF2}(u,\beta,\theta,C_j)]$. If Z is dichotomous, we use $\tilde{V}ar(U_f^{AF2}(\beta)) \equiv \tilde{V}ar\{U_f^{AF2}(\beta,r)\} = \tilde{E}[\{R(\beta) - \tilde{E}[R(\beta)]\}^2]\tilde{E}[\{Z-\tilde{E}(Z)\}^2]$.

Since (C,Z) is ancillary, $S_{eff}^{(F)} = U_f^{AF2}(h_{op},\theta_{op})$ is the efficient score for β_0 based on the C-full data in model (A.9) whether or not (A.7) is true, and, if (A.7) is true, whether or not (A.7) is known to be true *a priori*. Similarly, the efficient score S_{eff} and the solution D_{eff} to Eq. (4.5) based on the C-observed data in the model defined by (A.9), $K(X)>\sigma>0$ w.p.1, and (2.4a) do not depend on whether the restriction (A.7) is true. Thus the restriction (A.7) was useful only in that it allowed us to consistently estimate β_0 of (A.9) without requiring non-parametric estimation of the conditional law of either ϵ or Z given C. [$\Lambda_0^{(F),\perp}$ equals $\{U_f^{AF2}(h,\theta) + a(Z,C) - E[a(Z,C)\mid C] - E[a(Z,C)\mid Z]\}$, where a(Z,C) is any mean 0 function of Z and C, when (A.7) is known, and equals $\{U_f^{AF2}(h,\theta)\}$ when (A.7) is true but not known, although D_{eff} is of the form $U_f^{AF2}(h,\theta)$ in either case.]

Acknowledgement: This work was in part supported by grants K04-ES00180, 5-P30-ES00002, and R01-ES03405 from NIEHS. We are indebted to W. Newey for many helpful conversations concerning the subject matter of this paper. Z. Ying also provided helpful advice.

Bibliography

Andersen, P.K. and Gill, R.D. (1982). Cox's regression model for counting processes: A large sample study. Ann. Statist. 10:1100-1120.

Begun, J.M., Hall, W.J., Huang, W.M. and Wellner, J.A. (1983). Information and asymptotic efficiency in parametric-nonparametric models. Ann. Statist. 11:432-452.

Bickel, P., Klassen, C., Ritov, Y., and Wellner, J. (1990). Efficient and adaptive inferences in semiparametric models. (forthcoming)

Chamberlain, G. (1987). Asymptotic efficiency in estimation with conditional moment restrictions. J. Econometrics. 34:305-324.

Gray, R.J., and Tsiatis, A.A. (1989). The linear rank test for use when the main interest is in differences and cure rates. Biometrics 45:899-904.

Gill, R. (1980). Censoring and Stochastic Integrals, Mathematical Center Tract 124, Mathematische Centrum, Amsterdam.

Kalbfleisch, J.D. and Prentice, R.L. (1980). The Statistical Analysis of Failure Time Data. Wiley, New York.

Kress, R. (1990). Linear integral equations. Springer-Verlag Berlin.

Koul, H., Susarla, V. and Van Ryzin, J. (1981). Regression analysis with randomly right censored data. Ann. Statist. 9:1276-88.

Lagakos, S., Lim, L., and Robins, J.M. (1990). Adjusting for early treatment termination in comparative clinical trials. Statist. Med. 9:1417-1424.

Newey, W.K. (1990a). Semiparametric efficiency bounds. J Appl. Econom. 5:99-135.

Newey, W.K. (1990b). Efficient estimation of Tobit models under conditional symmetry in W. Barnett, J. Powell, and G. Tauchen, (eds), Semiparametric and Non-parametric Methods in Econometrics and Statistics, Cambridge Univ. Press, Cambridge, pp. 291-336.

Newey, W.K. (1992a). The variance of semiparametric estimators. Econometrica (forthcoming).

Newey, W.K. (1992b). Efficient estimation of semiparametric models via moment restrictions, manuscript, MIT.

Pakes, A. and Pollard, D. (1989). Simulation in the asymptotics of optimization estimators. Econometrica 57:1027-1057.

Prentice, R.L. (1978). Linear rank tests with right censored data. Biometrika 65:167-179.

Ritov, Y. and Wellner, J.A. (1988). Censoring, martingales, and the Cox model. Contemp. Math. Statist. Inf. Stoch. Pro. (N.U. Prabhu, ed.) 80:191-220. Amer. Math. Soc.

Ritov, Y. (1990). Estimation in a linear regression model with censored data. Ann. Statist. 18:303-328.

Robins, J.M. (1991). Estimating regression parameters in the presence of dependent censoring. (submitted)

Robins, J.M. and Tsiatis, A.A. (1991). Correcting for non-compliance in randomized trials using rank preserving structural failure time models. Commun. Statist.-Theory Meth. 20:2609-2631.

Robins, J.M., Rotnitzky, A., and Zhao, L.P. (1992). Analysis of semiparametric regression models for repeated outcomes under the presence of missing data. (submitted)

Robins, J.M., and Rotnitzky, A. (1992). Semiparametric efficiency in multivariate regression models with missing data. (submitted)

Robins, J.M., Zhao, L.P., Rotnitzky, A., and Lipsitz, S. (1991). Estimation of regression coefficients when a regressor is not always observed. (submitted).

Rubin, D.B. (1976). Inference and missing data. Biometrika 63:581-92.

Tsiatis, A.A. (1990). Estimating regression parameters using linear rank tests for censored data. Ann. Statist. 18:354-372.

Wei, L.J., Ying, Z., and Lin, D.Y. (1990). Linear regression analysis of censored survival data based on rank tests. Biometrika 77:845-852.

Departments of Epidemiology and Biostatistics, Harvard School of Public Health, 665 Huntington Ave., Boston, MA 02115. bjr/t2e.cr

Section 4
General Methodological Investigations

SEMI-PARAMETRIC ESTIMATION OF THE INCUBATION PERIOD OF AIDS

Jeremy M.G. Taylor and Yun Chon

Abstract

The incubation period distribution of AIDS is estimated from the grouped bivariate data which arises from a prevalent cohort study. A penalised likelihood approach is used to obtain smooth estimates of the incubation period distribution. We also examine how the individuals age at HIV infection and changes in the incubation period can be incorporated into the analysis.

1. Introduction

The scientific problem to be investigated in this article is to estimate the incubation period distribution of AIDS and to understand the effect of covariates on this distribution from the Multicenter AIDS Cohort Study of homosexual men recruited in Los Angeles in 1984–5. The incubation period is defined as the time interval from infection with the AIDS virus (HIV) to the onset of clinical symptoms (AIDS). In statistical terms, the problem is that of semi-parametrically estimating the joint bivariate distribution of two random variables conditional on covariates when the observed data is grouped. A similar analysis of an older version of this data set has been published in the medical literature (Taylor et al. 1991), and the basic approach used in analysing this particular dataset has been described in a statistical article (Taylor et al. 1991). This article is a continuation of these previous articles but with a focus on the statistical issues and the problems associated with introducing covariates into the analysis. The specific covariates which are discussed in this paper are treatment variables, which is essentially chronologic time, and age at HIV infection. In this article, we will describe the basic approach and then elaborate on parts of the analysis.

Previous work in this area using related methodology has been performed by others, both using parametric models (Brookmeyer et al. 1989, Kuo et al. 1991) and semi-parametric and non-parametric approaches (deGruttola et al. 1989, Bacchetti et al. 1991, Taylor et al. 1991).

2. Statistical Description of the Problem

There is a sample of n subjects, the observation on subject i consists of a known region B_i in the bivariate positive quadrant $\mathbb{R}^+ \times \mathbb{R}^+$. That is, there is a true unknown specific value $(x_i, y_i) \epsilon \mathbb{R}^+ \times \mathbb{R}^+$ for each subject, but this value is not observed. All that is known is that $(x_i, y_i) \epsilon B_i$. In addition, covariates Z_i, which could depend on (x, y), exist for each subject. The distribution of x and y may or may not be independent conditional on Z. Also, there is a truncated region T_i, disjoint from B_i such that if (x_i, y_i) had been in region T_i, then subject i would have been excluded from the sample, with no knowledge of his existence. The aim is to estimate the joint distribution of (x, y) given Z; denote the corresponding density indexed by parameter θ by

$$f(x, y; Z, \theta) \quad \text{where} \int_{\mathbb{R}^+}\int_{\mathbb{R}^+} f(x, y; Z, \theta)\, dxdy = 1$$

The likelihood of the observations is given by

$$L = \prod_{i=1}^{n} L_i(f) = \prod_{i=1}^{n} \left\{ \frac{\int_{B_i} f(x,y;Z_i,\theta)dxdy}{1 - \int_{T_i} f(x,y;Z_i,\theta)dxdy} \right\}.$$

In this article, we attempt a semi-parametric approach by making only weak assumptions concerning the bivariate distribution f, and we ensure that the estimate of f is "smooth" by maximizing a penalised likelihood (Green 1987). In particular, we maximize

$$\log L - P(f, \lambda)$$

where $P(f, \lambda)$ is a penalty function which is large if f is "rough" and small if f is "smooth". $P(f, \lambda)$ is a non-negative function for which $P(f, 0) = 0$, with the smoothing parameter vector λ controlling the degree of smoothness of the estimate of f. In these problems, the value of λ is usually chosen separately from the parameters of f.

As well as its obvious "smoothed" MLE interpretation, maximum penalised likelihood (MPL) has a Bayesian interpretation in which $\exp(-P(f, \lambda))$ is viewed as proportional to a, possibly improper, prior for f, then the MPL estimate is the posterior mode estimate.

3. Data Description

The data are from the 1637 homosexual men who enrolled in the Los Angeles portion of the Multicenter AIDS Cohort Study between April 1984 and February 1985 (Kaslow et al. 1987). All participants were AIDS-free at the time of their enrollment. Semi-annual follow-up visits are scheduled at which time HIV antibody testing is performed. Some subjects have stopped attending the scheduled 6 month visits but continue to be followed by telephone or mail. AIDS diagnosis information is obtained from the participants, their friends, their doctors, disease registries, death certificates and obituaries columns.

With these follow–up procedures, participants who have dropped out are likely to be found later only if they develop AIDS. To counter this potential bias, we assumed that anyone who dropped out of the study prior to January 1987, and who had not yet been reported to have AIDS by January 1991, did not have AIDS before January 1987.

As the definition of AIDS was changed in September 1987, we exclude AIDS diagnoses which were only applicable after this date to ensure homogeneity of the definition, i.e. only the pre September 1987 definition of AIDS is used in this analysis.

The bivariate ($\mathbb{R}^+ \times \mathbb{R}^+$) space which is fundamental to this analysis is (Date of HIV infection) x (Incubation period), denoted by (X,Y). Each subject has a true value of (x, y), which is not known exactly but is known to lie in a region B_i. Let $t = x + y$ be the date of AIDS. In our analysis $x = 0$ is taken to be 1 January, 1979, and we do not consider any information beyond 31 December 1989; i.e. t and x are censored at this date. The exact position and shape of the region B_i will be different for each subject, as both x and t could be known exactly, right censored or interval censored. Each of the 1637 participants can be classified into one of eight possible shapes for B_i. The boundaries which define the 8 shapes are (1) $x < I_0$, $t > A_4$, (2) $x < I_0$, $t = A_1$, (3) $x < I_0$, $A_2 < t \leq A_3$, (4) $I_1 < x \leq I_2$, $t > A_4$, (5) $I_1 < x \leq I_2$, $t = A_1$, (6) $I_1 < x \leq I_2$, $A_2 < t \leq A_3$, (7) $x > I_1$, $t > I_1$, (8) $x > I_1$, $t > A_4$. The above boundary dates are defined as follows. I_0 is the date of enrollment, I_1 is the date of the last HIV negative test, I_2 is the date of the first HIV positive test for seroconverters, A_1 is the date of AIDS diagnosis, A_2 and A_3 bound the date of AIDS when it is interval censored and A_4 is the last follow–up date at which AIDS is known not to be diagnosed. Note that the A's and I's depend on i. Groups 1, 2 and 3 are seropositive at enrollment; groups 4, 5 and 6 are seroconverters and groups 7 and 8 are seronegative. The number of subjects in the 8 groups are 545, 255, 9, 93, 12, 0, 589, and 134, respectively. The truncation region T_i is $\{(x, y)): x + y < I_0\}$.

Other AIDS studies have suggested that the incubation period distribution is influenced by the individuals' age at the time of infection (Darby et al. 1990, Biggar et al. 1990) and by the effect of treatments (Gail et al. 1990), specifically for this dataset the relevant treatments are AZT and aerosol pentamidine (AP). Both these variables present different problems when introduced into the analysis.

The exact age at HIV infection is unknown for nearly everyone in the cohort, however, it can be reasonably approximated by assuming the date of infection to be two years before enrollment for groups (1), (2) and (3), to be $\frac{1}{2}(I_1 + I_2)$ for groups (4), (5) and (6), to be 3 years after I_1 for groups (7) and (8). In addition, age–at–infection is treated as a binary variable, either 35 and older (n = 840), or 34 and younger (n = 797). We are primarily interested in how age effects the incubation period; however it should also be noted that the HIV infection distribution for the two age groups is likely to be different.

The treatments AZT and AP began in this cohort in approximately mid–1987 and increased in prevalence in later years. It is known when most but no all of the individuals in the study began therapy, however, we will not use this information because of the selection bias problems. In particular, subjects without AIDS choose therapy because of their greater risk of imminent AIDS due to their deteriorating immune system and ARC–like symptoms. If the actual treatment information for each individual was used in the analysis, it is quite possible that treatment would appear to be harmful rather than beneficial.

4. Discrete Bivariate Model

We adopt a semi–parametric approach for the estimation of f. The data are discretized into 6 month units, converting the $\mathbb{R}^+ \times \mathbb{R}^+$ bivariate space into a 23 x 23 contingency table. Let j denote the index of date of infection, where j = 1 indicates x ϵ[1 Jan 1979, 30 June 1979] and j = 23 indicates x > 31 Dec 1989. Similarly, k denotes the incubation period, k = 1 indicates y ϵ (0, 0.5], and k = 23 indicates y > 11 years.

The probability model for the ith subject in (j, k) cell is written as

$$P_{jk}(Z_i) = f_j \, g_{k|j}(Z_i) \text{ where } \sum_{j=1}^{23} f_j = 1 \text{ and } \sum_{k=1}^{23} g_{k|j}(Z_i) = 1 \text{ for all } j, i$$

where f_j is the marginal distribution for the date of HIV infection, and $g_{k|j}$ is the conditional distribution for the incubation period. Notice that we do not allow covariates to influence the infection distribution, although this generalisation could be easily incorporated. The likelihood of the observations is the same as described above, with sums replacing integrals in an obvious way.

We assume $f_j = c \dfrac{e^{j-4}}{1 + e^{j-4}}$ for j = 1,...,6, with the parameter c to be estimated. This parameterization for f_j was used to reduce instability problems in the estimation procedure, and is motivated by epidemiologic models for the growth of the HIV epidemic. In a sensitivity analysis, two other parametric forms of f_j for small j were considered. The results are reported elsewhere (Taylor et al. 1991), but in both cases the changes in the estimated infection and incubation period distribution were negligible.

The incubation period distribution g is parameterized in terms of the hazard h, that is

$$g_{k|j}(Z_i) = h_{k|j}(Z_i) \prod_{l=1}^{k-1} (1 - h_{l|j}(Z_i)) \quad k = 1,...,22;$$

$$\text{and} \quad g_{23|j}(Z_i) = 1 - \sum_{k=1}^{22} g_{k|j}(Z_i).$$

Individual level covariates can be introduced through a log-linear model

$$h_{k|j}(Z_i) = h^{\circ}_{k|j} \exp(\beta Z_i)$$

which generalises to a proportional hazard model in continuous time. For reasons explained below, we do not use this model for the individual level covariate age-at-infection. Also individual level therapy variables are not considered. So from here onwards we drop from the notation the dependence of the hazard on Z_i, although to investigate the effect of treatment on the incubation period a log-linear model for the hazard is used.

5. Penalty Function

The penalty function we used was

$$\frac{\lambda_1}{2} \sum_{j=5}^{20} (f_j + f_{j+2} - 2f_{j+1})^2 + \frac{\lambda_2}{2} \sum_{k=0}^{20} (h_k + h_{k+2} - 2h_{k+1})^2.$$

Note that very large values of λ_1 and λ_2 would force f and h to be linear. It is well known that the hazard of developing AIDS is very low in the first 2 years after infection and has frequently been modelled as a Weibull with shape parameter 2 to 2.5. For this reason and to assist in the computational instability problems, we defined $h_0 = 0$ and included it as part of the penalty function.

6. Confidence Intervals

Confidence intervals are based on 100 Bootstrap samples of the 1637 subjects in the cohort. Three approaches to obtaining Bootstrap confidence intervals were considered, the simple percentile method, the bias-corrected percentile method (Efron, 1982) and a method in which the 95% confidence intervals for a quantity of interest Q are of the form $(m^{-1}(\overline{m(Q)} - 2SD(m(Q))), m^{-1}(\overline{m(Q)} + 2SD(m(Q)))$, where m is a suitable chosen transformation to make the Bootstrap distribution approximately symmetric. As the quantities of interest are mainly probabilities or hazards we used a logit function for m. In nearly all cases the three methods gave very similar confidence intervals. The confidence intervals which are shown in some figures are for the bias corrected percentile method.

7. Computational Issues

All computations were performed using a Fortran program on an IBM 3090 with calls to IMSL program DBCONF for maximization of the penalized likelihood. The speed and convergence of the algorithm was unreliable if poor starting values were used or if the values of λ_1 and λ_2 were small. For small values of λ_1 and λ_2, there were multiple local maxima of the likelihood in some circumstances. With a good starting point and larger values of λ_1 and λ_2, the speed of convergence was substantially improved. Other authors (Bacchetti and Jewell, 1991) have extended the work of Turnbull (1976) on the EM algorithm to find the MPL estimates. This is an attractive alternative to our brute force approach which would enable one to consider a greater number of parameters.

8. Choice of Smoothing Parameters

One method of choosing a suitable value for λ is cross-validation. Let $\hat{f}(\lambda\ i)$ denote the MPL estimate of f when observation i is deleted, then we choose λ which maximizes $\prod_{i=1}^{n} L_i(\hat{f}(\lambda\ i))$. In our specific application, this is computationally too expensive, so instead we perform 20 fold cross-validation, in which we omit 1/20 of the data for each of 20 refittings.

An alternative to cross-validation is to choose the values of λ which give a "reasonable" amount smoothness to the solutions. This method, although subjective, will frequently be satisfactory.

Extensive cross-validation for a wide variety of values of λ_1 and λ_2 for the independence model suggested that good choices of λ_1 and λ_2 are 10^5 and 5×10^4, respectively (Taylor et al. 1991). Graphs of the estimates of f and h for these values of λ_1 and λ_2 are shown in Figures 1 and 2 together with 95% pointwise confidence intervals. Also shown in figure 2 without confidence intervals is the estimated hazard using only information up to mid-1987. The purpose of this analysis in which the data is censored in mid 1987 is to ensure

FIGURE 1
INFECTION DISTRIBUTION FOR INDEPENDENCE MODEL (β=0)
λ1=100,000, λ2=50,000

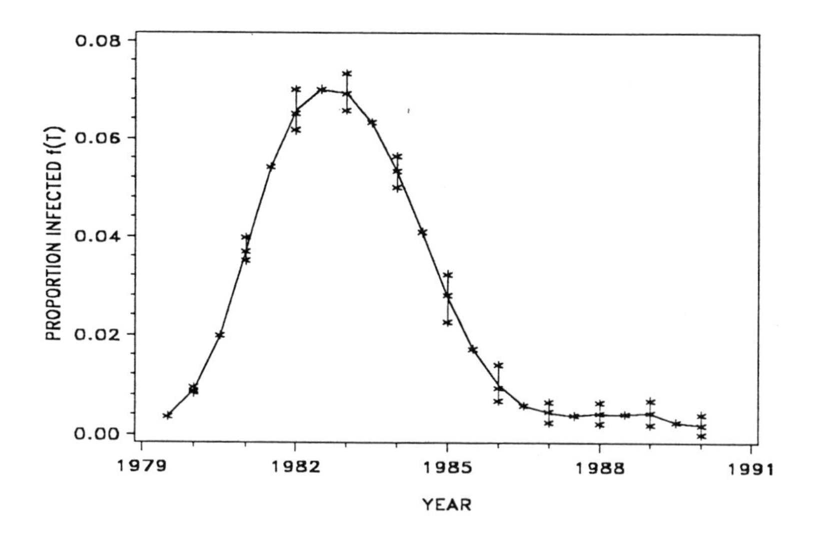

FIGURE 2
HAZARD FUNCTION FOR INDEPENDENCE MODEL (β=0)
λ1=100,000, λ2=50,000
O : HAZARD RATE USING DATA CENSORED JULY 87

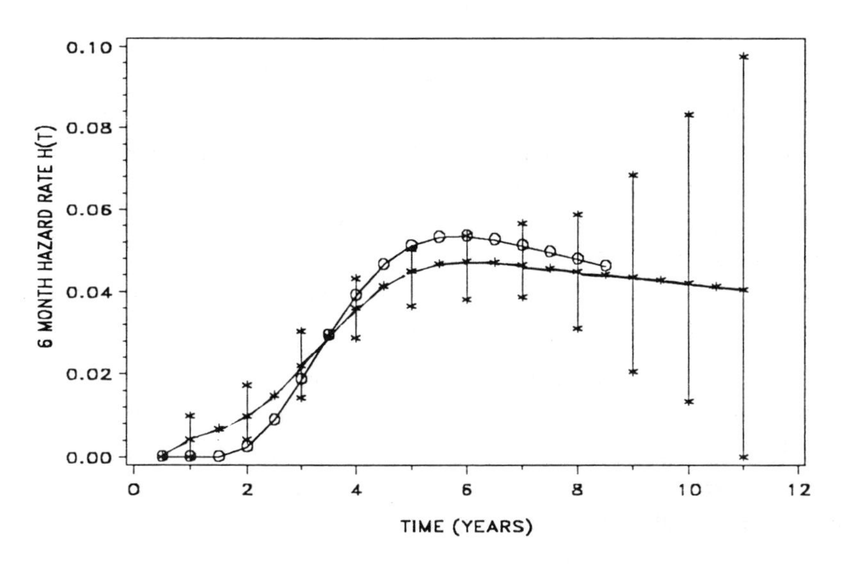

that the estimated hazard is not biased by AIDS therapy, which became widely available to pre–AIDS subjects in September 1987.

9. Influence of Age–at–Infection

It was obvious from examination of the data that the marginal distribution of the date of HIV infection was different for the two levels of the age–at–infection covariate. In particular, 73% of the under 35 group were seropositive at enrollment, whereas only 27% of the 35 and over group were seropositive. To investigate the effect of age, we simply divided the data into two groups and fit the independence model to each group separately.

Figure 3 shows the cumulative distribution of the incubation period with pointwise 95% confidence intervals for the two age groups. The results do suggest that older people are at greater risk for developing AIDS than younger people.

10. Non–stationarity of the Incubation Period

Non–independence of the incubation period and the infection date due to treatment effects or other changes in the incubation period is modelled either as

A. $h_{k|j} = \mathring{h}_k \exp(\beta(j + k - 1))$ or

B. $h_{k|j} = \mathring{h}_k \exp\{\beta(j + k - 17)\, I(j + k > 17)\, (1 - \frac{7-k}{7}\, I\,(k \leq 7))\}$.

The first model (A) corresponds to a gradual change in the incubation period with calendar time. The second model (B) corresponds to a treatment hypothesis in which effective therapy began in mid 1987 and the usage of therapy gradually increased from that time on. Also, model B incorporates the feature that therapy is most likely in individuals who have been infected at least $3\frac{1}{2}$ years and is increasingly less likely for shorter times since HIV infection. For model B the interpretation of the baseline hazard is that it is the hazard function of AIDS associated with the natural history of the disease. Both models A and B should be interpreted only as potentially plausible descriptions of the 2–dimension hazard surface, $h_{k|j}$, without any unrealistic discontinuities. For both A and B, we are using a single parameter β to model the non–independence of the infection and incubation distributions.

The results of model A suggested that the incubation period was possibly getting shorter ($\hat{\beta}$ = 0.040), but the confidence interval (–0.087, 0.096) included zero. Model A was not investigated further.

The estimates of β from model B were negative suggesting that treatment was possibly having a beneficial effect. This is reasonable because a significant number of the pre–AIDS cohort were taking AZT in 1988 and 1989 (Graham et al. 1991), and AZT has been shown to be effective in a randomized clinical trial setting. An alternative explanation is that there is a substantial reporting delay of AIDS cases in the study. We believe this is contributing very little to the negative estimate of β because the analysis is censored at 31 December 1989, but we use all information which was available in February 1991. So, although reporting delays of over a year have occurred, they are very rare. Table 1 presents estimates of β for different values of λ_2, notice that the choice of λ_2 is having a very considerable effect on the estimated treatment effect.

Figures 4 and 5 illustrate the change in hazard due to treatment as a function of the infection time for two values of λ_2, one which is too small (10^4) and one which is too large (5×10^5). Notice that the baseline hazard is essentially linear for the larger λ_2. The explanation of this phenomenon is that the inclusion of the extra parameter has

Table 1.

Influence of smoothing parameter on estimate of treatment effect.

λ_2	β	95% confidence interval
10^4	–.033	
2×10^4	–.036	(–.162, .068)
5×10^4	–.044	(–.181, .063)
10^5	–.052	(–.162, .058)
5×10^5	–.074	

released the baseline hazard at long times from its dependence on the data, and hence the estimate is linear because it is dominated by the penalty function. Thus, we have overestimated the baseline hazard and hence also overestimated β. The 95% confidence interval for 3 values of λ_2 are also given in table 1, notice that they all include zero. This suggested that the sample size was not sufficient to detect any treatment effect.

11. Simulation Study

To investigate the adequacy of the sample size and the magnitude of the biasing effect of the choice of λ_2 on β we undertook a small simulation study. Data, as would have been observed in the cohort, was simulated as follows. A date of infection (j) and incubation period (k) were generated according to the probability distribution P_{jk} defined on the 23 x 23 grid according to model

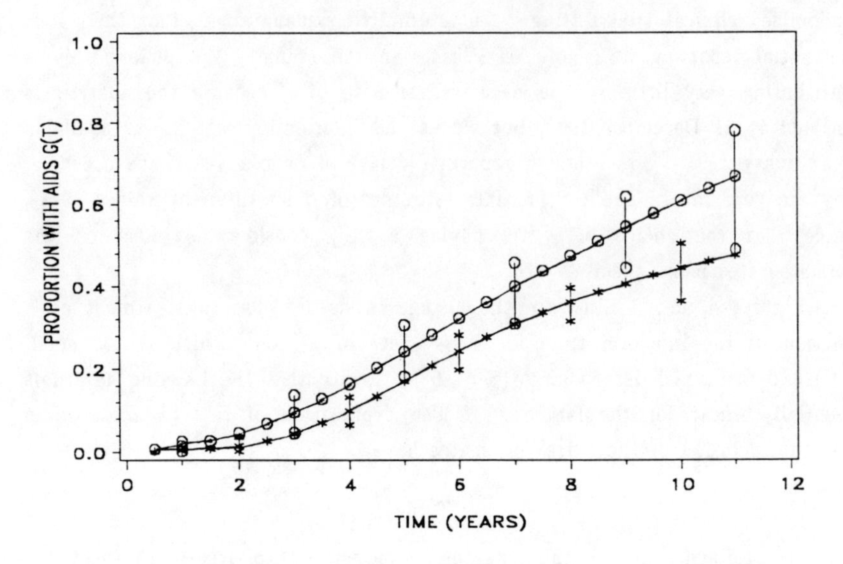
FIGURE 3
CUMULATIVE INCUBATION DISTRIBUTION INDEPENDENCE MODEL (β=0)
λ1=100,000, λ2=50000
o : AGE>=35, * : AGE<35
PROPORTION WITH AIDS G(T)
TIME (YEARS)

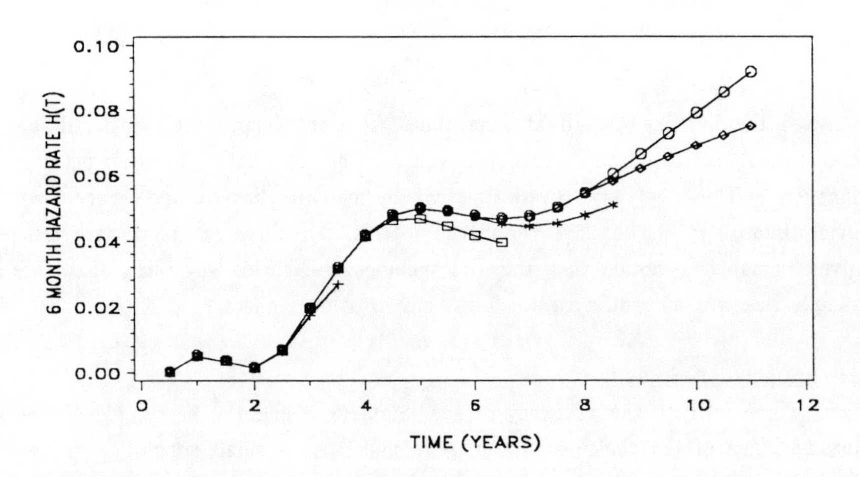
FIGURE 4
INCUBATION PERIOD HAZARD RATE, THERAPY MODEL B
UNDERSMOOTHED (λ1=100,000, λ2=10,000)
6 MONTH HAZARD RATE H(T)
TIME (YEARS)
CIRCLE : BASELINE HAZARD RATE
DIAMOND: INFECTED IN FIRST HALF OF 1979
STAR : INFECTED IN FIRST HALF OF 1981
SQUARE : INFECTED IN FIRST HALF OF 1983
PLUS : INFECTED IN FIRST HALF OF 1986

FIGURE 5
INCUBATION PERIOD HAZARD RATE, THERAPY MODEL B
OVERSMOOTHED ($\lambda 1=100{,}000$, $\lambda 2=500{,}000$)

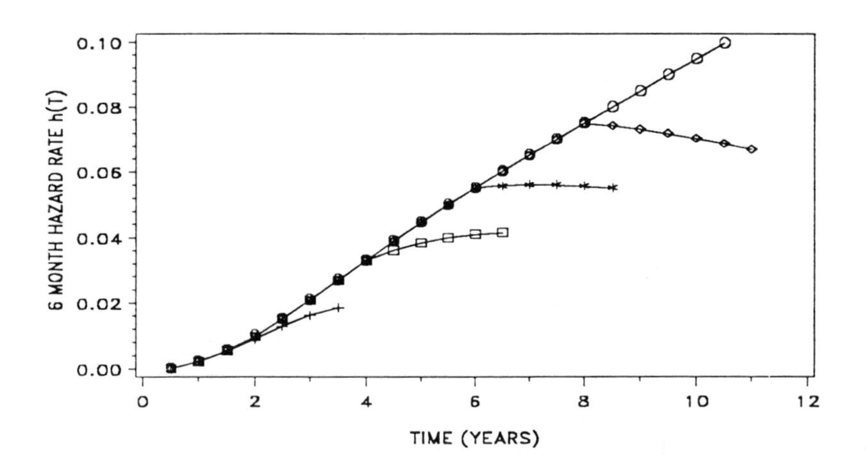

CIRCLE : BASELINE HAZARD RATE
DIAMOND: INFECTED IN FIRST HALF OF 1979 STAR : INFECTED IN FIRST HALF OF 1981
SQUARE : INFECTED IN FIRST HALF OF 1983 PLUS : INFECTED IN FIRST HALF OF 1986

FIGURE 6
MEAN OF ESTIMATED BASELINE HAZARD RATE
FROM SIMULATED DATA, THERAPY MODEL B

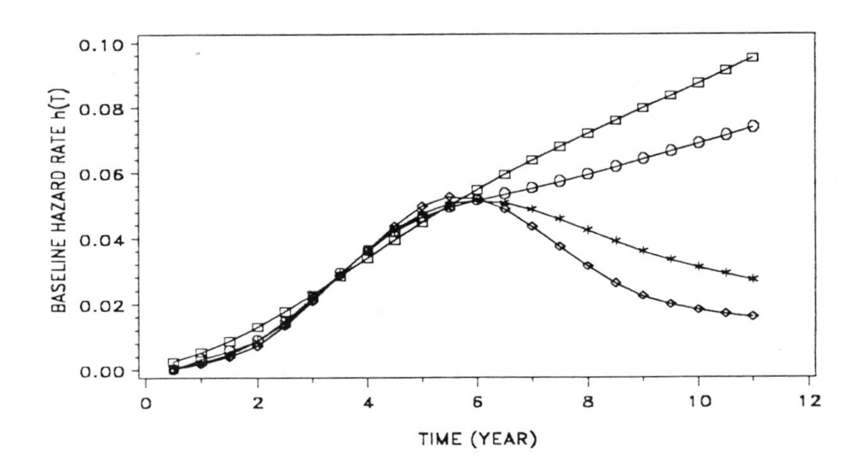

DIAMOND : $\lambda 1=100000$, $\lambda 2=10000$ STAR : $\lambda 1=100000$, $\lambda 2=50000$
SQUARE : $\lambda 1=100000$, $\lambda 2=500000$ CIRCLE : TRUE BASELINE HAZARD

B. The true value of β was −0.04. An interpretation of this value is that the hazard of AIDS is reduced by 15% eight years after infection for the cohort of individuals who were infected in the first half of 1981. The smooth curve in Figure 1 was used for the true infection distribution and a smooth hazard curve similar to that in Figure 2 was used for the true baseline hazard incubation period. An exact date of infection (x) was obtained from j by assuming that x was uniformly distributed over the 6 month interval defined by j. An exact incubation period (y) was obtained from k in a similar manner. For each of 1637 subjects, an exact date of enrollment was randomly chosen from the real enrollment time distribution. If the simulated (x,y) value fell into the truncation region defined by this enrollment date, a new (j,k) value was drawn. To mimic loss to follow-up, a disappearance date was generated for each subject. This disappearance date was January 1, 1990 with probability 0.86 and otherwise it was uniform between July 1, 1986 and January 1, 1990. For each person, the exact (x,y) value was converted into the region (B_i) which would have been observed if this was a real study. Fifty such datasets were generated and model B was fit to each one. We used $\lambda_1 = 10^5$ and three choices of λ_2, 10^4, 5×10^4, and 5×10^5. Table 2 presents the Monte Carlo averages and standard deviations of β. The table confirms the results of the data analysis that there is a considerable bias in the estimate of β, and that the bias is associated with the choice of λ_2. The magnitudes of the standard deviations are comparable to those associated with the confidence interval in Table 1, indicating that the Bootstrap procedure used to construct those confidence intervals is at least giving a reasonable approximation to the uncertainty associated with the estimates. The fact that the confidence intervals for β are so wide that they include zero indicates that there is not enough information in this data to be able to detect with certainty a treatment induced change in the hazard using only the AIDS diagnosis information.

Table 2.

Influence of smoothing parameter on estimate of treatment effect. Simulation study, true $\beta = -0.04$.

λ_2	Average β	SD(β)
10^4	.007	.081
5×10^4	−.019	.079
5×10^5	−.092	.052

Figure 6 depicts the Monte Carlo average of the baseline hazards. The graphs confirm that there is a bias in the estimate of the baseline hazard for times greater than about 7 years associated with the choice of λ_2.

12. Discussion

One validation of the numerical results is that they agree with other epidemiologic data. In particular, the infection curves in Figure 1 are consistent with what is known about the spread of the epidemic (Bacchetti, 1990). The results in Figure 2 are very similar to previous estimates, (see references listed in Taylor et al. 1991). The presence of an age effect and the suggestion of a treatment effect have been found by others (Gail et al. 1990, Darby et al. 1990, Biggar et al. 1990). These graphs in figure 2 and figure 6 indicate that it is only possible to obtain reliable estimates of the hazard function up to about 7 years after infection. At times longer than 7 years, it is impossible to obtain accurate values of the hazard, from the type of data described in this study, because of the possibility of contamination by treatment and the large statistical uncertainty associated with the estimates.

In this paper, we have illustrated some problems associated with trying to incorporate covariates into a procedure for smoothing grouped bivariate data. With regard to the age–at–infection covariate, we simply divided the sample into two parts and analysed each part separately. An alternative approach is to extend our model to include age as a time–varying covariate and then make the risk of infection be a function of age and calendar time. This is related to the Lexis diagram approach well known to demographers (Lexis, 1875), but only recently studied by statisticians (Keiding, 1990). For the analyses which were designed to model treatment effects, or essentially calendar time, some significant problems arose, these were selection bias, the lack of sample size to detect a treatment effect and the bias induced by the penalised likelihood approach. Perhaps a more fruitful approach would be just to smooth the bivariate P_{jk} distribution, rather than describing the lack of independence by one extra parameter. However the extremely large number of parameters necessary to specify the bivariate distribution may make this computationally prohibitive.

Acknowledgements

This work was partially supported by NIH grants and contracts AI29196 and AI72631. The data used in this paper is from the Los Angeles portion of the Multicenter AIDS Cohort Study. The authors thank the participants and personnel involved in that study for their cooperation.

References

Bacchetti, B. (1990). Estimating the incubation period of AIDS by comparing population infection and diagnosis patterns. *Journal of the American Statistical Association*, 85, 1002–1008.

Bacchetti, P. and Jewell, N.P. (1991). Non–parametric estimation of the incubation period from a prevalent cohort. *Biometrics*, 47, 947–960.

Biggar, R.J. and the International Registry of Seroconverters. (1990). AIDS incubation in 1891 HIV seroconverters from different exposure groups. AIDS 4, 1059–1066.

Brookmeyer, R. and Goedert, J.J. (1989). Censoring in an epidemic with an application to hemophilia–associated AIDS. *Biometrics* 45, 325–35.

Darby, S.C., Doll, R., Thakrar, B. et al. (1990). Time from infection with HIV to onset of AIDS in patients with haemophilia in the U.K. *Statistics in Medicine* 9, 681–9.

De Gruttola, V. and Lagakos, S.W. (1989). Analysis of doubly–censored survival data, with application to AIDS. *Biometrics* 45, 1–11.

B. Efron. (1982) The jackknife, the bootstrap and the other resampling plans. *Society for Industrial and Applied Mathematics.* Philadelphia.

Gail, M.H., Rosenberg, P.S. and Goedert, J.J. (1990). Therapy may explain recent deficits in AIDS incidence. *Journal of the Acquired Immune Deficiency Syndromes* 3, 296–306.

Graham, N.M.H., Zeger, S.L., Kuo, V. et al. (1991). Zidovidine use in AIDS–free HIV–1 seropositive homosexual men in the Multicenter AIDS Cohort Study (MACS), 1987 – 1989. *Journal of the Acquired Immune Deficiency Syndromes* 4, 267–76.

Green, P.J., (1987). Penalized likelihood for general semi–parametric regression models. *Int. Statist. Rev.* 55, 245–59.

Kaslow, R.A., Ostrow, D.G., Detels, R., Phair, J.P., Polk,B.F., Rinaldo, C.R. Jr. (1987). The Multicenter AIDS Cohort Study: rationale, organization, and selected characteristics of the participants. *American Journal of Epidemiology* 126, 310–18.

Keiding, N. (1990). Statistical inference in the Lexis diagram, Technical Report 90/4. Statistical Research Unit, University of Copenhagen.

Kuo, J–M., Taylor, J.M.G., and Detels, R. (1991). Estimating the AIDS incubation period from a prevalent cohort. *American Journal of Epidemiology* 133, 1050–57.

Lexis, W. (1875). *Einleitung in die Theorie der Bevölkerungsstatistik.* Trübner, Strassburg. Pp. 5–7 translated to English by N. Keyfitz and printed, with Fig. 1, in *Mathematical Demography* (ed. D. Smith & N. Keyfitz), Springer, Berlin (1977)

Taylor, J.M.B., Kuo, J–M., and Detels, R. (1991), Is the incubation period of AIDS lengthening?. *Journal of the Acquired Immune Deficiency Syndromes* 4, 69–75.

Taylor, J.M.G., Chon, Y. and Detels, R. (1991). Smoothing grouped bivariate data to obtain the incubation period distribution of AIDS. UCLA Statistics Series Technical Report.

Turnbull, B. (1976). The empirical distribution function with arbitrarily grouped, censored and truncated data. *Journal of the Royal Statistical Society* 38, 290–5.

Department of Biostatistics
UCLA School of Public Health
Los Angeles, CA 90024

USING SEMIPARAMETRIC RISK SETS FOR THE ANALYSIS OF CROSS-SECTIONAL DURATION DATA

Mei-Cheng Wang

Abstract

It is a common sampling scheme that individuals in a prospective cohort study are selected using a cross-sectional criterion. Suppose an epidemic process is characterized by three chronologically ordered events, termed event-A, -B, and -C. Suppose a prospective cohort only recruits individuals who have experienced event-A and have not experienced event-C. Therefore data from those who have experienced event-C prior to the time of recruitment are excluded from the analysis. In this paper we consider the situation when the time from event-A to event-B is treated as the major outcome variable, and interests are focused on nonparametric or semiparametric models for this variable. A class of semiparametric risk sets is introduced for constructing a variety of statistical methods. The general relationship between cross-sectional duration data and intercepted renewal data is characterized. The application of the proposed methods to intercepted renewal data is discussed. An example in which the event-ABC process corresponds to (HIV-infection, first diagnosis of AIDS, death) is presented.

1. Introduction

Suppose an epidemic process for a certain population is characterized by three chronologically ordered events, termed event-A, -B, and -C. For example, in epidemiological studies, the event-ABC process for an infectious disease could be (onset of infection, onset of disease, death), or (onset of infection, first diagnosis of disease, death). In general, event-B is naturally defined to be the onset of the disease when the onset time is detectable, and defined to be the first diagnosis of the disease when the onset time is not observable.

Let x, y and z represent the calendar time of event-A, the time from event-A to event-B, and the time from event-B to event-C, respectively. We shall treat y as the major outcome variable, even though other variables such as z or y + z could be of interest in some epidemiological studies. There is a variety of sampling schemes which are frequently used to derive observations from the target population. Here we give a brief description of these sampling techniques.

Sampling I. At a specified (calendar) time τ, retrospectively collect (x,y) from those individuals who have experienced both event-A and -B before or at τ. The observed data therefore include those (x, y)'s subject to the constraint $x + y \leq \tau$; see Figure 1. Well known examples in which this type of sampling is employed include the transfusion-related AIDS data and the reporting delay data from the Centers for Disease Control; see Jewell (1990) for a survey of statistical methods and applications subject to this type of data. Statistically, the observed y's are usually termed right truncated data.

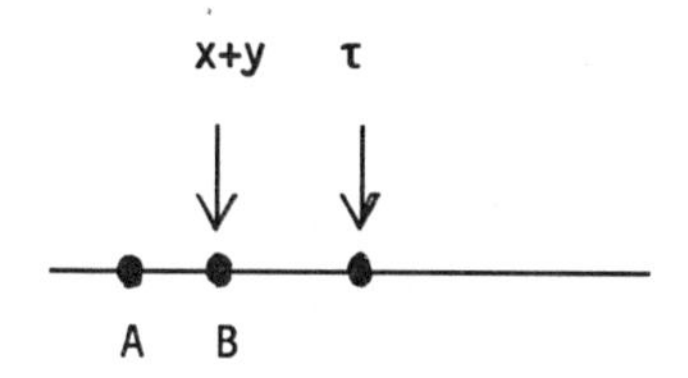

Figure 1. Sampling constraint: $X + Y \leq \tau$

Sampling II. At a specified time τ_i, an individual is randomly selected from those who have experienced event-A, but have not experienced event-B prior to τ_i. That is, the ith individual is observed under the constraint $x + y \geq \tau_i$. Follow-up for this individual is initiated at τ_i, ends at censoring or the occurrence of event-B. For example, in some cohort studies of AIDS. Event-A and -B correspond to the events of diagnosis of AIDS and death, and only those who have been diagnosed with AIDS and have not died are qualified for enrollment. Let x_i denote the calendar time of event-A, y_i the time from event-A to end of follow-up, and d_i the censoring indicator. The data then include (τ_i, x_i, y_i, d_i), $i = 1,\ldots,n$. The observed y's under this type of sampling are said to be left truncated and right censored; see Figure 2.

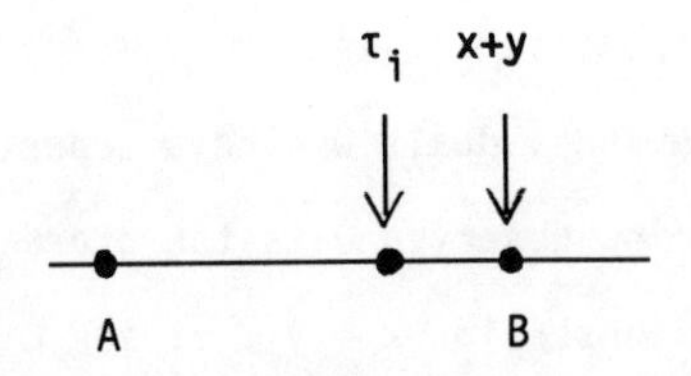

Figure 2. Sampling constraint: $X + Y \geq \tau_i$

Sampling III. At a specified time τ, retrospectively collect (x,y,z) from those individuals who have experienced event-A, -B and -C before or at τ. The observed data include those (x, y, z)'s subject to the sampling constraint $x + y + z \leq \tau$; see Figure 3 and Wang (1992). An example of this type of sampling is the CDC transfusion-related AIDS data with reporting delays. In this example, event-ABC corresponds to (HIV-infection, diagnosis of AIDS, report of AIDS). An AIDS case is not included in the data unless it is reported to the CDC before or at τ.

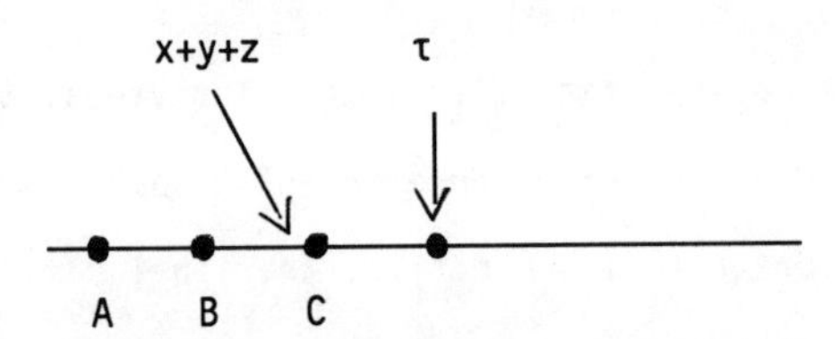

Figure 3. Sampling constraint: $X + Y + Z \leq \tau$

Sampling IV. Consider the following cross-sectional sampling for recruiting individuals into a prospective follow-up study. At a specified time τ_i, the ith individual is randomly selected from those who have experienced event-A during the time interval $[\tau_{i1}, \tau_{i2}]$, where $\tau_{i1} \leq \tau_{i2} \leq \tau_i$, and have not experienced event-C prior to τ_i, $i = 1,\ldots,n$. The ith individual is therefore observed subject to the constraint $x + y + z \geq \tau_i$. Follow-up is initiated at τ_i, and ends at censoring or the occurrence of event-C; see Figure 4. This type of sampling is the focus of the current paper. Notation for the observed data will be given and described in detail in Section 2.

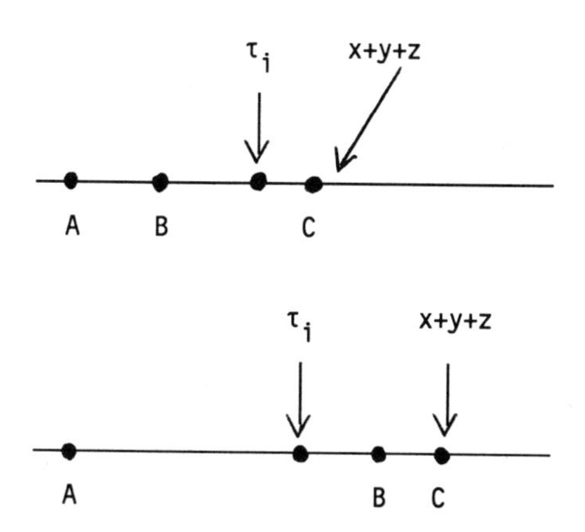

Figure 4. Sampling constraint: $X + Y + Z \geq \tau_i$

This paper has the following organization. A semiparametric model for the event-ABC process is introduced in Section 2. Section 3 gives a brief review of the risk sets for right censored data, and the risk sets for left truncated and right censored data. A class of semiparametric risk sets is introduced in Section 4. Section 5 includes a variety of statistical methods constructed on the basis of the semiparametric risk sets. The relationship between cross-sectional duration data and intercepted renewal data is characterized in Section 6. An example in which the event-ABC process corresponds to (HIV-infection, first diagnosis of AIDS, death) for an HIV-prevalent children's study is presented in Section 7.

2. A Semiparametric Model

Consider the following model assumptions:

M1. Event-A occurs at calendar time $X = x$, $0 \leq x < \infty$, according to a point process with intensity function $\phi(x)$. The point process has the following order statistic structure: Conditional upon τ and the total number of event-A's occurring before or at τ, the corresponding calendar times of event-A's are independently and identically distributed. Given the presence of event-A, the probability for the occurrences of event-B and -C is assumed to be one.

M2. The distribution of Y is independent of when event-A occurs, namely, Y is independent of X. Let $G(y) = P(Y \geq y)$ be the survival function of Y.

M3. The distribution of Z may depend on x and y. Let $H(z; x, y, \theta)$, $\theta \in \Theta \subset R^p$, be the parameterized conditional survival function of Z given x and y.

The above model M1~3 is the simple model for one-sample problems of Y. It is clearly a semiparametric model if the parameters ϕ and G are left as two nonparametric components. In a regression problem when the covariates $w \in R^d$ (where the calendar time x could be part of w) are present, model M1~3 can be extended by substituting $G(y; w)$, $H(z; w, y, \theta)$ for $G(y)$ and $H(z; x, y, \theta)$, respectively. Assume Sampling IV is used. Define

$$d_i = \begin{cases} 1 & \text{if event-B occurs before or at } \tau_i, \text{ or is observed during the follow-up period,} \\ 0 & \text{if event-B occurs after } \tau_i, \text{ and is censored,} \end{cases}$$

$$\delta_i = \begin{cases} 1 & \text{if event-C is observed during the follow-up period,} \\ 0 & \text{otherwise .} \end{cases}$$

Let x_i be the calendar time of event-A for the ith individual. Let y_i be the time from event-A to event-B when $d_i = 1$, and the time from event-A to end of follow-up when $d_i = 0$. Let z_i be the time from event-B to event-C when $\delta_i = 1$, zero when $d_i = 0$, and the time from event-B to end of follow-up otherwise. The observed data under Sampling IV can be represented as $(\tau_i, x_i, y_i, z_i, d_i, \delta_i)$, $i = 1,\ldots,n$.

3. Statistical Methods Based on Risk Sets

In survival analysis, the concept of "risk sets" plays an important role for the construction of a variety of statistical methods. Treating y as the outcome variable, we consider the following two types of risk sets.

3.1 Risk Sets for Right Censored Data

The familiar risk set at y is defined as

$$R(y) = \{y_j : y_j \geq y\} \qquad (3.1.1)$$

This type of risk set is, in general, appropriate for uncensored or right censored data (Kalbfleisch and Prentice, 1980), and inappropriate for data collected under Sampling II or Sampling IV. For example, using R(y) for the cross-sectional data under Sampling IV to construct the Kaplan-Meier estimator (1958) generally would lead to underestimation of the probability weight for shorter y's. In testing and regression problems, using R(y)'s to construct statistical methods in principle is inappropriate, the amount and direction of bias from these methods depend on distribution patterns of ϕ, G and H.

3.2 Risk Sets for Left Truncated and Right Censored Data

Risk sets for left truncated and right censored data generalize (3.1.1), and can be defined as

$$R(y) = \{y_j : \tau_j - x_j \leq y \leq y_j\} . \qquad (3.2.1)$$

Risk sets of this type are appropriate only for data subject to left truncation and right censoring, and therefore cannot be applied directly to the current data. However, if we are willing to exclude those observations which satisfy $x_i + y_i < \tau_i$ from analyzed data, in order to "make" the current data left truncated and right censored, then statistical methods based on (3.2.1) are applicable to the reduced data; see, for example, Wang (1991) for one-sample and bootstrapping problems, Cnaan and Ryan (1989) for application in natural history studies of disease, Lai and Ying (1991) for accelerated time regression, and Wang, Brookmeyer and Jewell (1992) for the comparison of incident and prevalent proportional hazards models. Excluding part of the data from analysis is in general not an attractive idea. Since the excluded data consist of uncensored y's and the excluded y's are likely to be the shorter ones, we may lose a substantial amount of information about the early incidences of event-B through using this data reduction procedure.

4. Semiparametric Risk Sets

4.1 When θ is Known

Assume θ is known. A class of semiparametric risk sets is introduced in this section. The motivation for a new risk set is its expected appropriateness, as compared with the inappropriateness of the risk set in (3.1.1), and the expected better efficiency from the corresponding statistical methods, when compared with methods based on (3.2.1).

Note that for given (τ, x), the subpopulation

$$D_{\tau,x} = \{(y, z): x + y + z < \tau\}$$

is excluded from the sampling population. However, for given (τ, x), the subpopulation

$$D^*_{\tau,x} = \{(y, z): x + y < \tau \text{ and } x + y + z \geq \tau\}$$

is part of the sampling population, and can be used to "recover" those belonging to $D_{\tau,x}$. Conditional on (τ, x, y) and $x + y < \tau$, the probability of an individual belonging to $D^*_{\tau,x}$ is $H(\tau\text{-}x\text{-}y;\ x,\ y,\ \theta)$, and the probability of the individual belonging to $D_{\tau,x}$ is $H(\bar{\tau}\text{-}x\text{-}y;\ x,\ y,\ \theta) = 1\text{-}H(\tau\text{-}x\text{-}y;\ x,\ y,\ \theta)$. Therefore, for an observed $(\tau_i,\ x_i,\ y_i)$ where $x_i + y_i < \tau_i$, the number of "unobserved" individuals with the same values of $(\tau_i,\ x_i,\ y_i)$ is projected to be $\bar{H}_i(\theta)/H_i(\theta)$, where $H_i(\theta) = H(\tau_i - x_i - y_i;\ x_i,\ y_i,\ \theta)$ and $\bar{H}_i = 1 - H_i(\theta)$. Thus, for each such observation, its unit count in $R(y)$ from (3.1.1) should be replaced by

$$\#[\text{observed}] + \#[\text{projected}] = 1 + [\bar{H}_i(\theta)/H_i(\theta)] = 1/H_i(\theta).$$

The projection method requires an assumption on H. That is, for each $(x,\ y,\ \theta)$, $H(\cdot;\ x,\ y,\ \theta)$ must be appropriately supported so that $H(\tau_i - x_i;\ x_i,\ y_i,\ \theta) > 0$ for each $i=1,\ldots,n$. This constraint is, however, satisfied for most of the commonly used parametric distributions. For the case $x_i + y_i \geq \tau_i$, clearly $H_i(\theta) = 1$ and the unit count $(= 1/H_i(\theta))$ remains the same for such cases. Now we may define the semiparametric risk set at y as

$$R(y;\ \theta) = \left\{ y_j,\ H_j^{-1}(\theta):\ y_j \geq y \right\}. \qquad (4.1.1)$$

The risk set (4.1.1) is semiparametric in that individuals at risk can be nonparametrically identified, but each individual's count, $H_j^{-1}(\theta)$, depends on the parametric assumption on H.

4.2 When θ is Unknown

In the situation when θ is unknown, the semiparametric risk set in (4.1.1) apparently cannot be used for constructing statistical methods. Though there may exist a variety of approaches for estimating θ, we note that z_i is observed subject to left truncation and right censoring and therefore consider deriving an estimator from the conditional likelihood on the basis of (z_i, δ_i)'s given (τ_i, x_i, y_i, d_i)'s,

$$L_c(\theta) \propto \prod_i \left[h(z_i; x_i, y_i, \theta)^{\delta_i} H(z_i; x_i, y_i, \theta)^{1-\delta_i} / H_i(\theta) \right] \tag{4.2.1}$$

Let $\hat{\theta}$ represent the maximum likelihood estimator (mℓe) derived from $L_c(\theta)$. Replacing θ in (4.1.1) by $\hat{\theta}$, we then derive a data-dependent risk set $R(y; \hat{\theta})$. There is an interesting characteristic of $R(\cdot; \hat{\theta})$ which is worth mentioning here. Note that the semiparametric risk set $R(\cdot; \theta)$ for known θ only depends on the random vectors (τ_i, x_i, y_i)'s, while $\hat{\theta}$ is derived from the conditional likelihood for given (τ_i, x_i, y_i, d_i)'s. Suppose a statistic $T(\hat{\theta}) = T(R(\cdot, \hat{\theta}), \underset{\sim}{d})$, $\underset{\sim}{d} = (d_1, \ldots, d_n)$, can be obtained as a function of $R(\cdot; \hat{\theta})$ and $\underset{\sim}{d}$. Through he decomposition $\hat{T}(\theta) = T(\theta) + [\hat{T}(\theta) - T(\theta)]$, the asymptotic covariance of $T(\hat{\theta})$ in a regular problem can then be expressed as the sum of (1) the asymptotic covariance from $T(\theta)$, (2) the asymptotic covariance from $T(\hat{\theta}) - T(\theta)$, and (3) twice the asymptotic covariance between $T(\theta)$ and $[\hat{T}(\theta) - T(\theta)]$. The components $T(\theta)$ and $[T(\hat{\theta}) - T(\theta)]$ in general are orthogonal to each other due to the conditioning structure, which implies (3) = 0. Therefore the asymptotic covariance of $T(\theta)$ has the general form (1)+(2). The asymptotic properties of $T(\hat{\theta})$ for different statistical problems may be explored via the probability structure of the semiparametric risk sets as well as the above decomposition.

5. Statistical Methods Based on Semiparametric Risk Sets

Using the semiparametric risk sets $R(y; \hat{\theta})$'s, we may construct a variety of statistical methods. This section gives a description of these methods. Some of the finite and large sample properties are developed and included in technical report #746, Department of Biostatistics, Johns Hopkins University.

Survival function estimation in one-sample problems

Define the "total count" of the risk set $R(y;\theta)$ as

$$R^*(y;\theta) = \sum_j H_j^{-1}(\theta) I(y_j \geq y) ,$$

and the count of the ties at y as

$$d^*(y;\theta) = \sum_j H_j^{-1}(\theta) I(y_j = y,\ d_j = 1) .$$

Let $y_{(1)} < \ldots < y_{(m)}$ be the distinct uncensored y's. A semiparametric estimator of G, in contrast with the Kaplan-Meier estimator (1958), can be constructed as

$$\hat{G}(y;\hat{\theta}) = \prod_{y_{(i)}<y} \left(1 - \frac{d^*(y_{(i)};\hat{\theta})}{R^*(y_{(i)};\hat{\theta})} \right) .$$

Weighted log rank test in two-sample problems

Let $w_i = 0$ and $w_i = 1$ represent two different groups. Let $\hat{\theta}$ be the conditional mℓe, from (4.2.1), derived on the basis of the density $h(z; w, y, \theta)$. Define

$$\bar{w}^*(y;\theta) = \left[\sum_j w_j H_j^{-1}(\theta) I(y_j \geq y) \right] / R^*(y;\theta) .$$

A two-sample log-rank statistic is then defined as

$$T(\hat{\theta}) = \frac{1}{n} \sum_i d_i v_i [w_i H_i^{-1}(\hat{\theta}) - \bar{w}^*(y_i;\hat{\theta})]$$

where v_i is the weight assigned to the ith observation.

Linear rank regression

Assume the log linear model

$$\log Y = w\beta + e \qquad (5.1)$$

where w is a 1×q vector of covariates, β is a q×1 vector of regression coefficients, and the residual e follows an unknown distribution F. Here the mean of e may not be zero. Let $\bar{w}^*(y;\theta)$ be defined as above. A weighted log-rank statistic can be given as

$$T(\beta;\hat{\theta}) = \frac{1}{n}\sum_i d_i\ \Psi(\hat{G}(e_i(\beta);\hat{\theta}))[w_i H_i^{-1}(\hat{\theta}) - \bar{w}^*(y_i;\hat{\theta})]$$

where $\Psi(\cdot)$ is a smooth function define on [0, 1] and $e_i(\beta) = \log y_i - w_i\beta$. Note that $T(\beta;\theta)$ reduces to the weighted log-rank statistic considered by Andersen, Borgan, Gill and Keiding (1981) when $H_i(\theta) \equiv 1$, or equivalently, when y's are observed subject only to right cencoring. An estimator of β in (5.1) can be derived by solving the equation $T(\beta;\hat{\theta}) = 0$; see Tsiatis (1990) for such an equation for the case $H_i(\theta) \equiv 1$.

Proportional hazards model

To be explored.

6. Cross-Sectional Duration Data vs. Intercepted Renewal Data

In Section 2, the population model is given. In this section, we explore the connection between a renewal process model, which is generated by pairwise dependent intervals, and the model M1~3 described in Section 2.

For each i = 1,...,n, let $(Y_{i1}, Z_{i1}), (Y_{i2}, Z_{i2}),\ldots$ be iid random vectors, where Y_{ij} and Z_{ij} are (possibly dependent) positive random variables. Assume Y_{ij} and Z_{ij} are distributed according to the survival function G(y) and the conditional survival function H(z; y), respectively. Let $V_{ij} = Y_{ij} + Z_{ij}$, j = 1,2,..., and let $K(\cdot)$ be the survival function of V_{ij}. The cumulative distribution function of V_{ij} is then $\bar{K}(v) = 1 - K(v) = \int_0^v \int_0^{v-y} d\bar{H}(z;y)d\bar{G}(y)$. Consider the ith renewal process $\{S_{ij}\}_{j=0}^{\infty}$, where $S_{io} = 0$ and $S_{im} = \sum_{j=1}^{m} V_{ij}$. Suppose the process starts at calendar time 0 and the triplet $(S_{i(j-1)}, y_{ij},$

z_{ij}) which satisfies $S_{i(j-1)} \le \tau_i < S_{ij}$ is observed, where τ_i is a constant independent of the ith renewal process. Let $N_i(x)$ be the number of renewal epochs occurring before x, that is, $N_i(x) = 1 + \max\{j: 0 \le S_{ij} < x\}$. Define the cumulative intensity function of renewal epochs as

$$\Phi(x) = E(N_i(x)) .$$

It follows from standard probability theory that

$$\Phi(x) = \sum_{j=1}^{\infty} j\, P(N_i(x) = j) = \sum_{j=1}^{\infty} P(N_i(x) \ge j)$$

$$= \sum_{j=0}^{\infty} P(0 \le S_{ij} < x) = \sum_{j=0}^{\infty} \overline{K}^{(x)j}(x)$$

where $\overline{K}^{(x)o}(x) = 1$ and for $j \ge 1$, $\overline{K}^{(x)j}$ denotes the convolution distribution of $V_1,\ldots,V_j$, or equivalently, the cdf of $V_1 +\ldots+ V_j$. Here note that, under appropriate continuity assumptions on G and H, the derivative of $\Phi(x)$ is $\phi(x)$, and which corresponds to the usual intensity function of a point process. Denote the observed random vector $(S_{i(j-1)}, Y_{ij}, Z_{ij})$ by (X_i, Y_i, Z_i). The observed data then include $(\tau_1, x_1, y_1, z_1),\ldots,(\tau_n, x_n, y_n, z_n)$. Now we consider two conditions (1) $\tau_i \approx \infty$, and (2) τ_i is an arbitrary constant. Condition (1) usually is referred to as the stationarity or equilibrium condition. Condition (2) in this section is referred to as the nonstationarity condition.

Suppose the distribution K is not arithmetic (Feller, 1971, chapter 5). Under (1), using the renewal theorem, one derives

$$\lim_{x\to\infty} [\Phi(x + \Delta x) - \Phi(x)]/\Delta x = 1/\mu \quad ,$$

where $\Delta x > 0$ and $\mu = E[V_{ij}]$. Let $T_i = \tau_i - X_i$ be the backward recurrence time. The marginal density of T_i is well known to be $K(t)/\mu$. Conditional on $T_i = t$, the density function of (Y_i, Z_i) is $[g(y)h(z;$

$y)/K(t)]I(y+z\geq t)$. Therefore the joint density of (T_i, Y_i, Z_i) is $[g(y)h(z; y)/\mu]I(y+z\geq t)$. Likelihood or density estimation methods for estimating the parameters of interest can then be developed using the specific structure of the above sampling distributions. References for the case $\text{Prob}(Z_{ij} = 0) = 1$ include Cox (1969) for uncensored renewal data, and Vardi (1989) for censored renewal data.

For the nonstationarity case (2), the joint density of (T_i, Y_i, Z_i) can be derived through standard probability arguments. However, interests here are focused on the conditional density for given (τ_i, x_i) rather than the unconditional one. Conditional upon (τ_i, x_i), the probability distribution of (y_i, z_i) can be shown to be the same as the conditional distribution under M1~3 as defined in Section 2 when censoring is absent, even though the population models for these two types of data are different. The unconditional distributions of (τ_i, x_i, y_i, z_i) under the two models are, however, different in view of the fact that in the renewal process model the intensity function for the occurrence of renewal epochs is generated by G and H, while the intensity function ϕ in M1~3 is regarded as a parameter independent of G and H. The use of the semiparametric risk sets for analyzing intercepted renewal data is generally appropriate here, since the methods only rely on the conditional probability structure rather than the unconditional one. Similar results hold when the intercepted renewal observations y_i and z_i are subject to right censoring.

7. An Example

An observational study of HIV-exposed young children in the School of Hygiene and Public Health, Johns Hopkins University, provides an example of the cross-sectional data under Sampling IV. The prevalent cohort for this study recruits any living child five years of age or younger from the Pediatric Intensity Primary Care Clinic in

Baltimore for a three year follow-up. All the children must have seropositive status at birth. Each child in the study is either seropositive or has been diagnosed with AIDS at the time of recruitment. The major goal of this study is to contribute to an understanding of the natural history as well as the psychosocial and medical impact of HIV-infection and AIDS on young children.

The event-ABC process in the study corresponds to (birth, first diagnosis of AIDS, death). The population of interest consists of young children who are born seropositive and prove to be truly HIV-infected within two years after birth. In the literature, it has been found that the incubation period of HIV-infection in children may vary depending upon the route of transmission. Initially, a child exposed through vertical transmission may test seropositive because the child has the mother's antibodies which can persist up to 18 months (The European Collaborative Study, 1988). An HIV-infected child is therefore not considered to be truly HIV-infected until approximately 18 to 24 months of age. It is estimated that approximately 70% of the seropositive infants will seroconvert to seronegative status within 24 months after birth (Fletcher et al., 1991). These seroconverted children can be identified during the course of the follow-up study if, for example, the only reason for censoring is due to the end of the study and the follow-up period for each individual is longer than two years.

Using the notation introduced in Section 2, the variables x, y and z correspond to the birth date of a truly HIV-infected child, the time from birth to diagnosis of AIDS, and the time from diagnosis of AIDS to death. Under the cross-sectional sampling design, a large proportion of the recruited HIV-infected children will develop or will have developed AIDS, during or before the follow-up study. Statistical methods des-cribed in earlier sections appear to be appropriate for the analysis, and will be applied to the study when data are available.

ACKNOWLEDGEMENTS. This research was supported in part by NIH grant R01-AI29197.

References

Andersen, P.K., Borgan, O., Gill, R.D., and Keiding, N. (1982). Linear nonparametric tests for comparison of counting processes, with applications to censored data. International Statistical Review, 50, 219-258.

Cnaan, A. and Ryan, L. (1989). Survival analysis in natural history studies of disease. Statistics in Medicine, 8, 1255-1268.

Cox, D. R. (1969). Some sampling problems in technology. In: New Developments in Survey Sampling, Johnson, N. L. and Smith, H., Jr. (eds.) New York: Wiley-Interscience, 506-527.

European Collaborative Study (1988). Mother-to-child transmission of HIV infection. Lancet i, 1039-1042.

Feller, W. (1971). An Introduction to Probability Theory and its Applications, Vol. 2. New York: John Wiley & Sons.

Fletcher, J.M., Francis, D.J., Pequegnat, W. et al. (1991). Neuro-development in HIV-1 infection and AIDS in infants and children: Application of growth curve models. Technical report, Department of Pediatrics, University of Texas Medical School of Houston.

Jewell, N. P. (1990). Some statistical issues in studies of the epidemiology of AIDS. Statistics in Medicine, 9, 1387-1416.

Kalbfleisch, J.D. and Prentice, R.L.(1980). The Statistical Analysis of Failure Time Data. New York: John Wiley.

Kaplan, E.L. and Meier, P. (1958). Nonparametric estimation from incomplete observations. Journal of the American Statistical Association, 53, 457-481.

Lai, T.L. and Ying, Z. (1991). Rank regression methods for left-truncated and right-censored data. The Annals of Statistics, 19, 531-556.

Tsiatis, A.A. (1990). Estimating regression parameters using linear rank tests for censored data. The Annals of Statistics, 18, 354-372.

Vardi, Y. (1989). Multiplicative censoring, renewal processes, deconvolution and decreasing density: Nonparametric estimation. Biometrika, 76, 751-761.

Wang, M.-C. (1991). Nonparametric estimation from cross-sectional survival data. Journal of the American Statistical Association, 86, 130-143.

Wang, M.-C. (1992). The analysis of retrospectively ascertained data in the presence of reporting delays. Journal of the American Statistical Association (to appear).

Wang, M.-C., Brookmeyer, R. and Jewell, N.P. (1992). Statistical models for prevalent cohort data. Biometrics (to appear).

Department of Biostatistics
Johns Hopkins University
School of Hygiene and Public Health
Baltimore, Maryland 21205

IS EARLIER BETTER FOR AZT THERAPY IN HIV INFECTION? A MATHEMATICAL MODEL

S. M. Berman and N. Dubin

Abstract

A mathematical model is proposed to determine the optimal level of the CD4-lymphocyte count at which to begin intervention therapy in Human Immunodeficiency Virus (HIV) infection. In the deterministic formulation of the model, the CD4 count for an untreated HIV-infected individual is assumed to decline linearly over time during the asymptomatic phase of the infection. Treatment with an antiviral such as zidovudine (AZT) is assumed to delay further decline in CD4 counts for a time period which may be constant or which functionally may depend upon the attained CD4 level. The optimal CD4 level for starting therapy is defined to be that which maximizes an individual's sojourn time above a predetermined critical level of CD4, below which serious health consequences are likely to occur. It is shown that earlier is better provided the duration of the effective therapeutic period increases with the starting CD4 level at a rate that is greater than or equal to the difference in the inverse CD4 slopes before and after treatment. The stochastic-model formulation of the CD4 count is defined as a time series which is the sum of the deterministic function and random errors which are independent and identically distributed at successive time points. An application is made to the specific case where the parameters of the deterministic model and of the (normal) error distribution were estimated from CD4 data obtained from intravenous drug users in New York City. The implications of the stochastic model are generally similar to the deterministic model. Whenever the deterministic model indicates that earlier is better, so does the stochastic model. For a logistic treatment-duration function ranging from a minimum of 12 months (for low starting levels) to a maximum of 30 months (for high starting levels), the model implies that an early start to AZT therapy is a good choice, unless the after-treatment slope is more than double the before-treatment slope.

1. Introduction.

In recent years two multi-institutional clinical trials sponsored by the AIDS Clinical Trials Group (ACTG) have provided evidence of a benefit to symptomatic HIV-infected individuals in being treated with the antiviral drug AZT (Fischl et al., 1987; Volberding, 1990). This drug is believed to result in increased numbers of a particular human lymphocyte called the CD4 cell, which generally is accepted by immunologists to be the principal target cell in HIV infection (McGrath, 1990; Crowe et al., 1990). The number of CD4 cells in uninfected individuals is variable, but frequently exceeds 1000 cells/ml (Yang and Dubin, 1990). Subsequent to infection with HIV, an individual's CD4 counts usually decline over time. It is anticipated that, if the CD4 count can be kept above some critical level, say 200 cells/ml, then the more serious health consequences of HIV infection can be avoided or, at least, delayed (Crowe et al., 1991). Unfortunately, there is evidence suggesting that the beneficial effects of AZT are of limited duration, after which the decline in CD4 levels recommences, perhaps at an accelerated pace. One source has suggested 18 months of benefit for symptomatic individuals (Fischl et al., 1989), whereas another has hypothesized that the duration of benefit should be longer among asymptomatic individuals whose immune systems are still relatively intact (Cotton, 1991). Another ACTG trial is currently under way to assess the benefits of AZT therapy for asymptomatic subjects (Volberding et al., 1990). Outside of clinical trials, HIV-infected subjects are generally considered to be eligible for AZT therapy when their CD4 counts have dropped to below 500 cells/ml on two closely consecutive readings, although by no means all eligible subjects to date have been treated with the drug (Rosenberg et al., 1991).

Determination of the optimal level at which to begin AZT intervention is amenable to mathematical modelling, provided some reasonable simplifying assumptions can be made. Suppose that, in the absence of intervention, the CD4 count for an untreated HIV-infected individual declines linearly over time subsequent to infection. Treatment with AZT is assumed to delay further decline in CD4 counts for a time period which may be constant or which functionally may depend upon the CD4 level at which therapy is commenced. The optimal point in time to begin therapy is defined to be that which maximizes the length of time an individual spends above a predetermined critical level of CD4, for example, 200 cells/ml, below which serious illness is likely to occur. It is implicitly assumed that keeping CD4 levels higher for a longer period of time is beneficial to the HIV-infected subject. Elsewhere in this volume, other authors (Jewell and Kalbfleisch, 1992; De Gruttola and Tu, 1992; Self and Pawitan, 1992; Robins and Rotnitzky, 1992) address issues related to modelling the relationship between a surrogate marker such as CD4 and clinical outcome.

The model developed below is given both a deterministic and stochastic formulation. It is then applied to data from intravenous drug users in New York City. It will be of particular interest to assess whether it is advantageous to begin AZT therapy at the earliest opportunity.

2. Deterministic Model.

Suppose the CD4 count is μ at time of infection $t=0$ and, in the absence of intervention, declines according to some function f to a critical level c. The CD4 count may be either in terms of absolute numbers of cells or some suitable monotonic transformation thereof. We assume that if there is intervention before the critical level is reached, then the therapy is effective in temporarily arresting the decline in CD4, for a time interval D. If therapy begins at $t=T_1$, CD4 is assumed to remain constant until T_1+D. Subsequently, CD4 resumes its decline, reaching the critical level c at time $t=T_1+D+T_2$. The model does not address what happens subsequent to $t=T_1+D+T_2$.

In mathematical terms, the CD4 count is considered to be a continuously measured variable represented by a real valued function $f(t)$, $t\geq 0$. Assume that $f(0)=\mu$, and that for some x, $c<x<\mu$, $f(t)$ decreases on an interval $[0,T_1]$ where $f(T_1)=x$. For a number $D>0$ it is assumed that $f(t)=x$ for all $T_1\leq t\leq T_1+D$. Finally, there is a number $T_2>0$ such that $f(t)$ is decreasing for $T_1+D\leq t\leq T_1+D+T_2$ and $f(T_1+D+T_2)=c$. Thus, T_1+D+T_2 represents the "time spent above c" or "positive sojourn time" of $f(t)$, $t\geq 0$. We will examine, under specific assumptions about the nature of the function $f(t)$, how the positive sojourn time varies with the level x, $c<x<\mu$, and, particularly, how to choose x so as to maximize the positive sojourn time.

More specifically, suppose that $f(t)$ is a continous piecewise linear function of the following form: It decreases linearly with negative slope $-m_1$ on the interval $[0,T_1]$, has constant value $x=\mu-m_1T_1$ during the effective treatment interval $[T_1, T_1+D]$, and resumes a linear decline with negative slope $-m_2$ on the interval $[T_1+D, T_1+D+T_2]$ (Fig. 1). Here D is assumed to be constant, and no assumptions have been made regarding the relative magnitudes of m_1 and m_2.

Since $m_1=(\mu-x)/T_1$ and $m_2=(x-c)/T_2$, the positive sojourn time T_1+D+T_2 is representable as

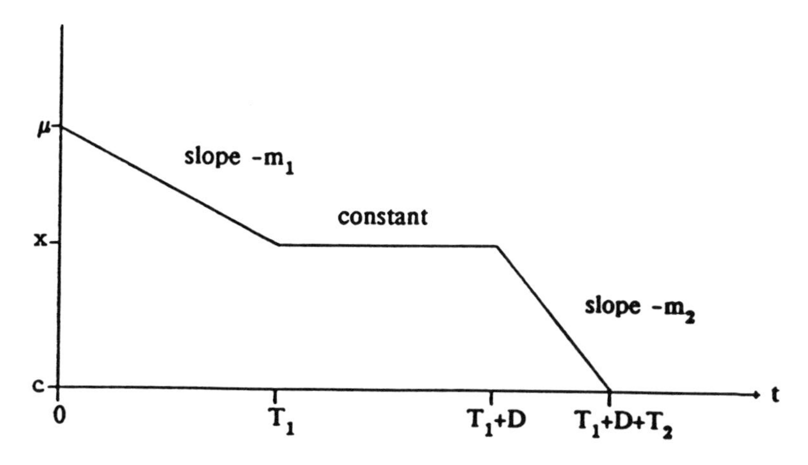

Figure 1. Hypothesized function f(t) for the effect of AZT therapy on the declining CD4 count during HIV infection.

$$J(x) = \frac{\mu - x}{m_1} + D + \frac{x-c}{m_2}, \qquad \text{for } c<x\leq\mu, \tag{2.1}$$
$$= \frac{\mu - c}{m_1}, \qquad \text{for } x=c.$$

Note that x=c corresponds to the situation in which there is no intervention prior to reaching the critical level. Suppose that

$$m_1 < m_2, \tag{2.2}$$

so that the decline in CD4 is faster after intervention than it is before. Then J(x) is a decreasing function of x for $c<x\leq\mu$, and

$$\lim_{x\to c} J(x) = \frac{\mu - c}{m_1} + D. \tag{2.3}$$

On the other hand $J(c) = (\mu-c)/m_1$, so that there is a jump discontinuity at x=c. This implies that there does not exist a value of x for which J(x) assumes its largest value for $c\leq x\leq\mu$: J(x) increases toward the value (2.3) as x decreases to c, but never attains that value. Hence, for the situation $m_1<m_2$, the positive sojourn time is maximized by delaying intervention until just before the critical level is reached. For $m_1>m_2$, the opposite holds; the positive sojourn time is maximized when intervention starts as early as possible. For $m_1=m_2$, the sojourn time does not depend upon x (and is maximized) provided x>c; in other words, the positive sojourn time is maximized provided therapy begins at any time prior to the patient's reaching the critical level.

The problem of maximizing the positive sojourn time becomes more interesting if is assumed that D is a function of x, so that (2.1) becomes

$$J(x) = \frac{\mu-x}{m_1} + D(x) + \frac{x-c}{m_2}, \qquad \text{for } c<x\leq\mu, \tag{2.4}$$
$$= \frac{\mu-c}{m_1}, \qquad \text{for } x=c.$$

Assume that $D(x)\geq 0$ for all $c<x\leq\mu$. For example, suppose that D(x) is the linear function $D(x)=\alpha x+\beta$ for some constants α and β; then

$$J(x) = (\alpha + \frac{1}{m_2} - \frac{1}{m_1})x + (\beta + \frac{\mu}{m_1} - \frac{c}{m_2}), \qquad \text{for } c<x\leq\mu, \tag{2.5}$$
$$= \frac{\mu-c}{m_1}, \qquad \text{for } x=c.$$

The positive sojourn time J(x) increases, decreases or is constant as a function of x accordingly as $\alpha+1/m_2-1/m_1$ is positive, negative or equal to 0. It follows that, for $D(x)=\alpha x+\beta$, if $\alpha>(1/m_1-1/m_2)$ the benefit is maximized when treatment starts as early as possible ($x=\mu$). If $\alpha<(1/m_1-1/m_2)$ the benefit is maximized when treatment starts as close as possible to the patient's reaching the critical level ($x=c$). If $\alpha=1/m_1-1/m_2$ the positive sojourn time is constant for all $c<x\leq\mu$, so that it is irrelevant when treatment is started, provided it is started prior to the critical level.

In general, if D(x) is not necessarily linear but continuously differentiable, then it is often possible to maximize J by finding the critical points, that is, points x where

$$D'(x) = \frac{1}{m_1} - \frac{1}{m_2}. \tag{2.6}$$

For example, if $D(x)= \alpha x^{\frac{1}{2}}+\beta$ for some constants α and β, then

$$J(x) = (\beta + \frac{\mu}{m_1} - \frac{c}{m_2}) + \alpha x^{\frac{1}{2}} - (\frac{1}{m_1} - \frac{1}{m_2})x, \qquad \text{for } c<x\leq\mu, \tag{2.7}$$
$$= \frac{\mu-c}{m_1}, \qquad \text{for } x=c.$$

If $m_1\geq m_2$, J(x) is monotonically increasing, attaining its maximum on $(c,\mu]$ at $x=\mu$, i.e. the positive sojourn time is maximized by starting therapy as early as possible. If $m_1<m_2$, J(x) has a single critical point

$$\frac{\alpha^2}{4}\left(\frac{1}{m_1}-\frac{1}{m_2}\right)^{-2}, \tag{2.8}$$

and it represents a relative maximum. Thus, if the critical point falls in the interval $(c,\mu]$, it represents a solution to the maximization problem. If the critical point exceeds μ, then the maximum of J(x) in (2.7) is assumed at the point $x=\mu$. If the critical point is less than or equal to c, then the maximum of J(x) in (2.7) is assumed in the limit as x approaches c.

Simple algebra shows that the critical point (2.8) falls in the open interval (c,μ) if and only if

$$2c^{\frac{1}{2}}\left(\frac{1}{m_1}-\frac{1}{m_2}\right) < \alpha < 2\mu^{\frac{1}{2}}\left(\frac{1}{m_1}-\frac{1}{m_2}\right), \tag{2.9}$$

whereas it assumes a value $\geq\mu$ if and only if

$$\alpha \geq 2\mu^{\frac{1}{2}}\left(\frac{1}{m_1}-\frac{1}{m_2}\right), \tag{2.10}$$

and assumes a value $\leq c$ if and only if

$$\alpha \leq 2c^{\frac{1}{2}}\left(\frac{1}{m_1}-\frac{1}{m_2}\right), \tag{2.11}$$

Therefore, if α satisfies (2.9), the x-level (2.8) yields the maximum sojourn time, while if it satisfies (2.10) the optimal policy is to start at $x=\mu$ (i.e., earlier is better) and if it satisfies (2.11) the optimal policy is to start at x as close as possible to c (i.e., later is better).

Consider the following question: For what class of functions D(x) is J(x) monotonically nondecreasing? In the latter case, the positive sojourn time increases with the level, so the rule is "Earlier is Better" (EIB). There is a simple criterion for a function D(x) to be associated with an EIB rule:

PROPOSITION. *D(x) is associated with an EIB rule if and only if*

$$D'(x) \geq \frac{1}{m_1}-\frac{1}{m_2}, \quad \text{for all } c<x\leq\mu. \tag{2.12}$$

PROOF. An EIB rule is always associated with a function J(x) in

(2.4) that is monotonically nondecreasing. This holds if and only if $J'(x) \geq 0$ for $c < x \leq \mu$, which, in turn, holds if and only if (2.12) holds.

The intuitive significance of the condition (2.12) is that it puts a lower bound on the growth of D(x). In other words, the function is required to increase at a prescribed rate over the whole interval of x-values, in order for the EIB rule to apply. Further, this lower bound is determined by the before- and after-treatment slopes, $-m_1$ and $-m_2$.

3. Stochastic model.

To introduce a stochastic formulation, we employ the following time series to represent the CD4 counts (or a suitable monotonic function of the counts) at equally spaced points on the time domain. The series can be viewed simply as the sum of f(t), as defined in the deterministic model, and random errors which are independent and identically distributed at successive time points. Note that this particular stochastic model, involving independent random errors, is mathematically well-defined only in the discrete time case. More precisely, let μ represent the expected CD4 count in an uninfected individual. Let $X_0, X_1, X_2, \ldots$ be independent random variables with mean 0 and common distribution function F; then, the successive CD4 readings for uninfected individuals are represented as $X_0+\mu, X_1+\mu, X_2+\mu, \ldots$.

Suppose an individual becomes infected with HIV at some time point which we take as time 0. Then the successive CD4 readings from that time are assumed to follow the linear model

$$\mu - nm_1 + X_n, \quad n=0,1,..., \tag{3.1}$$

for some $m_1>0$, where m_1 represents the average rate of decline of the CD4 level.

Let c be some number smaller than μ representing a critically low CD4 level, below which a patient is considered to be at risk of serious illness. Then the sojourn time of the series (3.1) above the level c is representable as

$$\sum_{n=0}^{\infty} \mathbf{1}[\ X_n > nm_1 + c - \mu\ ], \tag{3.2}$$

where $\mathbf{1}[\ ]$ is the indicator random variable. The expected sojourn time is obtained from this by replacing each indicator by its probability:

$$\sum_{n=0}^{\infty} [\ 1 - F(nm_1 + c - \mu)\ ]. \tag{3.3}$$

This is the expected sojourn time above c in the absence of any intervening AZT treatment.

Next we propose a modification of the series (3.1) to describe the process of intervention. Let x be some CD4 level between the "normal" level μ and the critical level c; that is, $c<x<\mu$. Suppose the AZT intervention at a particular level x is done in the following way: If, for the first time, an individual's CD4 falls below x, then a second reading is taken as soon as possible thereafter, and AZT treatment is initiated or not accordingly as the second reading is less than or at least equal to x, respectively. In other words, two closely spaced readings below x are assumed to lead to intervention.

Let the random variable N_1 represent the first index at which there are two readings below x. N_1 is formally defined in terms of two identical series of the form (3.1). Let $X_0, X_1, \ldots,$ $Y_0, Y_1, \ldots$ be independent random variables with mean 0 and common distribution function F; then N_1 is the smallest integer $n \geq 0$ for which both inequalities

$$X_n < x + nm_1 - \mu, \quad Y_n < x + nm_1 - \mu \tag{3.4}$$

hold. Note that the only terms of the sequence Y_n that are actually observed in practice are those for which $X_n < x+nm_1-\mu$ and $n \leq N_1$. The distribution of N_1 is characterized by the following relation: for $k \geq 0$,

$$P(N_1>k) = \Pi_{h=0}^{k} [\ 1 - F^2(hm_1+c-\mu)\ ]. \tag{3.5}$$

Indeed, the event $\{N_1>k\}$ is equal to the intersection of $\{X_h>hm_1+c-\mu\} \bigcup \{Y_h>hm_1+c-\mu\}$, for $0 \leq h \leq k$.

As soon as the (random) index N_1 is observed, AZT treatment is initiated, the Y-sequence is disregarded, and the next set of X's is observed. During treatment, we assume that the expected CD4 counts do not decline further. In mathematical terms, there is a number $D=D(x)$, depending on the level x, such that the CD4 levels at times $N_1+1, \ldots, N_1+D(x)$ are represented as (3.1) with N_1m_1 in the place of nm_1:

$$\mu - N_1m_1 + X_n, \quad n=N_1+1, \ldots, N_1+D(x). \tag{3.6}$$

These are the CD4 counts during AZT treatment. Let N_2 represent the number of these for which $\mu - Nm_1 + X_n > c$:

$$N_2 = \sum_{h=1}^{D(x)} 1[\ \mu - N_1m_1 + X_{h+N_1} > c]. \tag{3.7}$$

It can be shown that the random variables

$$N_1, X_{N_1+1}, X_{N_1+2}, \ldots$$

are mutually independent, and so

$$EN_2 = D(x) \sum_{n=0}^{\infty} P(N_1=n) [1 - F(nm_1+c-\mu)]. \tag{3.8}$$

Note that $P(N_1=n)=P(N_1>n-1)-P(N_1>n)$ for $n\geq 1$, and $P(N_1=0)= 1-P(N_1>0)$, so that the probabilities $P(N_1=n)$ in (3.8) can be computed from (3.5).

Under our model the beneficial effect of AZT intervention on the CD4 level is assumed to cease at the time point $N_1+D(x)$; thereafter, CD4 levels resume their decline (in expectation) and are represented by a time series like (3.1) but with m_1 replaced by m_2, and μ replaced by $\mu-N_1m_1$:

$$\mu - N_1m_1 - nm_2 + X_n, \quad \text{for } n\geq N_1+D(x)+1. \tag{3.9}$$

The sojourn time of the random variables (3.9) above the level c is defined as

$$N_3 = \sum_{h=1}^{\infty} 1[X_{N_1+D(x)+h} > N_1m_1+hm_2+c-\mu]. \tag{3.10}$$

By analogy to (3.8), we obtain

$$EN_3 = \sum_{n=0}^{\infty} P(N_1=n) \sum_{h=1}^{\infty} [1-F(nm_1+hm_2+c-\mu)]. \tag{3.11}$$

The total expected sojourn time above the critical level c is $EN_1+EN_2+EN_3$, and is given by the formula

$$\sum_{n=0}^{\infty} P(N_1=n) \{ n + D(x)[1-F(nm_1+c-\mu)] + \sum_{h=1}^{\infty}[1-F(nm_1+hm_2+c-\mu)] \}. \tag{3.12}$$

It is this quantity that one seeks to maximize by the optimal choice of the level x.

4. Application to Data Obtained from Intravenous Drug Users.

Berman (1990) used data from a cohort of intravenous drug users, previously described by Des Jarlais et al. (1987), Marmor et al. (1987) and Yang and Dubin (1990), to estimate the distribution of the natural logarithms of the CD4 counts (logCD4) among 191 subjects not infected with HIV. It was found to be approximately a normal distribution with mean μ=6.966 and standard deviation σ=0.354. Further, data from 59 HIV-infected subjects followed longitudinally in the same cohort, and not treated with AZT, indicated a linear decline in logCD4 with slope parameter m_1=0.0335 log cells/ml per month. Therefore, it is appropriate to use logCD4 in place of the untransformed count in defining the distribution F in our stochastic model. The mean μ=6.966 approximately corresponds to an untransformed CD4 of 1060 cells/ml among uninfected subjects. Analogously, the choice c=5.298 corresponds approximately to an untransformed critical level of 200 cells/ml. Under these parametric assumptions for the stochastic model, in the absence of intervention the expected sojourn time was calculated from (3.3) to be 50.28 months, or slightly over four years. This is similar to the deterministic sojourn time of 49.79 months calculated from (2.1).

Suppose that D(x) is constant for all x, and that the after-treatment slope is twice the before-treatment slope, $m_2=2m_1$. Note that x will be in units of logCD4 cells/ml. In Table 1 are given the expected sojourn times associated with a fixed treatment-effect duration D of six months to three years, in six month increments, and for various starting CD4 levels of treatment ranging from 250 to 800 cells/ml. Generally speaking, later

Table 1. Expected sojourn time above CD4=200, where $D(x)$ is a constant function and $m_2/m_1=2$.

		D(x)					
		6	12	18	24	30	36
x	e^x						
5.5215	250	49.89	54.70	59.52	64.33	69.14	73.95
5.7038	300	47.36	52.80	58.25	63.69	69.13	74.57
5.8579	350	45.19	50.94	56.68	62.43	68.17	73.92
5.9915	400	43.27	49.15	55.04	60.92	66.81	72.69
6.1092	450	41.54	47.49	53.44	59.39	65.33	71.28
6.2146	500	39.99	45.97	51.94	57.92	63.89	69.87
6.3099	550	38.59	44.58	50.56	56.55	62.54	68.53
6.3969	600	37.32	43.32	49.31	55.31	61.30	67.30
6.4770	650	36.19	42.19	48.18	54.18	60.18	66.18
6.5511	700	35.19	41.19	47.19	53.19	59.19	65.18
6.6201	750	34.33	40.33	46.32	52.32	58.32	64.32
6.6846	800	33.59	39.59	45.59	51.59	57.59	63.59

initiation of therapy here results in longer expected sojourns above 200, except for the longest fixed duration D=36 months, in which case it is best to start therapy at a level of approximately 300 cells/ml. For the deterministic model, since $m_1<m_2$, the sojourn time is maximized by delaying intervention until just prior to reaching 200 cells/ml. For D=18 months, for example, the maximum deterministic sojourn time is calculated from (2.3) to be 67.79 months. To illustrate the extent of agreement between the stochastic and deterministic models in the present example, the sojourn times may be compared: for D=18 and x=log250 one obtains a sojourn of 59.51 months from Table 1 and 64.45 months from (2.1), and for D=18 and x=log800 one obtains sojourns of 45.59 and 47.09 months, respectively.

Now suppose one fixes D at 18 months and varies the ratio of the slopes m_2/m_1. The deterministic model predicts that if the ratio is greater than 1 then later is better, whereas if the ratio is less than 1 then earlier is better, and if the ratio is equal to 1 then it doesn't matter when you start, as long as you start above CD4=200. In this particular situation the value $m_2/m_1=1$ constitutes a *transition point* between the domains in which "earlier is better" and "later is better," at which the deterministic sojourn of 67.79 months is independent of x. Results for the stochastic model are given in Table 2 for fixed D=18 and varying slope

Table 2. Expected sojourn time above CD4=200, where D(x)=18 is a constant.

		m_2/m_1					
		0.5	*1.0*	*1.5*	*2.0*	*3.0*	*5.0*
x	e^x						
5.5215	250	76.22	65.08	61.37	59.52	57.66	56.18
5.7038	300	81.96	66.15	60.88	58.25	55.61	53.51
5.8579	350	86.85	66.74	60.03	56.68	53.33	50.65
5.9915	400	91.01	67.03	59.03	55.04	51.04	47.84
6.1092	450	94.61	67.16	58.01	53.44	48.86	45.20
6.2146	500	97.80	67.23	57.04	51.94	46.85	42.77
6.3099	550	100.64	67.26	56.13	50.56	45.00	40.55
6.3969	600	103.19	67.27	55.30	49.31	43.32	38.54
6.4770	650	105.46	67.28	54.55	48.18	41.82	36.73
6.5511	700	107.46	67.28	53.88	47.19	40.49	35.13
6.6201	750	109.19	67.28	53.31	46.32	39.34	33.75
6.6846	800	110.66	67.28	52.82	45.59	38.36	32.58

ratios. The implications are the same as from the deterministic model, except that at the deterministic transition point $m_2/m_1=1$ there is a tendency for the stochastic model to favor an earlier start to treatment. Additional calculations (not tabulated) for the transitional region $1<m_2/m_1<1.5$ show that, as a function of the starting level x, the expected sojourn is relatively flat, with no clear advantage to later starting levels manifest until the ratio is at least 1.2. Note from Table 2 that the maximum expected sojourn changes very little as the slope ratio increases above $m_2/m_1=2$.

Now consider the situation in which D(x) is linear in x and the slope ratio is fixed at $m_2/m_1=2$. The choice of $D(x)=\alpha(x-\log 300)+18$, $\alpha>0$, has the following characteristics: (i) for all α, D=18 months when therapy starts at a CD4 level of 300 cells/ml, (ii) higher (earlier) starting levels are associated with a longer duration of treatment effect, and (iii) the rate of increase of the duration of treatment effect associated with higher (earlier) starting levels increases directly with α. For example, if $\alpha=12$ then if treatment is initiated at CD4=500, the duration of effective treatment is 24.1 months, more than six months greater than if 300 is the starting level. For $\alpha=36$ the relationship is steeper, $D(\log 500)=36.4$, whereas for $\alpha=4$ the relationship is flatter, $D(\log 500)=20.0$. The deterministic model predicts that earlier is

Table 3. Expected sojourn time above CD4=200, where $D(x)=\alpha(x-5.7038)+18$ and $m_2/m_1=2$.

		α					
		4	*6*	*12*	*14.93*	*24*	*36*
e	e^x						
5.5215	250	58.71	57.91	57.11	57.11	55.51	53.90
5.7038	300	57.34	57.34	57.34	57.34	57.34	57.34
5.8579	350	56.68	56.68	57.64	58.60	59.55	61.47
5.9915	400	56.02	56.02	57.98	58.96	60.92	64.85
6.1092	450	54.43	55.42	57.40	59.39	62.36	67.32
6.2146	500	53.93	54.93	57.92	58.91	63.89	69.87
6.3099	550	52.56	53.56	57.55	59.55	64.54	71.53
6.3969	600	51.31	53.31	57.30	59.30	65.30	73.29
6.4770	650	51.18	52.18	57.18	59.18	66.18	75.17
6.5511	700	50.19	52.19	57.19	59.19	67.18	77.18
6.6201	750	49.32	51.32	56.32	59.32	67.32	78.32
6.6846	800	48.59	50.59	56.59	59.59	68.59	80.59

better if $\alpha>1/2m_1=14.93$ and later is better if $\alpha<14.93$; there is a constant sojourn of 61.74 months at $\alpha=14.93$. One would expect $\alpha\approx15$ to be the transitional region between "later is better" and "earlier is better" for the stochastic model as well. Table 3 confirms that the implications of the stochastic and deterministic models are concordant in the "earlier is better" region. At precisely the transition point $\alpha=14.93$ (and to a lesser extent for smaller α), one again notes the tendency for the stochastic model to favor earlier starting levels, relative to the deterministic model.

Suppose $\alpha=12$ is fixed in the linear model, and the slope ratio is allowed to vary. The deterministic transition point occurs at $m_2/m_1=(1-\alpha m_1)^{-1}=1.67$, such that slope ratios smaller than 1.67 are associated with "earlier is better", and greater slope ratios with "later is better." As can be seen from Table 4, similar conclusions can be drawn from the stochastic model, provided one takes into account the relatively small tendency favoring earlier treatment.

Another possible choice for D(x) would be a function having an asymptotic maximum and a minimum over the range of x. The logistic function

$$D(x) = \frac{\gamma}{1 + \exp[\ -\delta(x-\log 200) + \kappa\ ]}$$

Table 4. Expected sojourn time above CD4=200, where D(x)=12(x-5.7038)+18.

		m_2/m_1						
		0.5	*1.0*	*1.5*	*1.67*	*2.0*	*3.0*	*5.0*
x	e^x							
5.5215	250	73.81	62.68	58.96	58.21	57.11	55.25	53.77
5.7038	300	81.06	65.24	59.97	58.90	57.34	54.70	52.60
5.8597	350	87.81	67.70	60.99	59.63	57.64	54.29	51.61
5.9915	400	93.95	69.97	61.98	60.35	57.98	53.98	50.78
6.1092	450	98.58	71.13	61.98	60.12	57.40	52.83	49.17
6.2146	500	103.77	73.20	63.01	60.94	57.92	52.82	48.75
6.3099	550	107.63	74.24	63.11	60.85	57.55	51.99	47.54
6.3969	600	111.18	75.26	63.29	60.85	57.30	51.32	46.53
6.4770	650	114.46	76.27	63.54	60.95	57.18	50.82	45.72
6.5511	700	117.46	77.28	63.88	61.16	57.19	50.49	45.13
6.6201	750	119.19	77.28	63.31	60.46	56.32	49.34	43.75
6.6846	800	121.66	78.28	63.82	60.88	56.59	49.36	43.58

is a good candidate, with asymptotic maximum

$$\lim_{x \to \infty} D(x) = \gamma$$

and minimum

$$D(\log 200) = \frac{\gamma}{1 + \exp(\kappa)} .$$

For example, with γ=30, δ=3 and κ=0.4, the maximum duration of treatment effect is 30 months, and the minimum is 12 months. If treatment is started as late as x=log300, then D=20.8, which increases to D=27.4 at x=log500, and to D=29.3 at x=log800. The largest increase is between log200 and log300. Because for the logistic function D′(x)>0 for all x, the deterministic EIB rule applies whenever $m_1 \geq m_2$. Table 5 contains results from the stochastic model for this choice of logistic function and varying slope ratio. For $m_2/m_1 \leq 1$ the stochastic model confirmed the deterministic EIB rule. That the EIB rule applies, however, does not necessarily mean that the expected sojourn increases substantially with x. Note that, for m_2/m_1=1, there is little to be gained from starting therapy prior to a patient's reaching a CD4 level of about 500. For m_2/m_1>1, the implications of the stochastic model

Table 5. Expected sojourn time above CD4=200, where $D(x)=\gamma/\{1+\exp[-\delta(x-\log 200)+\kappa]\}$, γ=30, δ=3, and κ=0.4.

		m_2/m_1					
		0.5	*1.0*	*1.5*	*2.0*	*3.0*	*5.0*
x	e^x						
5.5215	250	75.42	64.28	60.57	58.71	56.86	55.38
5.7038	300	83.78	67.96	62.69	60.06	57.43	55.32
5.8579	350	91.64	71.53	64.82	61.47	58.12	55.44
5.9915	400	97.88	73.89	65.90	61.90	57.91	54.71
6.1092	450	102.54	75.09	65.94	61.37	56.79	53.13
6.2146	500	106.76	76.19	66.00	60.91	55.81	51.74
6.3099	550	109.62	76.24	65.11	59.55	53.98	49.53
6.3969	600	113.18	77.26	65.29	59.30	53.32	48.53
6.4770	650	115.46	77.27	64.54	58.18	51.82	46.72
6.5511	700	117.46	77.28	63.88	57.19	50.49	45.13
6.6201	750	120.19	78.28	64.31	57.32	50.34	44.75
6.6846	800	121.66	78.28	63.82	56.59	49.36	43.58

move away from "earlier is better," but even when the after-treatment slope is twice the before-treatment slope ($m_2/m_1=2$), the expected sojourn is virtually flat as a function of x. Nonetheless, there is an optimal starting level at CD4≈400. This optimal starting level is quite insensitive to further increases in the slope ratio, decreasing only as far as 350 even when the slope ratio increases to 5.

5. Discussion.

Is earlier better when treating HIV-infected individuals with AZT? Well, it depends. In our model the crucial factors are the relative rates of decline of CD4 before and after the treatment period, m_1 and m_2, respectively, as well as the dependence of the duration function D on the CD4 level at which treatment is initiated. Some tentative generalizations emerge. When the deterministic EIB rule applies, the stochastic model is also EIB. Elsewhere, the stochastic model tends to modify the implications of the deterministic model in the direction of earlier being better. The magnitude of this effect is not necessarily large, but it depends in a complex fashion on the choice of parameters. To realistically predict the optimal level to start AZT therapy, one must have at least an approximate idea of all the parameter values and the form of the duration function D(x). For example, in our application to intravenous drug users, if one were to accept the logistic function for D(x) with $\gamma=30$, $\delta=3$ and $\kappa=0.4$ (Table 5), then one could conclude that an early start to therapy will be a good choice, unless the slope ratio exceeds 2.

There are several alternative formulations to the model which may prove useful. The CD4 count may not remain flat during the effective period of AZT therapy; there may be a discrete jump in CD4 at the initiation of therapy, or, alternatively, CD4 may continue to decrease during therapy, but at a slower rate. These modifications could be incorporated into our model without great difficulty. Another assumption made was that the after-treatment slope, m_2, was not dependent on the level x at which therapy is initiated. It has been suggested (Cotton, 1991) that the rate of CD4 decline after therapy may be slower if therapy begins earlier. This could be incorporated into the model by replacing m_2 by $m_2(x)$ in (2.4).

Specifically with respect to the stochastic formulation of the model, one posible modification would be to replace the deterministic duration function D(x) by a family of positive random variables D*(x) having distributions with parameters depending on x. An example might be exponential distributions with means b(x), for some function b. This would allow for individual variation in the duration of effectiveness of AZT. One situation in which such individual variation might manifest itself would be if drug-related toxicity resulting in treatment discontinuation occurs only in certain patients or after varying lengths of treatment. Another possible modification would be to substitute

$$D(Y_{N_1})$$

for D(x) in (3.6). In other words, the duration of treatment effect would reflect the actual CD4 level at the time treatment is started, rather than the criterion level x. However, this would result in an intractable mathematical formulation. The simpler formulation presented here is appropriate for the situation in which changes in CD4 over successive observations are small, so that

$$Y_{N_1} \approx x.$$

A related assumption in the stochastic model is that observations be equally spaced. If this assumption does not hold at least approximately, the model would have to be modified to accomodate such irregularities.

Conclusions drawn from data derived from intravenous drug users will not necessarily generalize to other risk groups. The overall poor health of intravenous drug users and, possibly, direct effects of continued drug use (Des Jarlais et al., 1987) may result in a faster CD4 decline among HIV-infected drug users than other risk groups. In most other risk groups we would expect the slope m_1 to be smaller and, consequently, the expected sojourn times to be longer.

Acknowledgments

The authors would like to thank Mr. Eugene Yuditsky for numerical calculations performed at the Courant Institute of Mathematical Sciences. This work was supported by grant DA-04722 from the National Institute on Drug Abuse and grants AI-29184 and AI-27742 from the National Institute of Allergy and Infectious Diseases.

References

Berman, S. M. (1990). A stochastic model for the distribution of HIV latency time based on T4 counts. *Biometrika* 77, 733-741.

Cotton, P. (1991). HIV surrogate markers weighed. *Journal of the*

American Medical Association **265**, 1357-1362.

Crowe, S., McGrath, M. S., and Volberding, P. A. (1990). Antiviral drug therapy for HIV infection: Rationale. In *The AIDS Knowledge Base: a textbook on HIV disease from the University of California, San Francisco, and the San Francisco General Hospital*, P. T. Cohen, M. A. Sande, and P. A. Volberding (eds), 3.2.5:1-9. Waltham, Massachusetts: The Medical Publishing Group.

Crowe, S. M., Carlin, J. B., Stewart, K. I., et al. (1991). Predictive value of CD4 lymphocyte numbers for the development of opportunistic infections and malignancies in HIV-infected persons. *Journal of AIDS* **4**, 770-776.

De Gruttola, V., and Tu, X. M. (1992). Modeling the relationship between disease progression and survival time. In *AIDS Epidemiology: Methodologic Issues*, N. P. Jewell, K. Dietz, and V. Farewell (eds). Boston: Birkhauser-Boston, 1992.

Des Jarlais, D. C., Friedman, S. R., Marmor, M., et al. (1987). Development of AIDS, HIV seroconversion, and potential cofactors for T4 cell loss in a cohort of intravenous drug users. *AIDS* **1**, 105-111.

Fischl, M. A., Richman, D. D., Grieco, M. H., et al. (1987). The efficacy of azidothymidine (AZT) in the treatment of patients with AIDS and AIDS-related complex. *New England Journal of Medicine* **317**, 185-191.

Fischl, M. A., Richman, D. D., Causey, D. M., et al. (1989). Prolonged zidovudine therapy in patients with AIDS and advanced AIDS-related complex. *Journal of the American Medical Association* **262**, 2405-2410.

Jewell, N. P., and Kalbfleisch, J. D. (1992). Marker processes in survival analysis. In *AIDS Epidemiology: Methodologic Issues*, N. P. Jewell, K. Dietz, and V. Farewell (eds). Boston: Birkhauser-Boston, 1992.

Marmor, M., Des Jarlais, D. C., Cohen, H., et al. (1987). Risk factors for infection with human immunodeficiency virus among intravenous drug abusers in New York City. *AIDS* **1**, 39-44.

McGrath, M. S. (1990). Immunology of AIDS: Overview. In *The AIDS Knowledge Base: a textbook on HIV disease from the University of California, San Francisco, and the San Francisco General Hospital*, P. T. Cohen, M. A. Sande, and P. A. Volberding (eds), 3.2.1:1-2. Waltham, Massachusetts: The Medical Publishing Group.

Robins, J. M., and Rotnitzky, A. (1992). Recovery of information and adjustment for dependent censoring using surrogate markers. In *AIDS Epidemiology: Methodologic Issues*, N. P. Jewell, K. Dietz, and V. Farewell (eds). Boston: Birkhauser-

Boston, 1992.

Rosenberg, P. S., Gail, M. H., Schrager, L. K., et al. (1991). National AIDS incidence trends and the extent of zidovudine therapy in selected demographic and transmission groups. *Journal of AIDS* **4**, 392-401.

Self, S., and Pawitan, Y. (1992). Modeling a marker of disease progression and onset of disease. In *AIDS Epidemiology: Methodologic Issues*, N. P. Jewell, K. Dietz, and V. Farewell (eds). Boston: Birkhauser-Boston, 1992.

Volberding, P. A. (1990). Clinical applications of antiviral therapy. In *The AIDS Knowledge Base: a textbook on HIV disease from the University of California, San Francisco, and the San Francisco General Hospital*, P. T. Cohen, M. A. Sande, and P. A. Volberding (eds), 4.2.5:1-5. Waltham, Massachusetts: The Medical Publishing Group.

Volberding, P. A., Lagakos, S. W., Koch, M. A., et al. (1990). Zidovudine in asymptomatic human immunodeficiency virus infection. A controlled trial in persons with fewer than 500 CD4-positive cells per cubic millimeter. *New England Journal of Medicine* **322**, 941-949.

Yang, T., and Dubin, N. (1990). Nonparametric density estimation for immunological measurements. *American Statistical Association 1989 Proceedings of the Section on Survey Research Methods*, 73-79.

Courant Institute of Mathematical Sciences, New York University, and Department of Environmental Medicine and Center for AIDS Research, New York University Medical Center.

ON THE ESTIMATION PROBLEM OF MIXING/PAIR FORMATION MATRICES WITH APPLICATIONS TO MODELS FOR SEXUALLY-TRANSMITTED DISEASES

Carlos Castillo-Chavez, Shwu-Fang Shyu, Gail Rubin and David Umbach

Abstract

A problem of considerable importance lying at the interface of social dynamics, demography, and epidemiology is determining and modeling who is mixing with whom. In this article we describe a general approach, using nonlinear mixing matrices, for modeling the process of pair-formation in heterogeneous populations. Determining who is mixing with whom is complicated by a variety of factors, including the problem of denominators, which is, in our context, equivalent to the nonexistence of closely interacting social/sexual networks. We describe the use of a mark-recapture model for estimating the sizes of the missing link, that is, the size of the population having sexual contact with a specified population and hence at risk for sexually-transmitted diseases. The need to estimate the size of the sexually-active subset before estimating the size of the population at risk introduces extra variability into the problem. An estimator of the variance of the estimated size of the population at risk that accounts for this extra variability and an expression for the bias of such an estimator have been derived. We illustrate our results with data collected from a population of university undergraduates, and make use of our axiomatic modeling approach for mixing/pair formation to compute specific mixing matrices. Complete details of this work will be published elsewhere.

1. Introduction

The importance of social and sexual interactions in the spread of sexually transmitted diseases, especially AIDS, has been well documented by sociologists, modelers, public health officials, etc. However, the development of methods for quantifying social dynamical processes in ways that allow different rates of mixing between subgroups in sexually-active populations has been quite difficult (but see Anderson *et al.*, 1986, 1989; Blythe *et al.*, 1991, 1992; Busenberg and Castillo-Chavez, 1991; Castillo-Chavez, 1989; Castillo-Chavez, ed., 1989; Castillo-Chavez and Busenberg, 1991; Castillo-Chavez *et al.*, 1991; Dietz, 1988; Dietz and Hadeler, 1988; Gupta *et al.*, 1989; Hethcote and Yorke, 1984; Hethcote and Van Ark, 1987, 1991; Hethcote *et al.*, 1991; Hyman and Stanley,

1988, 1989; Jacquez *et al.*, 1988; Rubin *et al.*, 1991; Sattenspiel and Castillo-Chavez, 1990; and references therein). Despite these efforts, work in this direction is still in its infancy in part because there is almost no adequate and/or sufficient data. Furthermore, the lack of substantial medical progress in dealing with HIV infections at the individual level has already had a strong impact on the dynamics of HIV at the population level. Dramatic changes of behavior have been observed in homosexually-active communities in San Francisco (Centers for Disease Control, 1985; McKusick et al., 1985a, 1985b; Shilts, 1987; Winkelstein, *et al.*, 1988), New York (Martin, 1986a; McFarland, 1972), and Boston (Saltzman *et al.*, 1987), demanding the development of dynamic models for the transmission of STDs that incorporate behavioral change. Unfortunately, epidemiological models that consider behavioral changes may not exhibit "typical" dynamics. In fact, multiple endemic equilibria may be quite common for models with state-dependent mixing/pair-formation processes, and control policies may have unpredictable results in these circumstances. For some recent efforts in this direction, the interested reader is referred to the work of Blythe *et al.* (1991), Castillo-Chavez (1989), Castillo-Chavez, ed. (1989), Huang *et al.* (1992) and Palmer *et al.* (1991).

This article is organized as follows: in Section 2, we describe a general axiomatic approach, using nonlinear mixing matrices for modeling the process of pair-formation in heterogeneous populations and explain their role in the transmission dynamics of STDs. Determining who is mixing with whom is complicated by a variety of factors including the problem of denominators which is, in our context, equivalent to the nonexistence of closely interacting social/sexual networks. In Section 3, we describe an axiomatic framework for modeling human interactions such as dating, mixing, or pair-formation (other interpretations are possible). In Section 4, we describe the use of a mark-recapture model for estimating the sizes of the missing link, that is, the size of the population having sexual contact with a specified population and hence at risk for sexually-transmitted diseases. One must estimate the size of the sexually-active subset before estimating the size of the population at risk, which introduces extra variability into the problem. An estimator of the variance of the estimated size of the population at risk that accounts for this extra variability and an expression for the bias of such an estimator have been derived (see Rubin *et al.*, 1991). In Section 5, we outline the possible use of these results with data collected from a population of university undergraduates, and by combining the results of Section 4 with our axiomatic modeling approach for mixing/pair formation we are able to compute specific mixing matrices (closed networks). In Section 6, we provide some conclusions and outline possible new directions.

2. Modeling of human epidemics

We begin with the description of a key component for a model of this type: the incidence rate (new cases of infection per unit time). To keep the level of discussion simple, we assume that we are dealing with a specific disease: gonorrhea. Therefore we have to consider, for a simple model, only two type of epidemiological classes: susceptibles and infecteds (here assumed infectious). The mixing probabilities, as well as other behavioral and epidemiological parameters, determine the rate at which new infections are generated. The incidence rate is given by a nonlinear function of the different interacting subpopulations and, in this context, we develop our approaches to estimating the social/sexual mixing structure of a population.

The data used in applying this modeling framework consists of a population of heterosexually-active college students and, consequently, we formulate our ideas in the context of two-sex heterosexually mixing populations (the description is considerably simplified when one deals with exclusively homosexually-active populations). Our heterosexually-active population is divided into classes or subpopulations which may be defined by sex, race, socio-economic background, average degree of sexual activity, etc. Models that incorporate factors such as chronological age, age of infection, variable infectivity, and partnership duration also have been formulated (see Busenberg and Castillo-Chavez, 1989, 1991).

For the purposes of this article, we consider only N-sexually active populations of females and L-sexually active populations of males, each divided into two epidemiological classes: $S_f^j(t)$ and $S_m^i(t)$ (susceptible females and males, i.e., uninfected and sexually active at time t); $I_f^j(t)$ and $I_m^i(t)$ (infected females and males at time t); for $j = 1,\cdots,N$ and $i = 1,\cdots,L$. Consequently, individuals at risk (sexually-active) of each sex and each subpopulation at time t are represented by $T_f^j(t) = S_f^j(t) + I_f^j(t)$ and $T_m^i(t) = S_m^i(t) + I_m^i(t)$. We obviously do not need to consider other individuals if our only concern is, as in this paper, the study of the dynamics of sexually-transmitted diseases.

Following the superscript notation, $B_f^j(t)$ and $B_m^i(t)$ denote the jth and ith incidence rates for females in group j and males in group i at time t, that is, the number of new infective cases in each subpopulation per unit time. As we shall see, $B_f^j(t)$ and $B_m^i(t)$ constitute a set of complicated expressions. In fact, they are functions of the frequency and type of sexual interactions that susceptible females of group j and susceptible males of group i have with all other sexually-active individuals (in this case, of the opposite sex, although this condition can be easily relaxed).

A dynamic model needs a source of new individuals; the modeling of this demographic process could be extremely complicated (see

Busenberg and Castillo-Chavez, 1989, 1991; Castillo-Chavez and Busenberg, 1991; Castillo-Chavez *et al.*, 1991). If one wishes, for example, to study the demographic consequences of a disease like HIV/AIDS, one needs to model carefully the "recruitment" of new individuals. Here we want to keep the demography simple and assume constant "recruitment" and constant per-capita mortality (removal from sexual activity) rates. Specifically, we let Λ_f^j and Λ_m^i denote the "recruitment" rates (assumed constant), μ_f^j and μ_m^i denote the (constant) per-capita removal rates from sexual activity, and γ_f^j and γ_m^i denote the (constant) per-capita recovery rates from gonorrhea infection. A simple model for the transmission dynamics of gonorrhea is given by the following set of differential equations:

$$\frac{dS_f^j(t)}{dt} = \Lambda_f^j - B_f^j(t) - \mu_f^j S_f^j(t) + \gamma_f^j I_f^j(t), \tag{1}$$

$$\frac{dI_f^j(t)}{dt} = B_f^j(t) - (\gamma_f^j + \mu_f^j) I_f^j(t), \tag{2}$$

$$\frac{dS_m^i(t)}{dt} = \Lambda_m^i - B_m^i(t) - \mu_m^i S_m^i(t) + \gamma_m^i I_m^i(t), \tag{3}$$

$$\frac{dI_m^i(t)}{dt} = B_m^i(t) - (\gamma_m^i + \mu_m^i) I_m^i(t), \tag{4}$$

$$i = 1,\cdots, L \text{ and } j = 1,\cdots,N.$$

Of course, this model is not fully specified until we provide explicit expressions for $B_f^j(t)$ and $B_m^i(t)$. The formulae are provided in two steps: first we provide expressions for the incidences in terms of a set of mixing probabilities $\{p_{ij}(t)$ and $q_{ji}(t)$: $i=1,\cdots,L$ and $j=1,\cdots,N\}$; and secondly, we describe these mixing probabilities (in the next section) in terms of an axiomatic system for social/sexual interactions. More definitions are needed:

$p_{ij}(t)$: fraction of partnerships of males in group i with females in group j at time t,

$q_{ji}(t)$: fraction of partnerships of females in group j with males in group i at time t,

$T_m^i(t)$: male population size of group i at time t,

$T_f^j(t)$: female population size of group j at time t,

c^i : average (constant) number of female partners per unit time of males in group i, or the ith-group rate of male pair-formation,

b^j : average (constant) number of male partners per unit time of females in group j, or the jth-group rate of female pair-formation,

β^i_m : transmission coefficient (constant) of males in group i,

β^j_f : transmission coefficient (constant) of females in group j.

The following expressions for the incidence rates are a direct consequence of these definitions:

$$B^i_m(t) = c^i S^i_m(t) \sum_{j=1}^{N} \beta^j_f p_{ij}(t) \frac{I^j_f(t)}{T^j_f(t)}, \tag{5}$$

and

$$B^j_f(t) = b^j S^j_f(t) \sum_{i=1}^{L} \beta^i_m q_{ji}(t) \frac{I^i_m(t)}{T^i_m(t)}. \tag{6}$$

The modeling of the mixing/pair-formation probabilities constitute the body of the next section.

3. Modeling of mixing/pair-formation probabilities

Solutions for one-sex mixing populations have been previously obtained by Anderson et al. (1989), Blythe and Castillo-Chavez (1989), Castillo-Chavez and Blythe (1989), Gupta *et al.* (1989), Hethcote and Yorke (1984), Hyman and Stanley (1988, 1989), Jacquez *et al.* (1988, 1989), Nold (1980), and many others. A representation theorem describing all mixing/pair-formation solutions as random perturbations of random (proportionate) mixing, based on the work of Blythe and Castillo-Chavez (op. cits.), was obtained by Busenberg and Castillo-Chavez (1989, 1991). Models that follow pairs of individuals (two-sex models) can be found (in a demographic context) in the works of Kendall (1949), Keyfitz (1949), Parlett (1972), and Pollard (1973). Formulations of the standard two-sex mixing pair-formation framework are found in the work of Fredrickson (1971) and Martin (1986b), while applications of the Fredrickson-McFarland framework to epidemiological models has been carried out by Castillo-Chavez (1989), Castillo-Chavez *et al.* (1991), Dietz (1988), Dietz and Hadeler (1988), Hadeler (1989a, 1989b), Hadeler and Ngoma (1990) and Waldstätter (1989). In this section we provide an alternative approach to modeling the process of pair-formation or social mixing. Like Fredrickson (1971), we use an axiomatic framework to describe the probabilities associated with possible interactions such as pair-formation, or social mixing (further details are found in Castillo-Chavez *et al.*, 1991, where some special solutions were given). Specifically, the set of mixing probabilities $\{p_{ij}(t)$ and $q_{ji}(t)$: $i = 1,\cdots,L$ and $j = 1,\cdots,N\}$ establishes the mixing/pair formation in a heterosexually-active population in agreement with the following (postulated) set of properties:

Def $(\mathcal{P}(t), \mathcal{Q}(t)) \equiv (p_{ij}(t), q_{ji}(t))$ is called a mixing/pair-formation matrix if and only if it satisfies the following properties at all times:

(A1) $0 \leq p_{ij} \leq 1, \qquad 0 \leq q_{ji} \leq 1,$

(A2) $\sum_{j=1}^{N} p_{ij} = 1 = \sum_{i=1}^{L} q_{ji}\,,$

(A3) $c^i T_m^i p_{ij} = b^j T_f^j q_{ji}, \qquad i = 1, \cdots, L, \quad j = 1, \cdots, N.$

(A4) If for some i, $1 \leq i \leq L$ and/or some j, $1 \leq j \leq N$, $c^i b^j T_m^i T_f^j = 0$, then we define $p_{ij} \equiv q_{ji} \equiv 0$.

Property (A3) can be interpreted as a conservation of partnerships law or a group reversibility property (applied to rates), while (A4) asserts, the obvious, that is, that the mixing of "non-existing" or non-sexually active subpopulations cannot be arbitrarily defined. A very useful solution is the Ross solution which corresponds to proportionate mixing when there are two clearly distinct sets of individuals who do not mix among themselves. Ross solutions naturally arise if we search for separable solutions.

Def A two-sex mixing/pair-formation function is called separable iff it is given by products of the form

$$p_{ij} = p_i \tilde{p}_j \quad \text{and} \quad q_{ji} = q_j \tilde{q}_i\,,$$

where p_i, $\tilde{p}_j$, q_j, $\tilde{q}_i$ are arbitrary functions subject to the mixing constraints, $i = 1, \cdots, L$ and $j = 1, \cdots, N$.

Theorem 1: The only separable solution is Ross solution given by $(\bar{p}^j, \bar{q}^i)$, which are featured by superscripts and bars, and

$$\bar{p}^j = \frac{b^j T_f^j}{\sum_{i=1}^{L} c^i T_m^i}\,, \quad \bar{q}^i = \frac{c^i T_m^i}{\sum_{j=1}^{N} b^j T_f^j}\,; \quad j = 1, \cdots, N \text{ and } i = 1, \cdots, L\,. \tag{7}$$

Remark: From (A3) it follows that

$$\frac{p_{ij}}{q_{ji}} = \frac{b^j T_f^j}{c^i T_m^i} = \frac{\bar{p}^j}{\bar{q}^i}\,, \tag{8}$$

and hence (A4) implies that the support of any two-sex mixing function is contained in the support of $(\bar{p}^j, \bar{q}^i)$.

We now use (7) to generate all solutions to axioms (A1)-(A4). We begin by introducing some new terms. Let

$(\phi_{ij}^m) \equiv$ males' structural covariance matrix $(0 \leq \phi_{ij}^m)$ denoting the degree of preference (i.e., the deviation from random mixing) that group i-males have from group j-females, $j = 1,\cdots,N$, $i = 1,\cdots,L$.

$$\ell_m^i \equiv \sum_{k=1}^{N} \bar{p}^k \phi_{ik}^m \equiv \text{weighted average preference of group } i \text{ males}, \quad i = 1,\cdots,L.$$

$$R_m^i \equiv 1 - \ell_m^i, \qquad i = 1, \cdots, L. \tag{9}$$

We require that $R_m^i \geq 0$, and that

$$\sum_{i=1}^{L} \ell_m^i \bar{p}^i = \sum_{i=1}^{L} \sum_{k=1}^{N} \bar{p}^k \phi_{ik}^m \bar{p}^i < 1\,. \tag{10}$$

Similarly, let

$(\phi_{ji}^f) \equiv$ females' structure covariance matrix $(0 \leq \phi_{ji}^f)$ denoting the degree of preference (i.e., the deviation from random mixing) that group j-females have for group i-males, $j = 1,\cdots,N$, $i = 1,\cdots,L$.

$$\ell_f^j \equiv \sum_{k=1}^{L} \bar{q}^k \phi_{jk}^f \equiv \text{weighted average preference of group } j\text{-females}, \quad i = 1,\cdots,N\,.$$

$$R_f^j \equiv 1 - \ell_f^j, \qquad j = 1, \cdots, N\,. \tag{11}$$

Again, we require that $R_f^j \geq 0$, and that

$$\sum_{j=1}^{N} \ell_f^j \bar{q}^j = \sum_{j=1}^{N} \sum_{k=1}^{L} \bar{q}^k \phi_{jk}^f \bar{q}^j < 1\,. \tag{12}$$

All solutions to axioms (A1) – (A4) are given (formally) by the following multiplicative perturbations to the separable mixing solution $(\bar{p}^j, \bar{q}^i)$:

$$p_{ij} = \bar{p}^j \left[\frac{R_f^j R_m^i}{\sum_{k=1}^{N} \bar{p}^k R_f^k} + \phi_{ij}^m \right], \qquad i = 1,\cdots,L; \quad j = 1,\cdots,N, \tag{13}$$

$$q_{ji} = \bar{q}^i \left[\frac{R_m^i R_f^j}{\sum_{k=1}^{L} \bar{q}^k R_m^k} + \phi_{ji}^f \right]. \tag{14}$$

The formal proof of this result can be found in Castillo-Chavez and Busenberg (1991). For future reference, we write down this theorem explicitly:

Theorem 2. Let $\{\phi_{ij}^m\}$ and $\{\phi_{ji}^f\}$ be two nonnegative matrices. Let $\ell_m^i \equiv \sum_{k=1}^{N} \bar{p}^k \phi_{ik}^m$ and $\ell_f^j \equiv \sum_{k=1}^{L} \bar{q}^k \phi_{jk}^f$, where $\left\{(\bar{p}^j, \bar{q}^i): j = 1,\cdots,N \text{ and } i = 1,\cdots,L\right\}$

denotes the set composed of Ross solutions. We also let $R_m^i \equiv 1 - \ell_m^i$, $i = 1, \cdots, L$ and $R_f^j \equiv 1 - \ell_f^j$, $j = 1, \cdots,N$, and assume that ϕ_{ij}^m and ϕ_{ji}^f are chosen in such a way that R_m^i and R_f^j remain nonnegative for all time. We further assume that

$$\sum_{i=1}^{L} \ell_m^i \bar{p}^i = \sum_{i=1}^{L} \sum_{k=1}^{N} \bar{p}^k \phi_{ik}^m \bar{p}^i < 1,$$

and

$$\sum_{j=1}^{N} \ell_f^j \bar{q}^j = \sum_{j=1}^{N} \sum_{k=1}^{L} \bar{q}^k \phi_{jk}^f \bar{q}^j < 1.$$

Then all the solutions to axioms (A1)-(A4) are given by Equations (13) and (14).

Remark: ϕ_{ij}^m and ϕ_{ji}^f can always be chosen in such a way that R_m^i and R_f^j remain nonnegative for all time (i.e., let them be in the interval [0,1]). However, there is no recipe for specifying necessary conditions for the nonnegativity of R_m^i and R_f^j because their values are intimately connected to the time-dependent values of Ross solutions and hence to the associated (and disease-dependent) dynamical system.

4. Estimation of sizes of mixing subpopulations

Our main purpose here is to compute *explicit examples* of mixing/pair-formation matrices from our data on mixing. These time-dependent matrices describe the network of interactions between groups of individuals (who is mixing with whom). Our examples (to be illustrated in Section 5), albeit for a single time, provide the first mixing matrices computed from data. Knowledge of these matrices over a period of time is essential to *any* type of long-term forecasting. Because our purposes are limited and our data is too specific, we do not need to use sophisticated approaches in the construction of these matrices. Mark-recapture methodology can be applied to survey data to estimate the number of different sexual partners from each of several groups that an individual has had in a fixed period of time, or to estimate the size of the population having sexual contact with members of a given group. Thus, one can apply this methodology to survey data to estimate the size of the population at risk for a sexually transmitted disease. Using data from our survey conducted at Cornell University in 1989 (see Crawford *et al.*, 1990), we use mark-recapture estimators to provide estimates of the size of the population that has sexual contact with Cornell undergraduates but are not Cornell undergraduates. We use these estimates and our one- and two-sex mixing framework to construct explicit mixing matrices (see Section 5). In our situation, prior to sampling, the population contains both marked and unmarked individuals: contacts (i.e., sexual partners) are either Cornell undergraduates or not and, obviously, we only have access to information about Cornell and non-Cornell partners from the Cornell students surveyed. It is appropriate to think of the students surveyed as observers in mark-recapture bird studies in which "recapture" is done by sighting. Because the nature of our population, we need not worry about loss of marks or marks being overlooked, which is a problem in many applications of mark-recapture to bird and mammalian populations. For each student surveyed, the contacts reported are distinct sexual partners. However, any two Cornell students that were surveyed may share one or more sexual partners, either from the Cornell undergraduate pool, from the greater Ithaca area, or from the world. Thus, the combined number may contain multiple counts of the same sexual partner; we are sampling *with replacement* with respect to sexual contacts when we combine information across the students surveyed. Hence the closed population single mark release model, which is based on sampling with replacement (Bailey 1951), gives an appropriate *first* estimate of the population size. We believe that given the current availability of data on mixing, this approximation is entirely appropriate for our purposes. Let the subscript k denote sex (k = male, female). S_k denotes the number of undergraduates of sex k registered at Cornell, and T_k of those (S_k) are sexually active. The total contacts with individuals (Cornell undergraduates, or not Cornell undergraduates) of sex k per unit time (two months) from respondents of the opposite sex is denoted by y_k, and x_k of those are contacts with Cornell undergraduates. Then the Lincoln-Petersen estimator $\hat{N}_k$ is given by

$$\hat{N}_k = T_k(y_k + 1) \Big/ (x_k + 1) \,, \tag{15}$$

which is a nearly unbiased estimator of the number of individuals of sex k at risk (N_k) (see Bailey, 1951), and

$$\hat{\mathrm{Var}}(\hat{N}_k \,|\, y_k, T_k) = T_k^2(y_k + 1)(y_k - x_k) \Big/ \left\{(x_k + 1)^2(x_k + 2)\right\} \tag{16}$$

is a nearly unbiased estimator of the variance of $\hat{N}_k$, when the number of sexually active students is known. Because a given sexual partner can be reported by more than one of the students surveyed, the total number of contacts (y_k) can be greater than N_k, thereby increasing the precision of the survey for N_k (see Seber, 1982).

However, we must estimate T_k from the survey data; T_k can be estimated with the maximum likelihood estimator under Bailey's approximate binomial model as

$$\hat{T}_k = S_k t_k \Big/ r_k \equiv S_k \hat{\pi}_k ,$$

where $\hat{\pi}_k$ estimates $\pi_k = T_k \;/\; S_k$, the probability of an individual of sex k in the surveyed population being sexually active, and r_k and t_k denote the number of Cornell undergraduates in the sample and the corresponding number that are sexually active. Hence, the corresponding estimator of N_k is

$$\tilde{N}_k = \hat{T}_k(y_k + 1) \Big/ (x_k + 1) , \tag{17}$$

which is a nearly unbiased estimator also, with proportional bias of order

$$\left[1 - \pi_k + \pi_k \exp\left\{-y_k S_k \Big/ (N_k r_k)\right\}\right]^{r_k} \equiv \left\{B(N_k)\right\}^{r_k} . \tag{18}$$

An estimator of the variance of $\tilde{N}_k$ that takes into account the additional variability due to estimation of T_k is given by

$$\hat{\mathrm{Var}}(\tilde{N}_k \,|\, y_k) = A(\hat{\pi}_k) \Big/ C(\hat{\pi}_k) + \tilde{N}_k^2\left[\left\{B(\tilde{N}_k/2)\right\}^{r_k} - \left\{B(\tilde{N}_k)\right\}^{2r_k}\right], \tag{19}$$

where

$$\begin{aligned} A(\hat{\pi}_k) = {} & S_k^3 y_k (y_k + 1)^2 (\tilde{N}_k r_k^3)^{-1} r_k \hat{\pi}_k [\{1 - a_k\} + \hat{\pi}_k (r_k - 1)\{3 - 7a_k\} \\ & + \hat{\pi}_k^2 (r_k - 1)(r_k - 2)\{1 - 6a_k\} - \hat{\pi}_k^3 (r_k - 1)(r_k - 2)(r_k - 3) a_k] , \end{aligned} \tag{20}$$

with $a_k = S_k / (\tilde{N}_k r_k)$, and

$$\begin{aligned} C(\hat{\pi}_k) = {} & \hat{\pi}_k^4 r_k (r_k - 1)(r_k - 2)(r_k - 3) y_k^4 a_k^4 + 2\hat{\pi}_k^3 r_k (r_k - 1)(r_k - 2) \\ & \times y_k^3 a_k^3 \left\{3 y_k a_k + 2\right\} + \hat{\pi}_k^2 r_k (r_k - 1) y_k^2 a_k^2 \left\{6(y_k a_k + 1)^2 + 1\right\} \\ & + \hat{\pi}_k r_k y_k a_k (y_k a_k + 2)\left\{2 + y_k a_k (y_k a_k + 2)\right\} + 1 . \end{aligned} \tag{21}$$

The bias of this variance estimator is given in Rubin *et al.* (1991).

We wish to estimate the size of the population that has sexual contact with Cornell undergraduates but are not Cornell undergraduates, that is, $O_k = N_k - T_k$. An estimate of O_k is given by

$$\begin{aligned} \hat{O}_k = \tilde{N}_k - \hat{T}_k &= \left\{\hat{T}_k (y_k + 1) \Big/ (x_k + 1)\right\} - \hat{T}_k \\ &= \hat{T}_k\left[\left\{(y_k + 1) \Big/ (x_k + 1)\right\} - 1\right]. \end{aligned} \tag{22}$$

The estimated variance of $N_k - T_k$ conditional on y_k contacts, is equal to the variance given in (19) plus

$$\hat{\text{Var}}(\hat{T}_k \mid y_k) = \hat{\pi}_k(1-\hat{\pi}_k)S_k^2 \Big/ (r_k-1) \ . \tag{23}$$

Mark-recapture estimators are design-based rather than model-based; they do not rely on a probabilistic model, such as exponential or Weibull, for the growth of the population whose size the researcher wishes to estimate. Therefore, mark-recapture population estimates can provide an independent benchmark against which to compare estimates based on different probabilistic models.

5. Mixing Matrices

We (Castillo-Chavez, Crawford, and Schwager, see Crawford *et al.*, 1990) found in our recent survey of social/sexual mixing among Cornell undergraduates (CUSSP) that over a period of two months a larger fraction of females (111/253) than males (21/249) reported sexual activity. Those males that reported sexual activity during this two-month period had an average of 2.5 sexual partners while females reported about 1.4 sexual-partners during the same period of time. Table 1 shows that female Cornell undergraduate respondents that were sexually active during September and October 1989 had about 50% of their sexual contacts with Cornell undergraduates, and the remaining 50% with "outsiders", which includes Cornell graduate students, staff, faculty (GSF), and indiviudals not affiliated with Cornell (non-CU). The diagonal elements in Table 1 are always larger; that is, we see a strong "like-with-like" component. Further, the upper triangular elements are larger than the lower triangular elements, that is, females mix more often with upperclassmen, usually older males. We further note that Table 1 is not a complete mixing matrix because the population is not closed. Estimates on the sizes and sexual activity of the external mixing populations are still required.

Using the mark-recapture methods described above in conjunction with our survey data and using the mixing axioms to input "missing" values, one can complete plausible mixing matrices (see Figures 1 and 2 below).

The two figures constitute a sample of the type of matrices that one may get as one closes the network with the help of the estimate of the size of the sexually-active population that has sexual or social contact with the Cornell undergraduate population and with the use of the axioms for mixing (that is we "force" the conservation of partners law). Of course, many other matrices are possible for the same data. However, the continued repetition of the above procedure yields the same qualitative picture if the number of groups is not too small or too large. The writing of this article had the purpose of describing the nature of the mixing problem and an outline of a possible solution. The specific details involved in the construction of these mixing matrices will be published elsewhere.

Total number of female respondents	Female respondent – male partners								
	Male Cornell undergraduate partners					Other male partners			
	Freshman	Sophomore	Junior	Senior	*Subtotal* ($x_{mj\cdot}$)	GSF	non-CU	*Subtotal* ($y_{mj\cdot}-x_{mj\cdot}$)	***Total Contacts*** ($y_{mj\cdot}$)
Freshman 20	5 (*17.2%*)	4 (*13.8%*)	4 (*13.8%*)	2 (*6.9%*)	15 (*51.7%*)	0 (*0%*)	14 (*48.3%*)	14 (*48.3%*)	29 (*100%*)
Sophomore 26	1 (*2.9%*)	12 (*34.3%*)	6 (*17.1%*)	2 (*5.7%*)	21 (*60.0%*)	5 (*14.3%*)	9 (*25.7%*)	14 (*40.0%*)	35 (*100%*)
Junior 36	1 (*2.4%*)	4 (*9.8%*)	11 (*26.8%*)	7 (*17.1%*)	23 (*56.1%*)	0 (*0%*)	18 (*43.9%*)	18 (*43.9%*)	41 (*100%*)
Senior 28	0 (*0%*)	0 (*0%*)	1 (*3.5%*)	7 (*24.1%*)	8 (*27.6%*)	9 (*31.0%*)	12 (*41.4%*)	21 (*72.4%*)	29 (*100%*)
Total 111	7 (*5.2%*)	20 (*15.0%*)	22 (*16.4%*)	18 (*13.4%*)	67 (*50.0%*)	14 (*10.4%*)	53 (*39.6%*)	67 (*50.0%*)	134 (*100%*)

Table 1. An extract from data derived from the sexual survey among Cornell undergraduates, Fall 1989. Data show the sexual mixing pattern of female respondents. All survey respondents classify their Cornell partners by college class. Therefore, three subscripts are required to tabulate Cornell sexual partners properly: k denotes the sex of the partner, j denotes the college class of the respondent and i denotes the college class of the partner. Above, $y_{kj\cdot}$ denotes the total number of sexual contacts with individuals of sex k during the two month period reported by individuals of class j, and $x_{kj\cdot}$ denotes the total number of sexual contacts with Cornell undergraduates of sex k reported by respondents of class j.

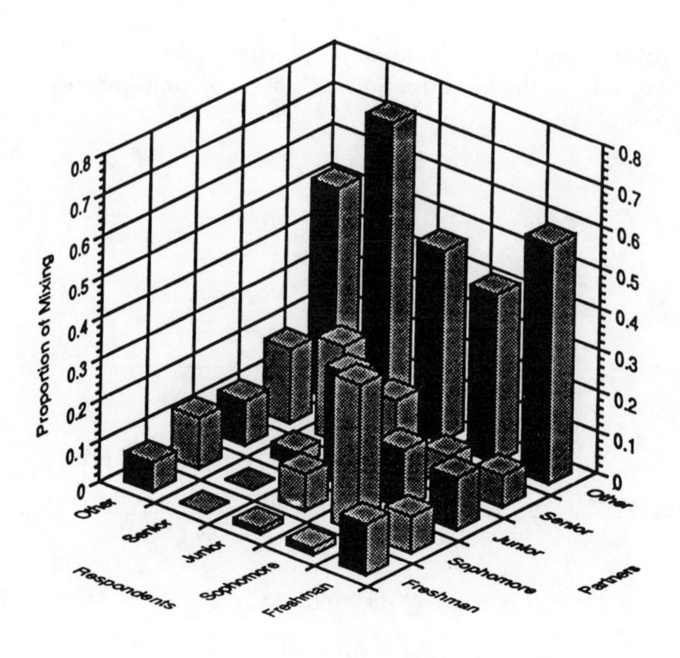

Fig. 1. Mixing matrices from survey data.

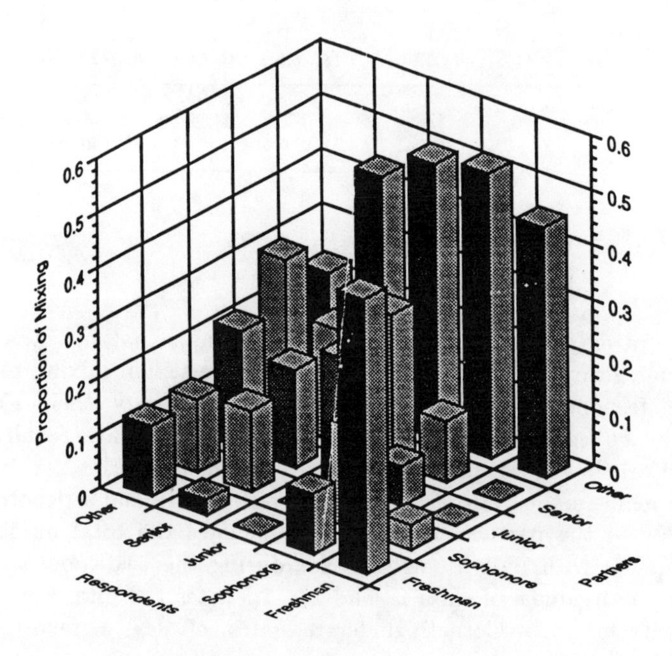

Fig. 2. Mixing matrices from survey data.

6. Conclusions

Several conclusions can be drawn from our preliminary efforts in estimating the contact structure of a heterosexually mixing population. A large number of groups will present very difficult estimation problems because of the large number of parameters involved, and because some of the mixing probabilities will be near zero. But a very small number of groups will not capture the level of heterogeneity needed to understand the consequences of extreme sexual behaviors. Given the difficulties involved in estimating mixing probabilities, levels of sexual activity, and group preferences or affinities from data, we see very little *practical* use of models that involve more than 8 groups, and strongly recommend the use of 4 to 6 groups for detailed epidemiological studies. Here the "correct" scale is determined by data. The selection of useful models for detailed epidemiological studies has to be guided by our clear understanding of the key features in HIV transmission. While very detailed epidemiological models may not be useful for specialized epidemiological investigations, their study is central to the theoretical understanding of the importance that several epidemiological and sociological factors – including long periods of incubation, variable infectivity, age-structure, and social mixing – may have on the dynamics of HIV/AIDS. Numerical and analytical studies (see Thieme and Castillo-Chavez, 1989, 1990) of detailed models provide the basis for the selection of the less detailed models that are required to address specific practical questions. In summary, theoretical studies in combination with data help us sort out the boundaries between practice and theory. Theoretical studies, through mathematical models, help us rank the importance of biological detail and guide us in choosing, *a priori*, the most appropriate scales at which to address specific biological questions.

7. Acknowledgements

This research has been partially supported by NSF grant DMS-8906580, NIAID Grant R01 A129178-02, and Hatch project grant NYC 151-409, USDA to CC-C. Also many thanks to Dr. K. Dietz for his valuable comments.

References

Anderson, R. M., May, R. M. and Medley, G. F. (1986). A preliminary study of the transmission dynamics of the human immunodeficiency virus (HIV), the causative agent of AIDS. *IMA J. Math. Med. Biol.* **3**, 229-263.

Anderson, R. M., Blythe, S. P., Gupta, S. and Konings, E. (1989). The transmission dynamics of the Human Immunodeficiency Virus Type 1 in the male homosexual community in the United Kingdom: the influence of changes in sexual behavior. *Phil. Trans. R. Soc. Lond.* **B 325**, 145-198.

Bailey, N. T. J. (1951). On estimating the size of mobile populations from recapture data. *Biometrika* **38**, 293-306.

Blythe, S. P. and Castillo-Chavez, C. (1989). Like-with-like preference and sexual mixing models. *Math. Biosci.* **96**, 221-238.

Blythe, S. P., Castillo-Chavez, C. and Casella, G. (1992). Empirical methods for the estimation of the mixing probabilities for socially-structured populations from a single survey sample. *Mathematical Population Studies* (in press).

Blythe, S. P., Castillo-Chavez, C., Palmer, J. and Cheng, M. (1991). Towards unified theory of mixing and pair formation. *Math. Biosci.* **107**: 379-405.

Blythe, S. P., Cooke, K. and Castillo-Chavez, C. (1991). Autonomous risk-behavior change, and non-linear incidence rate, in models of sexually transmitted diseases. *Biometrics Unit Technical Report* **BU-1048-M**, Cornell University, Ithaca, NY.

Busenberg, S. and Castillo-Chavez, C. (1989). Interaction, pair formation and force of infection terms in sexually-transmitted diseases. In *Mathematical and Statistical Approaches to AIDS Epidemiology,* C. Castillo-Chavez (ed.), Lecture Notes in Biomathematics 83, 289-300. Berlin, Heidelberg, New York, London, Paris, Tokyo, Hong Kong: Springer-Verlag.

Busenberg, S. and Castillo-Chavez, C. (1991). A general solution of the problem of mixing subpopulations, and its application to risk- and age-structured epidemic models for the spread of AIDS. *IMA J. of Mathematics Applied in Med. and Biol.* **8**, 1-29.

Castillo-Chavez, C. (1989). Review of recent models of HIV/AIDS transmission. In *Applied Mathematical Ecology,* S. A. Levin, T. G. Hallam and L. J. Gross (eds.), Biomathematics 18, 253-262. Berlin, Heidelberg, New York, London, Paris, Tokyo, Hong Kong: Springer-Verlag.

Castillo-Chavez, C. (ed.). (1989). *Mathematical and Statistical Approaches to* AIDS *Epidemiology,* Lecture Notes in Biomathematics 83. Berlin, Heidelberg, New York, London, Paris, Tokyo, Hong Kong: Springer-Verlag.

Castillo-Chavez, C. and Blythe, S. P. (1989). Mixing framework for social/sexual behavior. In *Mathematical and statistical approaches to AIDS epidemiology,* C. Castillo-Chavez (ed.), Lecture Notes in Biomathematics 83, 275-288. Berlin, Heidelberg, New York, London, Paris, Tokyo, Hong Kong: Springer-Verlag.

Castillo-Chavez, C. and Busenberg, S. (1991). On the solution of the two-sex moxong problem. In *Proceedings of the International Conference on Differential Equations and Applications to Biology and Population Dynamics*, S. Busenberg and M. Martelli (eds.), Lecture Notes in Biomathematics 92, 80-98. Berlin, Heidelberg, New York, London, Paris, Tokyo, Hong Kong, Barcelona, Budapest: Springer-Verlag.

Castillo-Chavez, C., Busenberg, S. and Gerow, K. (1991). Pair formation in structured populations. In *Differential Equations with Applications in Biology, Physics and Engineering*, J. Goldstein, F. Kappel and W. Schappacher (eds.), 47-65. New York: Marcel Dekker.

Castillo-Chavez, C., Cooke, K. L., Huang, W. and Levin, S. A. (1989a). Results on the dynamics for models for the sexual transmission of the human immunodeficiency virus. *Applied Math. Letters* 2, 327-331.

Castillo-Chavez, C., Cooke, K. L., Huang, W. and Levin, S. A. (1989b). On the role of long incubation periods in the dynamics of HIV/AIDS, Part 2: Multiple group models. In *Mathematical and Statistical Approaches to* AIDS *Epidemiology*, C. Castillo-Chavez (ed.), Lecture Notes in Biomathematics 83, 200-217. Berlin, Heidelberg, New York, London, Paris, Tokyo, Hong Kong: Springer-Verlag.

Centers for Disease Control. (1985). Self-reported behavioral change among gay and bisexual men, San Francisco. *MMWR* **34**, 613-615.

Crawford, C. M., Schwager, S. J. and Castillo-Chavez, C. (1990). A methodology for asking sensitive questions among college undergraduates. *Biometrics Unit Tech. Report* **BU-1105-M**, Cornell University, Ithaca, New York.

Dietz, K. (1988). On the transmission dynamics of HIV. *Math. Biosci.* **90**, 397-414.

Dietz, K. and Hadeler, K. P. (1988). Epidemiological models for sexually transmitted diseases. *J. Math. Biol.* **26**, 1-25.

Fredrickson, A. G. (1971). A mathematical theory of age structure in sexual populations: Random mating and monogamous marriage models. *Math. Biosci.* **20**, 117-143.

Gupta, S., Anderson, R. M. and May, R. M. (1989). Networks of sexual contacts: implications for the pattern of spread of HIV. *AIDS* **3**, 1-11.

Hadeler, K. P. (1989a). Pair formation in age-structured populations. *Acta Applicandae Mathematicae* **14**, 91-102.

Hadeler, K. P. (1989b). Modeling AIDS in structured populations. *47th Session of the International Statistical Institute, Paris, August /September.* Conference Proc. C1-2.1, 83-99.

Hadeler, K. P. and Ngoma, K. (1990). Homogeneous models for sexually transmitted diseases. *Rocky Mountain Journal of Mathematics* **20**, 967-986.

Hethcote, H. W. and Yorke, J. A. (1984). *Gonorrhea transmission dynamics and control*, Lect. Notes Biomath. 56. Berlin, Heidelberg, New York, London, Paris, Tokyo, Hong Kong: Springer-Verlag.

Hethcote, H. W. and Van Ark, J. W. (1987). Epidemiological models for heterogeneous populations: proportionate mixing, parameter estimation, and immunization programs. *Math. Biosci.* **84**, 85-111.

Hethcote, H. W., Van Ark, J. W. and Karon, J. M. (1991). A simulation model of AIDS in San Francisco, II. Simulations, therapy, and sensitivity analysis. *Math, Biosci.* **106**, 223-247.

Hethcote, H. W. and Van Ark, J. W. (1992). Weak linkage between HIV epidemics in homosexual men and intravenous drug users (in this volume).

Hyman, J. M. and Stanley, E. A. (1988). Using mathematical models to understand the AIDS epidemic. *Math. Biosci.* **90**, 415-473.

Hyman, J. M. and Stanley, E. A. (1989). The effect of social mixing patterns on the spread of AIDS. In *Mathematical Approaches to Problems in Resource Management and Epidemiology*, C. Castillo-Chavez, S. A. Levin and C. A. Shoemaker (eds.), Lect. Notes Biomath. 81, 190-219. Berlin, Heidelberg, New York, London, Paris, Tokyo, Hong Kong: Springer-Verlag.

Huang, W., Cooke, K. and Castillo-Chavez, C. (1992). Stability and bifurcation for a multiple group model for the dynamics of HIV/AIDS transmission. *SIAM J. of Applied Math.* (in press).

Jacquez, J. A., Simon, C. P., Koopman, J., Sattenspiel, L. and Perry, T. (1988). Modeling and analyzing HIV transmission: the effect of contact patterns. *Math. Biosci.* **92**, 119-199.

Jacqez, J. A., Simon, C. P. and Koopman, J. (1989). Structured mixing: heterogeneous mixing by the definition of mixing groups. In *Mathematical and Statistical Approaches to AIDS Epidemiology*, C. Castillo-Chavez (ed.), Lecture Notes in Biomathematics 83, 301-315. Berlin, Heidelberg, New York, London, Paris, Tokyo, Hong Kong: Springer-Verlag.

Kendall, D. G. (1949). Stochastic processes and population growth. *Roy. Statist. Soc., Ser.* **B 2**, 230-264.

Keyfitz, N. (1949). The mathematics of sex and marriage. In *Proceedings of the Sixth Berkeley Symposium on Mathematical Statistics and Probability, Vol. IV: Biology and Health*, 89-108.

McFarland, D. D. (1972). Comparison of alternative marriage models. In

Population Dynamics, T. N. E. Greville (ed.), 89-106. New York, London: Academic Press.

Martin, J. L. (1986a). AIDS risk reduction recommendations and sexual behavior patterns among gay men: a multifactorial categorical approach to assessing change. *Health Educ. Qtly.* **13**, 347-358.

Martin, J. L. (1986b). The impact of AIDS in gay male sexual behavior patterns in New York City. *Am. J. of Pub. Health* **77**, 578-581.

McKusick, L., Horstman, W. and Coates, T. J. (1985a). AIDS and sexual behavior reported by gay men in San Francisco. *Public Health Reports* **75**, 493-496.

McKusick, L., Wiley, J. A., Coates, T. J., Stall, R., Saika, B., Morin, S., Horstman, C. K. and Conant, M. A. (1985b). Reported changes in the sexual behavior of men at risk for AIDS, San Francisco, 1983-1984: the AIDS behavioral research project. *Public Health Reports* **100**, 622-629.

Nold, A. (1980). Heterogeneity in disease-transmission modeling. *Math. Biosci.* **52**, 227–240.

Palmer, J. S., Castillo-Chavez, C. and Blythe, S. P. (1991). State-dependent mixing and state-dependent contact rates in epidemiological models. *Biometrics Unit Technical Report* **BU-1122-M**, Cornell University, Ithaca, NY.

Parlett, B. (1972). Can there be a marriage function?. In *Population Dynamics*, T. N. E. Greville (ed.), 107-135. New York, London: Academic Press.

Pollard, J. H. (1973). The two-sex problem. In *Mathematical Models for the Growth of Human Populations*, Chapter 7. Cambridge University Press.

Rubin, G., Umbach, D., Shyu, S-F. and Castillo-Chavez, C. (1991). Application of capture-recapture methodology to estimation of size of population at risk of AIDS and/or other sexually-transmitted diseases. *Biometrics Unit Technical Report* **BU-1112-M**, Cornell University, Ithaca, NY.

Saltzman, S. P., Stoddard, A. M., McCusker, J., Moon, M. W. and Mayer, K. H. (1987). Reliability of self-reported sexual behavior risk factors for HIV infection in homosexual men. *Public Health Reports* **102**, 692-697.

Sattenspiel, L. and Castillo-Chavez, C. (1990). Environmental context, social interactions, and the spread of HIV. *American Journal of Human Biology* **2**, 397-417.

Seber, G. A. F. (1082). *The estimation of animal abundance and related parameters.* New York: MacMillan.

Shilts, R. (1987). *And the band played on.* New York: St. Martin's Press.

Thieme, H. R. and Castillo-Chavez, C. (1989). On the role of variable infectivity in the dynamics of the human immunodeficiency virus epidemic. In *Mathematical and Statistical Approaches to* AIDS *Epidemiology*, C. Castillo-Chavez (ed.), Lecture Notes in Biomathematics 83, 157-176. Berlin, Heidelberg, New York, London, Paris, Tokyo, Hong Kong: Springer-Verlag.

Thieme, H. R. and Castillo-Chavez, C. (1990). On the possible effects of infection-age-dependent infectivity in the dynamics of HIV/AIDS. *Biometrics Unit Technical Report* **BU-1102-M**, Cornell University, Ithaca, NY.

Waldstatter, R. (1989). Pair formation in sexually transmitted diseases. In *Mathematical and Statistical Approaches to AIDS Epidemiology*, C. Castillo-Chavez (ed.), Lecture Notes in Biomathematics 83, 260-274. Berlin, Heidelberg, New York, London, Paris, Tokyo, Hong Kong: Springer-Verlag.

Winkelstein, W. Jr., Wiley, J. A., Padian, N. S., *et al.* (1988). The San Francisco Men's Health Study, continued decline in HIV seroconversion rates among homosexual/bisexual men. *Am. J. Pub. Health* **78**, 1472-1474.

Carlos Castillo-Chavez, Shwu-Fang Shyu and Gail Rubin

Biometrics Unit,
337 Warren Hall, Cornell University
Ithaca, NY 14853

David Umbach

National Institute of Environmental Health Sci.
P. O. Box 12233
Research Triangle Park, NC 27709